T0315257

PHYTOCHEMICALS IN FOOD AND HEALTH

Perspectives for Research and Technological Development

PHYTOCHEMICALS IN FOOD AND HEALTH

Perspectives for Research and Technological Development

Edited by
Deepak Kumar Verma, PhD
Mamta Thakur, PhD

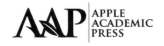

First edition published 2022

Apple Academic Press Inc.
1265 Goldenrod Circle, NE,
Palm Bay, FL 32905 USA
4164 Lakeshore Road, Burlington,
ON, L7L 1A4 Canada

CRC Press
6000 Broken Sound Parkway NW,
Suite 300, Boca Raton, FL 33487-2742 USA
2 Park Square, Milton Park,
Abingdon, Oxon, OX14 4RN UK

© 2022 Apple Academic Press, Inc.

Apple Academic Press exclusively co-publishes with CRC Press, an imprint of Taylor & Francis Group, LLC

Library and Archives Canada Cataloguing in Publication

Title: Phytochemicals in food and health : perspectives for research and technological development / edited by Deepak Kumar Verma, PhD, Mamta Thakur, PhD.

Names: Verma, Deepak Kumar, 1986- editor. | Thakur, Mamta, editor.

Description: First edition. | Includes bibliographical references and index.

Identifiers: Canadiana (print) 20210156929 | Canadiana (ebook) 20210156996 | ISBN 9781771889360 (hardcover) | ISBN 9781774638149 (softcover) | ISBN 9781003082125 (ebook)

Subjects: LCSH: Phytochemicals. | LCSH: Grain—Composition. | LCSH: Legumes—Composition. | LCSH: Medicinal plants—Composition. | LCSH: Botanical chemistry.

Classification: LCC QK861 .P65 2022 | DDC 572/.2—dc23

Library of Congress Cataloging-in-Publication Data

CIP data on file with US Library of Congress

ISBN: 978-1-77188-936-0 (hbk)
ISBN: 978-1-77463-814-9 (pbk)
ISBN: 978-1-00308-212-5 (ebk)

About the Editors

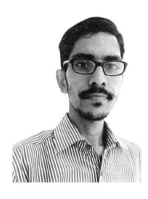

Deepak Kumar Verma, PhD
Department of Agricultural and Food Engineering, Indian Institute of Technology, West Bengal, India

Deepak Kumar Verma, PhD, is an agricultural science professional with specialization in food processing engineering Dr. Verma is currently assigned for research on "Aroma Volatile and Flavoring Compounds from Indian Rice Cultivars," whereas during master's degree, his research focused on "Physico-Chemical and Cooking Characteristics of Azad Basmati (CSAR 839-3): A Newly Evolved Variety of Basmati Rice (*Oryza Sativa* L.)." Dr. Verma has edited over a dozen books on topics pertaining to plant biochemistry, plant physiology, microbiology, plant pathology, genetics and plant breeding, plant biotechnology and genetic engineering, seed science and technology, food science and technology. He is a member of several professional bodies, and his activities and accomplishments include conferences, seminars, workshops, training, and also the publication of research articles, books, and book chapters.

He earned his BSc degree in agricultural science from the Faculty of Agriculture, Gorakhpur University, Gorakhpur, and MSc (Agriculture) in Agricultural Biochemistry with the first rank and also received a department topper award from the Department of Agricultural Biochemistry, Chandra Shekhar Azad University of Agricultural and Technology, Kanpur, India. He earned his PhD degree at the Agricultural and Food Engineering Department, Indian Institute of Technology Kharagpur (West Bengal). He received a DST–INSPIRE Fellowship for PhD study from the Department of Science & Technology (DST), Ministry of Science and Technology, Government of India.

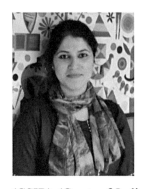

Mamta Thakur, PhD
Department of Food Engineering and Technology,
Sant Longowal Institute of Engineering and
Technology (Deemed-to-be-University),
Longowal (Punjab) India

Mamta Thakur, PhD, is a Food Technologist with special interest in Functional Foods. She has been awarded Senior Research Fellowship (SRF) by Council of Scientific and Industrial Research (CSIR) (Govt. of India), PBC fellowship for summer training by Govt. of Israel, and "Best Popular Science Story" award under "Augmenting Writing Skills for Articulating Research (AWSAR)" by Department of Science and Technology (Govt. of India). She provided the teaching services in the Department of Food Science, Nutrition and Technology, Chaudhary Sarwan Kumar Himachal Pradesh Krishi Vishvavidyalaya (CSKHPKV), Palampur (Himachal Pradesh) India for one academic semester. Dr. Thakur received her doctoral degree with a specialization in Food Technology from the Department of Food Engineering and Technology, Sant Longowal Institute of Engineering and Technology (Deemed University), Longowal (Punjab), India. Her PhD research project is focused on "Characterization and Utilization of Bee Pollen to Develop Functional Milk Powder." She earned her master's degree in Food Technology at Vasantrao Naik Marathwada Krishi Vidyapeeth, Parbhani, Maharashtra, India, and her BTech degree in Food Science and Technology from CSKHPKV, Palampur in 2014. Her master's research focused on the development of non-dairy probiotic beverage based on pomegranate juice using the lactobacilli strains possessing the functional characteristics. She has also formulated the Bitter Gourd Lemon Juice Concentrated Drink for Zain Natural Agro India Pvt. Ltd., Parbhani (Maharashtra) with a special focus on diabetic people. Her research reflects an intense interest in developing and characterizing health and functional foods carrying the bioactive components. She has published research papers in international peer-reviewed journals and has authored two book chapters as well as review articles. She has participated in many national and international conferences, seminars, and workshops. She has been awarded Best Paper Award at the 3rd International Conference on Food Properties (iCFP2018) held at Sharjah, UAE

Contents

Contributors

Cristobal Noe Aguilar
Bioprocesses Research Group, Food Research Department, School of Chemistry,
Universidad Autonoma de Coahuila, Unidad Saltillo, 25280, Coahuila, México.
E-mail: cristobal.aguilar@uadec.edu.mx

Afroze Alam
Narayan Institute of Pharmacy, Jamuhar, Sasaram (ROHTAS) 821305, Bihar India.
School of Pharmaceutical Sciences, Shoolini University, Bajhol, Solan 173229,
Himachal Pradesh, India. E-mail: afrozepharma@gmail.com, afrozalam@niop.in

Bavita Asthir
Department of Biochemistry, College of Basic Sciences and Humanities,
Punjab Agriculture University, Ludhiana 141004, Punjab, India. E-mail: b.asthir@rediffmail.com

Ashish Baldi
Department of Pharmaceutical Sciences & Technology, Maharaja Ranjit Singh Punjab Technical
University, Bathinda 151001, Punjab, India. E-mail: baldiashish@gmail.com

Sankhadip Bose
NSHM Knowledge Campus, Kolkata—Group of Institutions, 124 B. L. Saha Road, Kolkata, India,
E-mail: sankha.bose@gmail.com

Ana Veronica Charles
Department of Food Science and Technology, Universidad Autónoma Agraria Antonio Narro. Saltillo,
25000, Coahuila, Mexico. E-mail: anavero06@hotmail.com

Mónica L. Chávez-González
Bioprocesses and Bioproducts Group and Nanobioscience Group, Food Research Department,
School of Chemistry. Autonomous University of Coahuila, Saltillo Campus. 25280. Coahuila, México.
E-mail: monicachavez@uadec.edu.mx, monlizchg@gmail.com

Karina Cruz
Bioingenio LifeTech SA de CV, 25280, Saltillo, Coahuila, México. E-mail: kcruzald@gmail.com

K. L. Dhar
School of Pharmaceutical Sciences, Shoolini University, Bajhol, Solan 173229, Himachal Pradesh,
India. E-mail: dharkl@yahoo.com

Subhajit Dutta
Division of Pharmacognosy, Department of Pharmaceutical Technology, Jadavpur University,
Kolkata-700032, India, E-mail: subhajitdutta1919@gmail.com

Umar Farooq
Faculty of Dentistry, Taif University, Taif, Kingdom of Saudi Arabia, E-mail: ufarooq8@gmail.com

Alessandra Gambero
UNICAMP—State University of Campinas, Chemical, Biological and Agricultural Pluridisciplinary
Research Center (CPQBA), Av. Alexandre Cazellato, 999, CEP 13148-218, Paulínia, São Paulo, Brazil.
E-mail: alegambero@cpqba.unicamp.br

Heliodoro de la Garza
Department of Food Science and Technology, Universidad Autónoma Agraria Antonio Narro. Saltillo, 25000, Coahuila, Mexico. E-mail: hegarza_2000@yahoo.com.mx

Joaquin Hernandez-Escamilla
Department of Food Science and Technology, Universidad Autónoma Agraria Antonio Narro. Saltillo, 25000, Coahuila, Mexico. E-mail: joakin_hdez_es08@hotmail.com

Clélia Akiko Hiruma-Lima
UNESP—São Paulo State University, Department of Physiology, Biosciences Institute, R. Prof. Dr. Antonio Celso Wagner Zanin, 250, CEP 18618-689, Botucatu, São Paulo, Brazil. E-mail: clelia.hiruma@unesp.br

Jose Luis Martinez Hernandez
NanoBioscience Research Group, Food Research Department, School of Chemistry, Universidad Autonoma de Coahuila, Unidad Saltillo, 25280, Coahuila, México. E-mail: jose-martinez@uadec.edu.mx

Khushdeep Kaur
Department of Biochemistry, College of Basic Sciences and Humanities, Punjab Agriculture University, Ludhiana 141004, Punjab, India. E-mail: khushbrar731@gmail.com

Maninder Kaur
Department of Food Science & Technology, Guru Nanak Dev University, Amritsar 143 001, Punjab, India. E-mail: mandyvirk@rediffmail.com

G. Kimmy
Department of Food Engineering & Technology, Sant Longowal Institute of Engineering and Technology Longowal, Sangrur 148106, Punjab, India. E-mail: kishorigoyal09@gmail.com

Pinderpal Kaur
Department of Food Science & Technology, Chaudhary Devi Lal University, Sirsa 125055, Haryana, India. E-mail: pinderpal94@gmail.com

Pradyuman Kumar
Department of Food Engineering & Technology, Sant Longowal Institute of Engineering and Technology Longowal, Sangrur 148106, Punjab, India. E-mail: pradyuman2002@hotmail.com

Shailendra Kumar
Govt. Pharmacy Institute, Agam Kuan, Gulzar Bagh Patna 800007, Bihar, India. E-mail: profshailendrakumar@yahoo.com

Subhash C Mandal
Division of Pharmacognosy, Department of Pharmaceutical Technology, Jadavpur University, Kolkata 700032, India. E-mail: scmandal1963@gmail.com

Miguel Medina
Research and Development Staff, Bioingenio LifeTech SA de CV, 25280, Saltillo, Coahuila, México. E-mail: miguelmem84@gmail.com

Kamlesh Kumar Naik
Nandha College of Pharmacy, Perundurai Main Road, Erode, Tamil Nadu-638052, India. E-mail: kuman17@gmail.com

Emilio Ochoa
Department of Food Science and Technology, Universidad Autónoma Agraria Antonio Narro. Saltillo, 25000, Coahuila, Mexico. E-mail: eorochoa@gmail.com

Larissa Lucena Périco
UNESP—São Paulo State University, Department of Physiology, Biosciences Institute,
R. Prof. Dr. Antonio Celso Wagner Zanin, 250, CEP 18618-689, Botucatu, São Paulo, Brazil.
E-mail: larissalucenaperico@gmail.com

Sukhvinder Singh Purewal
Department of Food Science & Technology, Maharaja Ranjit Singh Punjab Technical University,
Bathinda 151001, Punjab, India. E-mail: purewal.0029@gmail.com

Daniel Rinaldo
UNESP—São Paulo State University, School of Sciences, Eng. Luiz Edmundo Carrijo Coube Ave,
CEP 17033-360, Bauru, São Paulo, Brazil. E-mail: daniel.rinaldo@unesp.br

Raul Rodriguez
Food Research Department, School of Chemistry, Universidad Autonoma de Coahuila, Unidad Saltillo,
25280, Coahuila, México. E-mail: raul.rodriguez@uadec.edu.mx

Kawaljit Singh Sandhu
Department of Food Science & Technology, Maharaja Ranjit Singh Punjab Technical University,
Bathinda 151 001, Punjab, India. E-mail: kawsandhu@rediffmail.com; kawsandhu5@gmail.com

Lourdes Campaner dos Santos
UNESP—São Paulo State University, Inst Chem, Dept Organ Chem, Av. Prof. Francisco Degni,
55, Jardim Quitandinha, CEP 14800-900, Araraquara, São Paulo, Brazil.
E-mail: loursant@gmail.com

Marcelo Aparecido da Silva
UNIFAL—Univ Federal de Alfenas, Faculty of Pharmaceutical Sciences,
Rua Gabriel Monteiro da Silva, 714, Centro, CEP 37130-000, Alfenas,
Minas Gerias, Brazil. E-mail: marcelo.silva@unifal-mg.edu.br

Marcelo J. Dias Silva
UNESP—São Paulo State University, Biosciences Institute, Coastal Campus of São Vicente,
Praça Infante Dom Henrique, s/n, CEP 11330-900, São Vicente, São Paulo, Brazil,
E-mail: marcelofarmadias@gmail.com

Smita Singh
Department of Life Sciences (Food Technology), Graphic Era (Deemed to be) University,
Dehradun, Uttarakhand 248002, India. E-mail: sweetsmita1004@gmail.com

Prem Prakash Srivastav
Agricultural and Food Engineering Department, Indian Institute of Technology Kharagpur,
Kharagpur 721302, West Bengal, India. E-mail: pps@agfe.iitkgp.ernet.in

Mamta Thakur
Department of Food Engineering and Technology, Sant Longowal Institute of Engineering and
Technology, Longowal 148106, Punjab, India. E-mail: thakurmamtafoodtech@gmail.com

Soubhagya Tripathy
Agricultural and Food Engineering Department, Indian Institute of Technology Kharagpur,
Kharagpur 721 302, West Bengal, India. E-mail: mr.soubhagyatripathy@gmail.com

Deepak Kumar Verma
Agricultural and Food Engineering Department, Indian Institute of Technology Kharagpur, Kharagpur 721302, West Bengal, India.
E-mail: deepak.verma@agfe.iitkgp.ernet.in, rajadkv@rediffmail.com

Wagner Vilegas
UNESP—São Paulo State University, Biosciences Institute, Coastal Campus of São Vicente, Praça Infante Dom Henrique, s/n, CEP 11330-900, São Vicente, São Paulo, Brazil.
E-mail: vilegasw@gmail.com

Abbreviations

AD	Alzheimer's disease
ANFs	antinutritional factors
ANSs	antinutritional substances
AOA	antioxidant activity
ARE	antioxidant responsive element
BBI	Bowman–Birk trypsin chymotrypsin inhibitor
CGA	chlorogenic acid
CTC	condensed tannin content
CVD	cardiovascular disease
DPPH-RS	DPPH radical scavenging
DPPHRSP	DPPH [2,2-diphenyl-1-picrylhydrazyl] radical scavenging potential
EA	ethyl acetate
ER	estrogen receptor
ESI-MS	electrospray ionization mass spectrometry
FAOUN	Food and Agriculture Organization of United Nation
FDA	Food and Drug Administration
FOS	fructo-oligosaccharide
FRAP	ferric reducing antioxidant power
G-5-P	ribulose-5-phosphate
G6PD	glucose-6-phosphate dehydrogenase
GA	gallic acid
GAE	gallic acid equivalents
GC-MS	gas chromatography-mass spectrometry
GI	gastrointestinal tract
GSH	glutathione
HCN	hydrogen cyanide
HDLC	HDL cholesterol
HPLC	high-performance liquid chromatography
HT	hydrolysable
IBD	inflammatory bowel disease
LDL	low density lipoprotein
LDLC	LDL cholesterol

MAPK   mitogen-activated protein kinases
MRP1   multidrug resistance protein
MS   mass spectrometer
NADPH   nicotinamide adenine dinucleotide phosphate
NMT   N-myristoyltransferase
NSAIDs   nonsteroidal anti-inflammatory drugs
ODPA   3-N-oxalyl-l-2,3-diaminopropanoic acid
PAD   photodiode array detector
PD   Parkinson's disease
PDA   photodiode array
PI3K   phosphatidylinositol 3-kinase
PKC   protein kinase C
PNPMF   National Policy of Medicinal and Phytotherapeutic Plants
POX   peroxidase
PPCs   polyphenolic compounds
ppm   parts per million
PPO   polyphenol oxidase
PPOA   polyphenol oxidase activity
PPP   pentose phosphate pathway
QAs   quinolizidine alkaloids
RNS   reactive nitrogen species
ROS   reactive oxygen species
RPA   reducing power activity
RP-HPLC   reversed-phase high-performance liquid chromatography
RSM   response surface methodology
SDF   soluble dietary fiber
SG   sorghum grain
SRS   superoxide radical scavenging
SSF   solid state fermentation
TAAs   toxic amino acids
TC   total cholesterol
TEAC   Trolox equivalent antioxidant capacity
TFC   total flavonoids content
TNBS   trinitrobenzenesulfonic acid
TPC   total phenolic content
UPLC   ultra-performance liquid chromatography
UV   ultraviolet

Preface

Phytochemistry is the study of nonnutritional chemicals (refered to as phytochemicals) commonly produced by plants (such as fruits, vegetables, cereals, legumes, herbs, spices, and other medicinal plants), particularly the secondary metabolites, which are synthesized for self-defense. Phytochemistry takes into account the structural compositions of these metabolites, the biosynthetic pathways, functions, mechanisms of actions in the living systems, and their medicinal, industrial, and commercial applications. The proper understanding of plant-derived chemicals, that is, phytochemicals, is essential for developing novel disease preventive properties. Different phytochemicals have different pharmaceutical properties, such as antioxidant properties, hormonal action, stimulation of enzymes, interference with DNA replication, antimicrobial properties, etc. They protects the cells from the oxidative damage by free radicals, thus assisting in the reduction of oxidative stress.

Based on such developments, the applications of phytochemistry are expanding in different disciplines, especially in food science and technology. Food is a significant source of nutrients in diet including the phytochemicals, which has been gaining attention throughout the world due to their contribution in human wellness. Phytochemicals including the flavonoids, carotenoids, allicin, polyphenols, hydrolyzable tannins, lignans, and phytosterols provide flavor and color to vegetables, fruits, and herbs. Among the broad groups of phytochemicals, the food products usually contain anthocyanidins, isoflavones, flavonoids, carotenoids, etc. The importance of polyphenols in human health and their existence in food products has been explained in many studies. The phytochemicals that have different chemical structures are metabolized differently in the body, thereby consequently resulting in different health impacts. A remarked increase in the consumption of functional foods containing bioactive compounds has been observed for a decade. Only 1% of phytochemicals have been identified, and researchers claim that there will be many more to discover in the foods we consume.

Phytochemistry involves the resourceful utilization of available or newly emerging technologies of biological matters, like biomolecules obtained from them to carry out a commercial, medical or scientific progression. Phytochemicals are diminutive entities with enormous potential applications that may play a beneficial or harmful role in our life. There is variety of phytochemicals, some of which are classic examples of industrially significant compounds. New emerging technologies have broadened our knowledge and understanding of how phytochemicals are linked to food, health, and social well-being.

The entitled book *Phytochemicals in Food and Health: Perspectives for Research and Technological Development* contains nine chapters that are divided into three main parts: *Part 1* Phytochemistry of Cereals and Legumes, *Part 2* Phytochemistry of Medicinal Plants, and *Part 3* Technological Advances in Phytochemical Study.

Several newly emerged techniques have significantly changed the scenario of the food and health sector by making the processes more stable and economically viable. Chapter 1 highlights the role of antinutritional substances of legumes in human health and focuses on recent research on the elimination of such antinutrients through technological processing. Information on sorghum phytochemicals, their processing and the development of food products, as well as their application to human health, is discussed in Chapter 2. While, knowledge of the proximate composition and bioactive profile of sorghum phytochemicals to assist the food and pharmaceutical industries is the focus in Chapter 3, on the production of nutraceuticals and functional foods of pharmaceutical importance. Chapter 4 focuses on the knowledge of *T. cordifolia* and more on the development of its therapeutic use in the food, health, and pharmacology industries. Chapter 5 describes the phytomedicine of Brazilian medicinal plants because they have the potential to treat chronic diseases. Chapter 6 presents a comparative study on polyphenolic content and antibacterial capacity, which has shown that the reflux method used as an extractor agent by ethanol is a good alternative for the production of vegetable extracts rich in phenolic compounds. Chapter 7 relates to the relationship between the isoflavone quality as a functional food and the structure–function relationship as described in the butterfly model. Chapter 8 addresses the plants' polyphenolic compounds, including their biosynthesis process, their classification, function, and role as bioactive compounds. Chapter 9 deals with the scientific exploration of food and health diets and many powerful health-related healing properties.

We have brought together a group of excellent national and international contributors in the forefront of food bioprocessing technology in context to produce an outstanding reference book that is expected to be a valuable resource for researchers, academicians, students, food, nutrition and health practitioners, and all those working in the food and health industry. I extend my sincere thanks to all the authors who have contributed with dedication, persistence, and cooperation in completing their chapters in a timely manner to this book and whose cooperation has made our task as editors a pleasure. We hope that this book will have enlightening and inspiring action to readers.

—Editors

Part I
Phytochemistry of Cereals and Legumes

CHAPTER 1

The Emphasis of Effect of Cooking and Processing Methods on Antinutritional Phytochemical of Legumes and Their Significance in Human Health

DEEPAK KUMAR VERMA*, MAMTA THAKUR, SMITA SINGH, SOUBHAGYA TRIPATHY, KAWALJIT SINGH SANDHU, MANINDER KAUR, and PREM PRAKASH SRIVASTAV

Agricultural and Food Engineering Department, Indian Institute of Technology Kharagpur, Kharagpur 721 302, West Bengal, India

Corresponding author.
E-mails: deepak.verma@agfe.iitkgp.ernet.in, rajadkv@rediffmail.com

ABSTRACT

Legumes are important source of nutrients in human diet, particularly from low-income group of developing nations. They are rich in proteins and good source of polyphenolic compounds which result in several positive effects on health. However, their nutritional value is adversely impacted by the presence of many antinutritional factors, such as amylase inhibitors, chlorogenic acid, cyanogenic glycosides, goitrogens, gossypol, isoflavones, lectins (phytohemagglutinins), oligosaccharides, oxalates, phytic acid (phytates), protease inhibitors (trypsin inhibitors), saponins, tannins, etc. These antinutritional substances can be removed or minimized to an acceptable level by simple and inexpensive processing techniques like boiling, dehulling, fermentation, extrusion, soaking, and pressure cooking which are discussed in detail. The present chapter will also highlight the significance of antinutritional substances in human health. Recent researches carried out to eliminate these antinutrients using technological processing are also emphasized in the study.

1.1 INTRODUCTION

Legumes are the fruits or seeds of such a plant, namely, various type of beans, chickpeas (*Cicer arietinum*), faba beans or broad beans (*Vicia faba*), lentils (*Lens culinaris*), mung beans (*Vigna radiata*), peas (*Pisum sativm*) and others which belong to the family *Fabaceae* and used for human consumption (Figure 1.1) (Duke, 1981; Gupta, 1987; Graham and Vance, 2003; Tucker, 2003; Gepts et al., 2005; Lewis et al., 2005). They are an important source of a wide range of carbohydrate (sugars and starches), dietary fiber, protein, unsaturated fat, vitamins, and minerals, as well as antinutritional substances (Vijayakumari et al., 1993; Graham and Vance, 2003; Bhat and Karim, 2009).

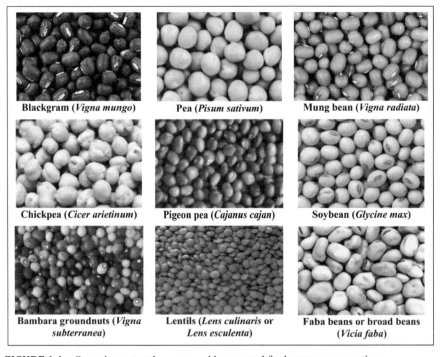

FIGURE 1.1   Some important legumes and beans used for human consumption.

Antinutritional substances (ANSs) are produced naturally involving various processes that have adverse effects on the nutritional value of foods. In other words, ANSs are those which affect our normal metabolism and nutritional conditions adversely but are derived from the natural sources of food and are referred to as antinutritional factors (ANFs) (Liener, 1975, 1980; Pusztai, 1989; Belmar et al., 1999; D'Mello, 2000; Jain et al., 2009; Akande et al., 2010). The presence of ANFs contained by important leguminous food sources is summarized in Table 1.1.

TABLE 1.1 Antinutritional Factors of Certain Leguminous Food Sources

ANF(s) Type	Leguminous Food Source	Botanical Name	Amount (mg/g, Unless Otherwise Stated)
Phytate	Chickpea (cooked)	*C. arietinum*	2.9–11.7
	Cowpea (cooked)	*Vigna unguiculata*	3.9–13.2
	Kidney beans (cooked)	*Proteus vulgaris*	8.3–13.4
	Lentils (cooked)	*L. culinaris*	2.1–10.1
	Peanuts	*Arachis hypogaea*	9.2–19.7
	Soybeans	*Glycine max*	9.2–16.7
Tannins	Bambara groundnuts	*Vigna subterranea*	0.02
	Cowpea	*V. unguiculata*	2.47
	Indian bean (Lablab)	*Lablab purpureus*	85 (d. w.)
	Red kidney bean	*Phaseolus* spp.	11
	White kidney beans		9.80
Trypsin inhibitor	Bean	*P. vulgaris*	18.1 (TIU/mg)
	Cowpea	*V. unguiculata*	13.9–46
	Lentil	*L. culinaris*	28.3 (d. w.)
	Pea	*P. sativm*	1.4 (TIU/mg)
α-Amylase inhibitor	Rice bean	*V. umbellata*	1100.1
	Black gram	*V. radiate*	120.1
Oxalate	Bambara groundnuts	*V. subterranea*	0.01
Lectin	Pea	*P. sativm*	0.6
Saponins	Chickpea	*C. arietinum*	3.6
	Lupine	*Lupinus* spp.	1.5
	Soybeans	*G. max*	56 (d. w.)

d.w.: dry weight, TIU: trypsin inhibitor unit.

Sources: Nikmarama (2017) [Reprinted from Nikmarama, N.; Leong, S. Y.; Koubaa, M.; Zhu, Z.; Barba, F. J.; Greiner, R.; Oey, I.; Roohinejad, S. Effect of extrusion on the anti-nutritional factors of food products: an overview. *Food Control*, 2017, *79*, 62–73. © 2017 Elsevier with permission]

Legume seeds in food and feed possess an ample amount of protein but their utilization is usually limited and not that simple and easy due to the deficiency of sulfur-containing amino acids, low protein digestibility and the presence of certain ANFs like amylase inhibitors, chlorogenic acid (CGA), cyanogenic glycosides, goitrogens, gossypol, isoflavones and polyphenols, lectins (phytohemagglutinins), oligosaccharides, oxalates, phytic acid (phytates), protease inhibitors (trypsin inhibitors), pyrimidine glycosides, quinolizidine alkaloids (QAs), saponins, tannins, toxic amino acids (TAAs), etc. (Abd El-Hady and Habiba, 2003; Khattab et al., 2009; Kalogeropoulos et al., 2010; Nagabhushana Rao and Shrivastava, 2011; Pedrosa et al., 2012).

ANFs affect the nutritional value of food. They adversely affect the digestibility and nutritional value of the food and feed. These factors interfere with the digestion and absorption process and even cause various undesirable physiological side effects like flatulence (Pedrosa et al., 2012). Interestingly only a few legumes may contain all these ANFs and many others contain a few of them. Tannin and cyanogen are reported to be present in almost all the legumes (Nagabhushana Rao and Shrivastava, 2011). There is a high demand for safe food with the maximum retention of nutritional components. Therefore, reduction or complete elimination of these antinutrients is essential to ensure the consumers' safety. The effects of processing on ANFs depend on the time, temperature, and moisture content of the commodity and the processing techniques improve the nutritional aspects of legumes shown in Table 1.2 (Alonso et al., 1998). Therefore, this chapter is aimed to investigate and focus on the overview of the current evidence of the antinutritional phytochemicals of legumes, and its health potential as well as the effects of processing methods on the phytochemicals.

1.2   MAJOR ANTINUTRITIONAL FACTORS (ANFSS) PRESENT IN LEGUMES

1.2.1   AMYLASE INHIBITORS

The presence of α-amylase inhibitors in legume species was first reported by Bowman (1945). These are present in pigeon pea (*Cajanus cajan*) and interfere with starch digestion. Chickpea (*C. arietinum*) and field bean contain low amount of amylase inhibitors while adzuki bean known as red mung bean (*Vigna angularis*), lentil (*L. culinaris*), lima bean (*Phaseolus lunatus*), pea (*P. sativm*), soybean (*G. max*), and winged bean also known as the Goa bean (*Psophocarpus tetragonolobus*) have been reported to contain no amylase activity (Grant et al., 1995). These are heat-labile and active between 4.5 and 9.5 pH range.

TABLE 1.2 Antinutritional Factors Inactivation in Certain Leguminous Food through Food Processing with Special Reference to Extrusion

Food Type	Botanical Name	Process Condition	ANF Type(s)	Positive Effects of Extrusion Processing
Lentil	*L. culinaris Medik*	Twin screw extruder, Four independent heating zones: Conveying zone (95, 115, and 135 °C), Mixing zone (110, 130, and 150 °C), Cooking zone (125, 145, and 165 °C), High pressure zone (die) (140, 160, and 180 °C), Feed rate: 20.4 kg/h, Feed moisture content: 14%, 18%, and 22%, Screw speed: 150, 200, and 250 rpm	Trypsin inhibitors Phytate Tannins	Reduction of trypsin inhibitors, phytate and tannin levels for up to 99.54%, 99.30%, and 98.83%, respectively, in extruded product obtained at 18% feed moisture content, 160 °C die temperature and 200 rpm of screw speed
Pinto beans	*P. vulgaris*	Presoaking: 8 h in water followed by oven-drying at 65 ± 2 °C for 12 h, Twin-screw extruder, Temperature: 85, 100, and 120 °C (die end), Feed rate: 120 g/min, Feed moisture content: 36%	Phytohemagglutinin (Lectins)	Combined extrusion processing and steam-cooking reduced the lectin in bean flour by 85%–95% compared to raw bean flours
Bean	*P. vulgaris*	Single screw extruder, Temperature: 150 °C, Feed moisture content: 20%, Screw speed: 25 rpm, Compression ratio: 1:6	Lectin Trypsin inhibitors	Trypsin inhibitors and lectin were totally inactivated
Cotyledons	*P. vulgaris*	Single screw extruder, Temperature: 150, 154, 164, 174, and 178 °C, Feed moisture content: 12.3%, 14%, 18%, 22%, and 23.7%, Screw speed: 414 rpm	Trypsin inhibitors α-amylase inhibitors and hemagglutinins	The activities of the trypsin and α-amylase inhibitors and hemagglutinins were completely eliminated
Kidney bean	*P. vulgaris var. Pinto*	Twin-screw extruder, Temperature: 150 °C, Feed rate: 350 g/min, Feed moisture content: 25%, Screw speed: 100 rpm	Phytate Tannins Lectins Trypsin inhibitors Chymotrypsin inhibitors α-amylase inhibitors	The contents of phytate, tannins, lectins and trypsin, chymotrypsin, and α-amylase inhibitory activities were reduced. Rats fed with raw beans had lower growth rate and food intake compared to those fed with extruded legumes

TABLE 1.2 *(Continued)*

Food Type	Botanical Name	Process Condition	ANF Type(s)	Positive Effects of Extrusion Processing
Field pea	*Pisum sativum*	Precooked in single-step conditioner (350 rpm), Preconditioner temperature: 70, 90, and 100 °C, Twin-screw extruder, Barrel temperature: 70 °C (middle), 95 °C (front), and 110 °C (outlet die), Feed rate: 107–116 g/min, Screw speed: 380 rpm, Two drying treatments (low treatment: from 120 to 90 °C, high treatment: from 150 to 120 °C)	Phytate Tannins Trypsin inhibitors	Phytate and total tannin were greatly reduced
Chickpea	*C. arietinum*			
Faba pea	*V. faba*			
Hard-to-cook common beans	*P. vulgaris* L.	Single screw extruder, Central temperature: 150 °C, Feed moisture content: 20%, Screw speed: 150 rpm	Phytate Hemagglutinins (lectin) α-amylase inhibitors Trypsin inhibitors	The inhibitory activity of trypsin in the BRS pontal (71%) and BRS grafite (69%) flours were reduced The α-amylase inhibitory activity and hemagglutination activity were eliminated The phytate was reduced by 17% and 26%, respectively, in pontal and grafite cultivars
Lathyrus seeds	*Lathyrus sativus*	Twin-screw extruder, Temperature: zone 1: 90–140 °C, zone 2: 100–180 °C, zone 3: 120–220 °C, and zone 4: 100–200 °C, Feed moisture content: 14%, 18%, 22%, 26%, or 30%	Trypsin inhibitors Phytate phosphorus Tannins β-ODAP	The content of β-ODAP and tannins were reduced while the activity of trypsin inhibitors was completely inhibited. Reduction/inactivation effect on ANFs was enhanced with an increase of moisture content in seeds (from 14% to 30%) before extrusion and with an increase of barrel temperature from 90/100/120/100 °C to 140/180/220/200 °C.

TABLE 1.2 (Continued)

Food Type	Botanical Name	Process Condition	ANF Type(s)	Positive Effects of Extrusion Processing
Kidney beans	*P. vulgaris* var. Athropurpurea	Twin-screw extruder, Die temperature: 152 and 156 °C, Feed moisture content: 25%, Feed rate: 383 and 385 g/min, Screw speed: 100 rpm	Phytate Tannins Trypsin inhibitors Chymotrypsin inhibitors	Inhibitors of trypsin, chymotrypsin, and α-amylase were all eliminated and inhibition of hemagglutinins activity was possible without modifying the protein content.
Faba bean	*V. faba* L. var. Equina		α-amylase inhibitors Hemagglutinins	
Peas	*P. sativm*	Twin-screw extruder, Die temperature: 145 °C, Feed rate: 21.5 kg/h, Feed moisture content: 25%, Screw speed: 100 rpm	Tannins Protease inhibitors Lectins Phytate	Polyphenols were lowered but not completely eliminated.
				Trypsin inhibitory and lectin activities were completely inhibited.
				Chymotrypsin inhibitory activity was reduced.
				A minor reduction in the phytate content of peas was found.

Sources: Nikmarama (2017) (Reprinted from Nikmarama, N.; Leong, S. Y.; Koubaa, M.; Zhu, Z.; Barba, F. J.; Greiner, R.; Oey, I.; Roohinejad, S. Effect of extrusion on the anti-nutritional factors of food products: an overview. *Food Control*, 2017, 79, 62–73. © 2017 Elsevier with permission).

These inhibitors form complexes with amylase that is being affected by the concentration of the inhibitors, ionic strength, pH, temperature, and time. Amylase is responsible for breakdown of starch into glucose and maltose and the presence of amylase inhibitors reduces polysaccharides hydrolysis including glycogen and starch due to which reduced growth is seen in chickpeas (*C. arietinum*). They act as starch blockers and cause symptoms like diarrhea in human. These inhibitors are also known for their therapeutic value, as they decrease carbohydrate absorption in diabetic patients and in the obese (Garcia-Olmedo et al., 1987; Menezes and Laljo, 1987). Amylase inhibitors block the starch from being absorbed by the body. Starch is broken down in the presence of digestive enzyme amylase prior to their absorption (Marshall and Lauda, 1975; Choudhury et al., 1996). Pigeon pea contains amylase inhibitors that are active in the pH range of 4.5–9.5 and are also heat-labile. The synthesis and degradation of these inhibitors are taken place during late development and late germination of seed, respectively (Giri and Kachole, 1998).

1.2.1.1   EFFECT OF COOKING AND PROCESSING METHODS

The effect of soaking and cooking is nonsignificant for the removal of activities of the α-amylase and α-glucosidase inhibition in the seeds of sesban (*Sesbania sesban*) but significantly high α-amylase inhibition (72.97%) was reported in the processed samples. The losses of activities of the α-amylase and α-glucosidase inhibition in the underutilized legume grain after sprouting and oil-frying show similar behavior to seeds of velvet bean (*Mucuna pruriens*) during germination (Randhir et al., 2009). In contrast to this, Randhir et al. (2008) report that the inhibition property of these enzymes increased in certain cereals during the sprouting and autoclave treatment. On the other hand, the levels of α-amylase and α-glucosidase inhibition during the sprouting of seeds and after frying were comparable with the acarbose which is known as synthetic antidiabetic agent. Similarly, open-pan roasting was effective for the activities of α-amylase and α-glucosidase inhibition in *S. sesban* seeds as well as the most suitable method for the preservation of phenolic compounds and their enzyme inhibition properties.

1.2.1.2   SIGNIFICANCE IN HUMAN HEALTH

Even though the biological significance of α-amylase inhibitors has not been fully understood, it is believed to play some role in the pest and disease-resistance mechanisms of plants. A positive correlation has been observed between the α-amylase inhibitor present in pigeon peas with the insect resistance (Giri, 1964; Ambekar et al., 1996). The ingestion of α-amylase inhibitor in the diet can cause celiac disease (Strumeyer, 1972) and pancreatic hypertrophy (Puls and Keup, 1973). The α-amylase inhibitor extracted from kidney beans (*Phaseolus vulgaris*) are used for the treatment of obesity (Marshall and Lauda, 1975). Besides this, the inhibitors of pancreatic α-amylase restrict the breakdown and absorption of starch that ultimately decreases the postprandial glucose levels and is responsible for the loss of weight in humans as well (Bailey, 2003; Tarling et al., 2008).

1.2.2 CHLOROGENIC ACIDS

CGAs are phenolic compounds (Figure 1.2A) present in legumes (Herrmann, 1976; Kuhnau, 1976). Coffee is the major source and other sources include apples (*Malus pumila*), artichoke (*Cynara cardunculus*), berries, pears (*Pyrus* spp.), and eggplant (*Solanum melongena*) also known as aubergine (*Solanum melongena*) (Clifford, 1999). CGA (5-caffeoylquinic acid) in foods is found in the form of caffeic acid as an ester with quinic acid. Caffeic acid is the main representative of hydroxycinnamic acids (Boerjan et al., 2003).

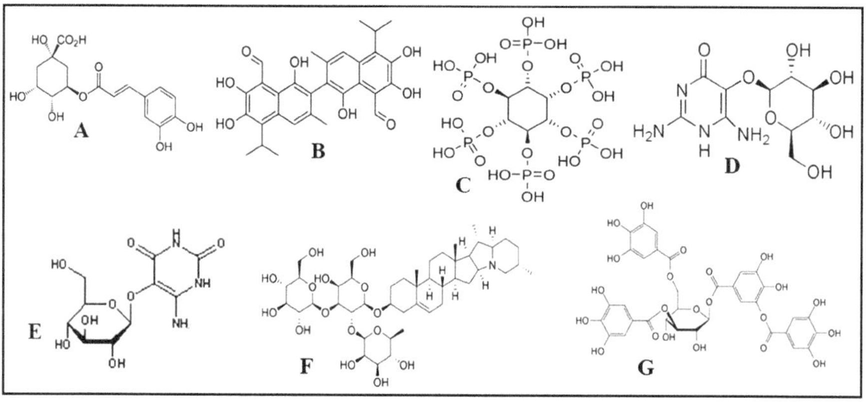

FIGURE 1.2 Chemical structure of antinutritional compounds. (A) Chlorogenic acids, (B) Gossypol, (C) Phytic acid, (D) Vicine, (E) Convicine, (F) Saponin, and (G) Tannin.

1.2.2.1 EFFECT OF COOKING AND PROCESSING METHODS

Generally, green beans are heated up to 200–240 °C during roasting (Andriot et al., 2004). It leads to severe changes in the nutritional components along with the decrease in the content of CGA. This happens mainly due to the Maillard reaction that takes place after condensation of sugars with free amino acids, peptides, or proteins which leads and responsible to form a wide range of chemical compounds that are reported to retain the antioxidant activity or even to have prooxidant properties (Nicoli et al., 1999). The chlorogenic acid gets oxidized by polyphenol oxidases and interacts with the NH_2 groups of amino acids that ultimately lowers the nutritional value. It is significantly reduced with the cooking process of the legumes (Lee et al., 2011; Rauter et al., 2012).

1.2.2.2 SIGNIFICANCE IN HUMAN HEALTH

Chlorogenic acid causes biological effects after entering into the blood circulation and those not absorbed will enter into the colon and cause the same effects. CGAs are antioxidants *in vitro* (Castelluccio et al., 1995; Rice-Evans et al., 1996). CGA also inhibits DNA damage (Shibata et al., 1999; Kasai et al., 2000) and oxidation of low-density lipoprotein (LDL) (Laranjinha et al., 1994; Nardini et al., 1995) *in vitro*. CGA has been found to prevent Alzheimer's disease by reducing apoptosis induced by the amyloid β-cells (Kwon et al., 2010). In addition, it has anticholinesterase, antiamnesic, antiinflammatory, and antioxidant activities (Howes et al., 2003; Santos et al., 2006; Orhan et al., 2007; Kwon et al., 2010). It enhances plasma homocysteine levels that are responsible for the onset of cardiovascular diseases. It has weak antimicrobial activity and is active against the polio virus at low concentrations. It even causes dissipation of the sodium electrochemical gradient to enhance the passage of glucose through the bowel (Stacewicz-Sapuntzakis et al., 2001). Neochlorogenic acid and CGA fractions have been reported with chemopreventative and chemotherapeutic activities. They decrease cancer risk by protecting scavenging reactive oxygen species (ROS), enhancing DNA (deoxyribonucleic acid) repair, detoxification and modification of carcinogen uptake and metabolism. The *in vivo* studies have shown that 33% of CGA is absorbed in the small intestine, and the rest is transported to the colon, where the bioavailability depends on the metabolism of certain microflora (Noratto et al., 2009). It has been proven that CGA has the ability to inhibit tumors formation in the bowel and liver (Stacewicz-Sapuntzakis et al., 2001). Similarly, the *in vitro* studies have shown that the CGA and neochlorogenic acid at respective concentrations of 17 and 10 mg/L suppress breast cancer cell growth (MD-MGA-435) without affecting the normal breast epithelial cells (MCF-10A) (Noratto et al., 2009).

1.2.3 CYANOGENIC GLYCOSIDES

Cyanogens are glycosides of 2-hydroxynitriles present in Leguminosae (e.g., in *P. lunatus* and *Vicia sativa*) (Bell and Charlwood, 1980; Conn, 1981; Bisby et al., 1994). The chemical structure of some the cyanogenic glycosides (Figure 1.3) and its main sources are shown in Table 1.3. β-Glucosidase hydrolyzes cyanogenic glycosides into 2-hydroxynitrile which is further broken into aldehyde or ketone and hydrogen cyanide (HCN) by hydroxynitrilelyase. HCN inhibits cytochrome oxidase enzymes that are found in mitochondrial respiratory chain. Leguminos plants, namely, *P. lunatus*, *P. vulgaris*, and the *C. cajan* (red gram) release HCN by hydrolysis while only from *P lunatus*, liberation of HCN is due to enzyme action reported, especially during grinding or chewing or under damp conditions (Purseglove, 1991).

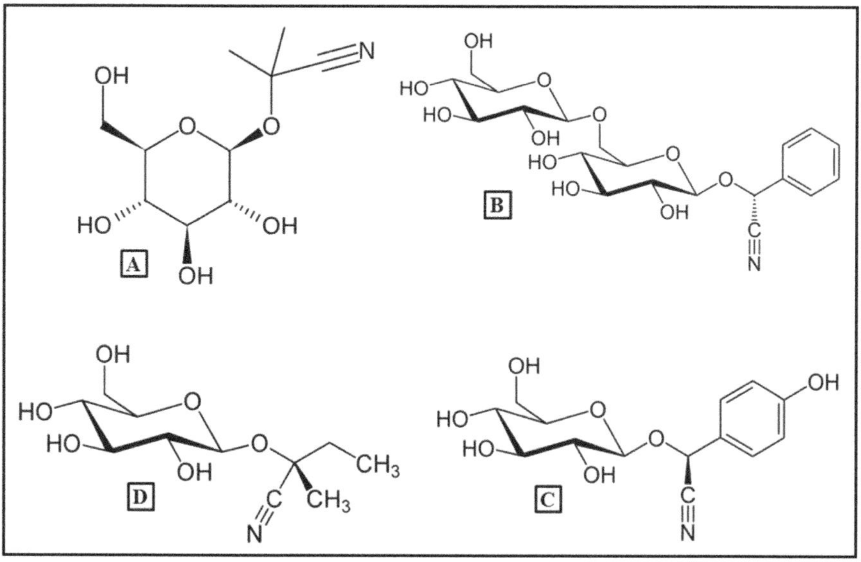

FIGURE 1.3 Major cyanogenic glycosides present in legumes. (A) Linamarin, (B) Amygdalin, (C) Lotaustralin, and (D) Dhurrin.

TABLE 1.3   Cyanogenic Glycosides and Its Major Sources

Cyanogenic Glycosides	Chemical Formula	Plant Sources
Linamarin	$C_{10}H_{17}NO_6$	*Manihot esculenta* (cassava), *P. lunatus* (lima bean), and *Linum usitatissimum* (flax)
Amygdalin	$C_{20}H_{27}NO_{11}$	Seeds (kernels) of legumes, apricot, bitter almonds, apple, peach, and plum
Lotaustralin	$C_{11}H_{19}NO_6$	*Lotus australis* trefoil (Austral), *M. esculenta*, *P. lunatus*, *Rhodiola rosea* (roseroot), and *Trifolium repens* (white clover)
Dhurrin	$C_{14}H_{17}NO_7$	*Sorghum bicolor* (Sorghum)

1.2.3.1   EFFECT OF COOKING AND PROCESSING METHODS

The processing of legumes ruptures the cells and releases the degrading enzymes to the bound and inactive forms of the cyanogens (Bainbridge et al., 1998). The extent of removal of cyanogens depends upon the amount of cyanogen present and type of processing employed (Nambisan, 1994; Cardoso et al., 2005). As per World Health Organization, the initial cyanide (HCN) should not exceed 250 µg/g for efficient processing (Cardoso et al., 2005). In Table 1.4, the presence of HCN in different leguminous plants is shown. The cells are ruptured during cooking at 60–70 °C followed by removal linamarase. This leads to inadequate detoxification and retention of cyanogenic glycosides (Jansz and Uluwaduge, 1997) and hence the extent of reduction of cyanogenic glycosides is temperature dependent (Hidayat et al., 2002). Jansz and Uluwaduge (1997) reported the reduction of cyanogen by cooking up to 50%–70% in Southern Asia. On the other hand, Fukuba et al. (1982) observed that the soaking and squeezing stage prior to cooking reduced cyanogen up to 70%. Similarly, cooking of cassava leaves has resulted in 75% reduction (Hidayat et al., 2002) and in some cases more than 90% reduction in HCN level (Ngudi et al., 2003).

TABLE 1.4   Cyanide Presence Certain Leguminous Plants

Leguminous Plants	Botanical Name	HCN Yield (mg/100 g)
Lima bean	*P. lunatus*	210–312.0
Black-eyed pea	*Vigna sinensis*	2.1
Garden pea	*P. sativum*	2.3
Kidney bean	*P. vulgaris*	2.0
Bengal gram	*C. arietinum*	0.8
Red gram	*C. cajan*	0.5

Sources: Gupta (1987) [Reprinted from Gupta, Y. P. Anti-nutritional and toxic factors in food legumes: a review. *Plant Foods for Human Nutrition*, 1987, *37* (3), 201–228. © 1987 Springer with permission]

1.2.3.2 SIGNIFICANCE IN HUMAN HEALTH

The cyanogenic glycosides liberates HCN that exerts both acute and chronic effects on human health. The potential toxicity of cyanoglycosides is due to enzymatic degradation that releases HCN, the cause for acute poisoning. The symptoms of acute toxicity include convulsions, diarrhea, dizziness, drop in blood pressure, headache, mental confusion, rapid pulse, rapid respiration, stomach pains, twitching, and vomiting, while the chronic effects are associated with the long-term poor nutrition.

1.2.4 GOITROGENS

Goitrogens are responsible for the enlargement of thyroid gland. They are common in legumes like soybean (*G. max*) and groundnut. They restrict the synthesis and secretion of thyroid hormones that regulate the body metabolism, growth, and reproductive system. The soybeans exert goitrogenic effect as well. Legumes like common bean, pea, peanut (*A. hypogaea*), and soybean (*G. max*) inhibit iodine absorption with the help of thyroid. Arachidoside is a compound reported to have goitrogenic effect, generally found in the outer layer of shells of *A. hypogaea* (peanut). Such leguminous plants secrete goitrogen, if fed by livestock it passes to the children through their milk (Ramadoss and Shunmugam, 2014).

1.2.4.1 EFFECT OF COOKING AND PROCESSING METHODS

Microwave irradiation has been reported to inactivate myrosinase enzyme and decomposes glucosinolates that cause goitrogenic in nature. In different meals, the decomposition of glucosinolate reported in the range of 70–254 mol/mmol (Maheshwari et al., 1980; Aumaitre et al., 1989). The decomposition of glucosinolates increases with the increase in moisture content and time of exposure to microwave heating. The extrusion cooking is rather more effective in removing glucosinolates from legumes than by microwave treatment. Dry extrusion has been found to reduce in the range from 193 to 428 mol/mmol of total glucosinolates (Smithard and Eyre, 1986; Aumaitre et al., 1989; Fenwick et al., 1986). On the other hand, wet extrusion of high glucosinolate rapeseed meal with ammonia (150 °C, 200 rpm, with 2% ammonia) resulted into a significant reduction (670 mol/mmol) (Huang et al., 1995).

1.2.4.2   SIGNIFICANCE IN HUMAN HEALTH

The glucosinolates induce goiter in animals, but their role in humans is not fully understood. They are anticarcinogenic and cancer-promoting, based on the species and circumstances of administration (Cassidy et al., 1994). Genistein is one of the major isoflavones synthesized by the soybean (*G. max*) that has both estrogenic and goitrogenic activities (Sheehan, 1997, 1998). Besides this, genistein has been tested in various experimental setups for the chemoprevention of breast and prostate cancer, relief of postmeno-pausal symptoms, and prevention or slowing of osteoporosis. In humans, it was found that the goiter in infants is prevented by the supplementation with iodine (Shepard et al., 1960). The hypothyroid is caused by the biochemical impairment of hormone synthesis and metabolism, and exposure to environ-mental goitrogens, such as cyanogenic glycosides, flavonoids glucosinolates, and sulphonamides (Gaitan et al., 1989). The incidence of goiter and other hypothyroid conditions have been reported in humans even in the absence of iodine deficiency (Ishizuki et al., 1991).

1.2.5   GOSSYPOL

Gossypol is a chemical compound (Figure 1.2B) which displays the toxicity symptoms like irregular heartbeat, labored breathing, loss of appetite, and loss of body weight. Death can occur with reduced oxygen-carrying capacity of the blood, hemolytic effects on erythrocytes, and circulatory failure. Dietary gossypol even leads olive-green discoloration of egg yolks (Church, 1991; McDonald et al., 1995). The gossypol binds to reactive epsilon amino group of lysine upon heating (Wilson et al., 1981; Robinson, 1991; Church, 1991).

1.2.5.1   EFFECT OF COOKING AND PROCESSING METHODS

Solvent extraction is one among the various methods for the removal of gossypol from legumes. Others are calcium hydroxide treatment (Nagalak-shmi et al., 2002, 2003), ferrous sulfate treatment (Barraza et al., 1991; Taba-tabai et al., 2002), microbes fermentation (Shi et al., 1998; Wu and Chen, 1989), and so on may also use. In addition, the fermentation for 48 h was found to reduce the gossypol level to 45.44 mg/kg and the detoxification rate was about 91.72%. It was also observed that the high temperature augmented the formation of stable bonds between gossypol and other molecules and the bound form of gossypol is physiologically inactive (Randel et al., 1992).

2.5.2 SIGNIFICANCE IN HUMAN HEALTH

Gossypol and its derivatives have potential therapeutic use. These compounds showed *in vitro* action against some viruses, such as human immunodeficiency virus (Polsky et al., 1989; Yang et al., 2012), H5N1 influenza virus (Yang et al., 2012, 2013), and several bacteria and yeasts (Yildirim-Aksoy et al., 2004; Turco et al., 2004; Anna et al., 2012). Gossypol is a promising treatment for leukemia (Balakrishnan et al., 2008), lymphoma (Johnson, 2008), colon carcinoma (Wang et al., 2000), breast cancer (Van Poznak et al., 2001; Weiping et al., 2007), myoma (Han et al., 1987), prostate cancer (Jiang et al., 2012), and other malignancies (Badawy et al., 2007; Chien et al., 2012; Hsiao et al., 2012). In animals, their effects include growth, reproduction, intestine, and other internal organs' abnormalities (Berardi and Goldblatt, 1980; Francis et al., 2001; Robinson et al., 2001). In free form, it reduces the oxygen-carrying capacity of the blood and causes breathing problems and edema of the lungs in monogastric animals (Alford et al., 1996), while in male ruminants, nonruminants, and preruminants, it causes labored breathing, dyspnea, reduced growth rate, formation of edema, congestion of lungs, and liver along with degeneration of heart fibers (Randel et al., 1992).

1.2.6 ISOFLAVONES

Isoflavones mainly reported from the Fabaceae/Leguminosae are chemically phenylchromen-4-one. Among the various phenolic compounds in the seeds of chickpea (*C. arietinum*), the two major ones are the isoflavones, biochanin A [5,7-dihydroxy-4′-methoxyisoflavone] and formononetin [7-hydroxy-4′-methoxyisoflavone] (Wood and Grusak, 2007). The other phenolics reported in chickpea oil are daidzein, genistein, matairesinol, and secoisolariciresinol (Champ, 2002; Dixon, 2004).

1.2.6.1 EFFECT OF COOKING AND PROCESSING METHODS

The processing of soybeans has significant effects on its nutritional content (Wang and Murphy, 1994, 1996). Some soybean varieties and soy foods are suggested and reported that processing affect their isoflavone content (Murphy, 1981; Farmakalidis and Murphy, 1985; Jackson et al., 1999). The heat processing, enzymatic hydrolysis, and fermentation process have profound effect on the distribution of the soy foods isoflavone components (Wang and Murphy, 1994). Certain processing methods like boiling, milling, and protein coagulation do not destroy the daidzein or genistein significantly in tofu production, while 15%–21% loss of daidzein and genistein, respectively reported in other methods such as roasting (Franke et al., 1995). Defoaming is also reported to eliminate isoflavones from the soy beverage (Okubo et al., 1983).

1.2.6.2   SIGNIFICANCE IN HUMAN HEALTH

Isoflavones are heterocyclic phenols found in soybean (G. max) having several health promoting effects like cardiovascular disease, prevention of cancer, and reduction in osteoporosis. These are recommended to relieve for menopausal women from menopause symptoms instead of hormonal replacement therapy (HRT) (Beck et al., 2005). The HRT of isoflavones is due to the estrogenic effects of the metabolites. There is potential risk of breast cancer reported in using HRT. *In vivo* and *in vitro* experiments have suggested that genistein and daidzein encourage to the growth of estrogen-dependent human breast tumor (Allred et al., 2001; Ju et al., 2001, 2006). The isoflavones exert both estrogen agonist and antagonist activities (Wood et al., 2006). Isoflavones are diphenolic and responsible for lowering the incidence of heart disease by different mechanisms (Figure 1.4), some of them are as following:

1. Inhibition of LDL-C oxidation (Tikkanen et al., 1998; Tikkanen and Adlercreutz, 2000),
2. Inhibition of proliferation of aortic smooth muscle cells (Pan et al., 2001), and
3. Maintenance of physical properties of arterial walls (van der Schouw et al., 2002).

1.2.7   LECTINS (PHYTOHEMAGGLUTININS)

Lectins (proteinaceous in nature) found in legumes vary from 0.6% in garden pea (P. sativum), 2.4%–5% in P. vulgaris (kidney bean), and 0.8% in P. lunatus (lima bean) and G. max (soya bean) with respect to total protein content (TPC) (Zhang et al., 2009). The lectins from mung bean (V. radiata) have been found to be nontoxic, whereas the lectins obtained from immature seeds of pigeon pea and rice bean are toxic and harmful. They reduce the bioavailability of nutrients by directly acting on the digestive enzymes. So, the higher doses of lectins in diet lead to nutritional deficiencies and immune (allergic) reactions. Lectins cause gastrointestinal distress through interaction with the gut epithelial cells (Oliveira et al., 1989). The extracts

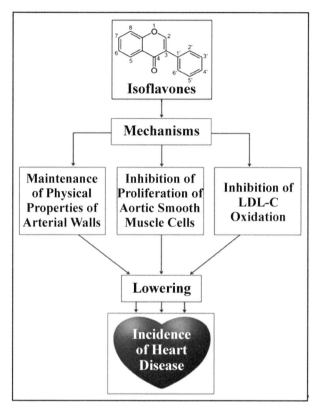

FIGURE 1.4 Isoflavones mechanisms lower heart disease incidence.

from many edible crude bean seeds cause agglutination of red cells and have affinity for certain sugar molecules. Lectins reduce the bioavailability of nutrients by acting on the digestive enzymes. It is reported that soaking prior to autoclaving or cooking is required for complete elimination of the toxicity of lectins (Jain et al., 2009).

1.2.7.1 EFFECT OF COOKING AND PROCESSING METHODS

The processing methods like soaking, sprouting, cooking, and fermenting inactivate the lectins but not completely (Pusztai et al., 1991). It has been found that many legume lectins are resistant to high temperature, that is, have a relatively high thermal stability (70 °C), while some are relatively resistant to proteolytic enzymes and stomach acid (Kilpatrick et al., 1985). It has been observed that preliminary soaking before autoclaving or cooking completely eliminates the toxicity lectins. Presoaking beans at suitable conditions followed by cooking above 80 °C eliminate lectins and make the product safe.

2.7.2   SIGNIFICANCE IN HUMAN HEALTH

The study of Jönsson et al. (2005) reported that an increase in uptake of dietary lectin affects weight gain by means of lectin resistance. It is a key hormone in regulating energy intake and energy expenditure and lectin resistance with the malfunctioning lectin receptors reduces satiation signals from the brain. A reduced feeling of satiation mediates overeating that result into obesity (Enriori et al., 2012; Spreadbury, 2012). On the other hand, plant lectins have gained attention due to their antitumor properties. Lectins can bind to cancer cells which have been reported for their beneficial effects in cancer patients (Abdullaev and Gonzalez de Mejia, 1997). The consumption of plant lectins has beneficial effects on colorectal cancer patients but the mechanism is still unknown (Evans et al., 2002).

1.2.8   OLIGOSACCHARIDES

Legumes are rich sources of oligosaccharides (around up to 20%) in the form of stachyose and raffinose (Bisby et al., 1994). The galacto-oligosaccharides are a family of short chain carbohydrates related to sucrose. Pea contains total oligosaccharides (3.73% of total solids). Stachyose is the most abundant among the oligosaccharides even in cooked and soaked pulses (Han and Baik, 2006). Verbascose is a galacto-oligosaccharide having highest molecular weight and is present abundantly in peas but absent in chickpeas (*C. arietinum*) (Han and Baik, 2006). The arabinose, galactose, rhamnose, and uronic acids are known as the main of pectins and the sum of these sugars reported 10.8%, 9.3%, and 9.5% in chickpeas (*C. arietinum*), lentils (*L. culinaris*), and peas, respectively. Raffinose, stachyose, and verbascose are soluble carbohydrates which are not affected by digestive enzymes (Guillon and Champ, 2002; Campos-Vega et al., 2009). Along with other by-products like gases it leads to flatulence and other disturbances.

1.2.8.1   EFFECT OF COOKING AND PROCESSING METHODS

The process like dehulling, soaking, and soaking/cooking which have shown a significant effect on sucrose, raffinose, and stachyose in one variety of tropical African yam bean (*Sphenostylis stenocarpa*) and mature dry seeds of nine varieties of cowpea (*V. unguiculata*). Soaking of these seeds for 12 h followed by cooking for 30 min eliminated most of the oligosaccharides (Nwinuka et al., 1997). Similarly, cooking reduces total β-galactosides in brown pigeon peas and by 21% and 67%, respectively, as compared to the raw samples. Cooking in presence of 0.1% alkaline solution has shown better reduction due to heat induced hydrolysis of the oligosaccharides into simple disaccharides and monosaccharides (Onigbinde and Akinyele, 1983). The combined effect of soaking and cooking has been reported by Uzogara et al. (1996) as well.

1.2.8.2   SIGNIFICANCE IN HUMAN HEALTH

Various experiments have been conducted to study the effects of oligosaccharides on commensal bacteria and health of young animals and human infants (Gibson and Wang, 1994). Fructo-oligosaccharide (FOS) has been observed to escape the enzymatic digestion in the small intestine and forms a substrate for the gastrointestinal microflora (Tokunaga et al., 1989). The FOS, on the other hand, enhances the growth of *Bifidobacterium* and *Lactobacillus*, but prevent *Escherichia coli* in the large intestine (Hidaka et al., 1986, 1991; Bunce et al., 1995; Roberfroid et al., 1998). This leads to increase fecal bile acid excretion and decrease in its intestinal concentration (Delzenne, 1993; Kim and Shin, 1998).

1.2.9   OXALATES

Oxalic acid is found in legumes as free acid and soluble salts of potassium (K) and sodium (Na), and insoluble salts of calcium (Ca), magnesium (Mg), and iron (Fe) (Noonan and Savage, 1999). The oxalate contents usually present in legumes such as lentils (*L. culinaris*), red kidney beans, and white kidney beans which are shown in Table 1.5. The highest oxalate content is present in Anasazi beans (80 mg/100 g wet weight) while lowest in black-eyed peas (4 mg/100 g wet weight) (Honow and Hesse, 2002; Massey et al., 2001). Oxalate salts are negligibly soluble at intestinal pH and oxalic acid is known to decrease Ca absorption in monogastric animals (Allen, 1982). Oxalate content (0.39%) in raw chickpea (*C. arietinum*) was reduced up to 71.79% after it was pressure cooked (Apata and Ologhobo, 1997).

TABLE 1.5   Oxalate Content Present in Different Legumes

Legumes	Oxalate Content (mg 100/g Wet Weight)
Beans	
Anasazi	80
Azuki	25
Black	72
Garbanzo	9
Great northern	75
Large lima	8
Mung	8
Navy	57
October	28
Pink	75
Pinto	27
Red kidney	16
Small red	35
Small white	78
Peas	
Black-eyed	4
Green split	6
Yellow split	5

Sources: Chai and Liebman (2005) [Reprinted from Chai, W.; Liebman, M. Oxalate content of legumes, nuts, and grain-based flours. *Journal of Food Composition and Analysis*, 2005, *53*(8): 723–729. © 2005 Elsevier with permission]

1.2.9.1   EFFECT OF COOKING AND PROCESSING METHODS

Several methods are being applied to reduce oxalate content in legumes and vegetables. The processing method severely affect the content of oxalate during the vegetable preparation. The discarding water used in boiling prior to cooking of vegetables reduces the level of oxalate content (Cleveland and Soleri, 1991). It has also been seen that freezing and controlled boiling of legumes and vegetables followed by discarding the water considerably reduces the oxalate content. The controlled preservation and processing methods also completely eliminate the potential dangers of oxalate toxicity (Oyenuga and Fetuga, 1975; Cleveland and Soleri, 1991).

1.2.9.2   SIGNIFICANCE IN HUMAN HEALTH

The consumption of soluble oxalates in diet causes an excessive urination of oxalate (hyperoxaluria) with an increased risk of developing kidney stones. Therefore, people are recommended to reduce the intake of foods with high oxalate content (Massey, 2003). It elevates the risk of kidney stone formation but decreases the Ca availability in the digestive tract. As the insoluble oxalate is unlikely to be absorbed from the intestinal tract (Simpson et al., 2009), these have to be removed by different processing and cooking methods.

1.2.10   PHYTIC ACID (PHYTATES)

Phytic acid (Figure 1.2C) present in legumes like chickpea (*C. arietinum*), lentil (*L. culinaris*), pea (*P. sativm*), and soybean (*G. max*) is responsible for mineral bioavailability. Phytic acid level varies from 100 to 313.4 mg/100 g (Jain et al., 2009). It is known as chelating agent for cations, and a form for storage of cations as well as phosphorous in many seeds (Oberleas, 1973). It chelates minerals like Ca, Mg, copper (Cu), and iron (Fe^{2+} and Fe^{3+}) (Sharpley et al., 1994). It even interferes with metabolic processes causing reduced solubility of the metals (Oberleas and Prasad, 1969; Oberleas, 1973). Low absorption of minerals causes reduced weight in livestock.

1.2.10.1   EFFECT OF COOKING AND PROCESSING METHODS

Phytic acid content decreases significantly after soaking, cooking, roasting, and autoclaving (Jain et al., 2009). The reason behind this is leaching out of this compound into water. Similarly, roasting and autoclaving decrease the phytic acid content in dry bean (Tabekhia and Luh, 1980), chickpea (*C. arietinum*), and black gram (*Vigna mungo*) (Duhan, 1989), cowpea (*V. unguiculata*) (Akinyele, 1989), and black bean (Sievwright and Shipe, 1986). There is greater reduction of phytic acid in roasted samples as compared to other methods.

1.2.10.2   SIGNIFICANCE IN HUMAN HEALTH

With regard to human health, dietary phytic acid exerts both negative and positive effects (Harland and Morris, 1995). The excretion of mixed phytate salts contribute to mineral deficiency in totally relying on grains and legumes as staple foods. The dietary phytic acid shows anticancer agent and antioxidant properties (Graf, 1987; Harland and Morris, 1995). The adverse impact of dietary phytic acid is on youth of developing world, whereas the positive impact is in the developed countries with the concern of oxidative damage and cancer.

1.2.11   PROTEASE INHIBITORS (TRYPSIN INHIBITORS)

Trypsin inhibitors are proteinous compounds known to inhibit the proteolytic enzymes. Its activity increases with the seed maturation (Jain et al., 2009). The trypsin activity in different leguminous plants is shown in Table 1.6. The factors like partial size, moisture content, time, temperature, and pressure affect the cooking rates and inactivates the trypsin inhibitor which ultimately enhances nutritive value of protein. Inactivation of trypsin inhibitors is essential for use in animal and human food (Gomes et al., 1979; Genovese and Lajolo, 1996). The Kunitz soybean trypsin inhibitor (STI) is responsible for induction of the pancreatic enlargement while Bowman–Birk trypsin chymotrypsin inhibitor from soybeans (*G. max*) and from chickpeas (*C. arietinum*) inhibits insect midgut proteinases, thus defends seeds against insects.

TABLE 1.6   Trypsin Activity in Certain Leguminous Plants

Leguminous Plants	Botanical Name	HCN Yield (Units/mg Protein)
Hyacinth	*Dolichos lablab* L.	16.97
Lathyrus	*L. sativus*	11.88
Soybean	*G. max*	38.57
Cowpea	*V. unguiculata*	19.00
Bengal gram	*C. arietinum*	8.57
Red gram	*C. cajan*	7.77
Black gram	*Vigna* spp.	7.56
Green gram		5.36
Cluster bean	*Cyamopsis tetragonoloba*	2.45

Sources: Gupta (1987) [Reprinted from Gupta, Y. P. Anti-nutritional and toxic factors in food legumes: a review. *Plant Foods for Human Nutrition*, 1987, *37* (3), 201–228. © 1987 Elsevier with permission]

1.2.11.1   EFFECT OF COOKING AND PROCESSING METHODS

Moist heat destroys trypsin inhibitor activity in pulses. Dry heat is not effective against trypsin and chymotrypsin inhibitor in pigeon pea, but soaking (24 h) followed by cooking (20 min) destroys trypsin activity. Autoclaving for 15–20 min at 120 °C, extrusion cooking at 150 °C, or microwave radiation at 107 °C for 30 min is equally effective for the purpose (Jain et al., 2009). Similarly, the heating for 60 min at 100 °C was found to eliminate over 90% of the trypsin in *P. vulgaris* (Trugo et al., 1990).

1.2.11.2   SIGNIFICANCE IN HUMAN HEALTH

The trypsin inhibitory substances can induce pancreatic enlargement through stimulation of cholecystokinin release (Melmed and Bouchier, 1969; Folsch et al., 1974). The enlarged pancreas is responsible for the secretion of pancreatic enzymes that causes the loss of endogenous protein through the pancreas. It also causes indigestion of dietary protein that hinders the growth retardation of growing animals. The rats fed with the 53.9% TI activity in jojoba meal showed growth retardation (Flo et al., 1997). The plant protease inhibitor STI has been reported to alter the hemostasis in humans (Walsh and Ahmad, 2002).

1.2.12   PYRIMIDINE GLYCOSIDES

Vicine (Figure 1.2D) and convicine (Figure 1.2E) are β-glycosides of the pyrimidines divicine and isouramil found in the seeds of *V. sativa* and *V. faba*. The seeds of *V. faba* leads to an acute hemolytic disease known as favism (Mager et al., 1980; Cheeke, 1989). The unstable hydrolysis products of vicine form radicals that deplete the reduced glutathione (GSH) in glucose-6-phosphate dehydrogenase (G6PD) deficient red blood cells. Due to the insufficient nicotinamide adenine dinucleotide phosphate G6PD deficiency leads to the GSH replenishment causing the predisposal of the red blood cells to oxidative damage finally resulting in a hemolytic crisis. It is prevalent in Mediterranean and Southwest Asian populations (Belsey, 1973). Antioxidants are responsible for the removal of the effects of vicine from animal diets (Mager et al., 1980; Cheeke, 1989).

1.2.12.1   EFFECT OF COOKING AND PROCESSING METHODS

The roasting process severely affect the vicine content in the legume seeds of different varieties. An average of 6.06% decrease in vicine content was observed upon roasting. The boiling was found to be more effective in reducing glycosides than roasting because of the solubility of glycosides in water (Abd Allah et al., 1988). The convicine content of *V. faba* diminished from 1.53 to 0.48 mg/g upon roasting and from 1.52 to 0.23 mg/g upon boiling. The average decrease in the content of vicine and convicine was higher by boiling (18.86% and 22.53%, respectively) than by roasting (6.06% and 22.53%, respectively) (Cardador-Martínez et al., 2012). Similar results were observed by Jamalian (1999) in the cotyledons and flour of broad beans (*V. faba*). Khalil and Mansour (1995), on the other hand, reported a decrease of 35% and 37% in the content of vicine and convicine by cooking and autoclaving of broad beans (*V. faba*), respectively.

1.2.12.2   *SIGNIFICANCE IN HUMAN HEALTH*

The vicine and convicine are hydrolyzed by β-glycosidase into aglycone derivatives namely divicine and isouramil that cause favism and ultimately an acute hemolytic anemia (Mckay 1992). Favism occurs after consumption of broad beans (*V. faba*), in 10%–20% of patients with G6PD deficiency in their red blood cells (Cappellini and Fiorelli, 2008; Schuurman et al., 2009). The favism symptoms are seen after 6–24 h of ingestion by broad beans (*V. faba*) which include abdominal and lumbar pain, dizziness, fever headache, nausea, paleness, shiver, tiredness, and vomiting (Luzzatto et al., 2001). In contrast to this, they are beneficial in preventing cardiac arrhythmia and controlling the growth of the malaria parasite (Golenser et al., 1983; Roth et al., 1983). It also shows antitumor property (Cowden et al., 1987).

1.2.13   *QUINOLIZIDINE ALKALOIDS (QAS)*

QAs comprise major group of legume alkaloids (Figure 1.5) mainly produced by members of the Sophoreae. They are more restricted to the more primitive tribes of the Fabaceae (Kinghorn and Balandrin, 1984). These alkaloids have toxic and repellent property (Wink, 1992, 2000). Some of the QAs like sparteine and lupanine show antiarrhythmic activity. The use of sparteine as a uterus-contracting drug has been discontinued. Besides this, they act as hypotensive, CNS-depressant, and antidiabetic agents. These are degraded by daylight as well as during seed germination (Wink and Witte, 1985).

1.2.13.1   *EFFECT OF COOKING AND PROCESSING METHODS*

The influence of roasting, extrusion cooking, aqueous thermal treatment, and alkaline thermal treatment in reducing the levels of QAs in the *Lupinus albus* seeds grown in Ethiopia was studied by Habtie et al. (2009). It was found that the alkaloids exhibited linear reduction in each of roasting, extrusion cooking,

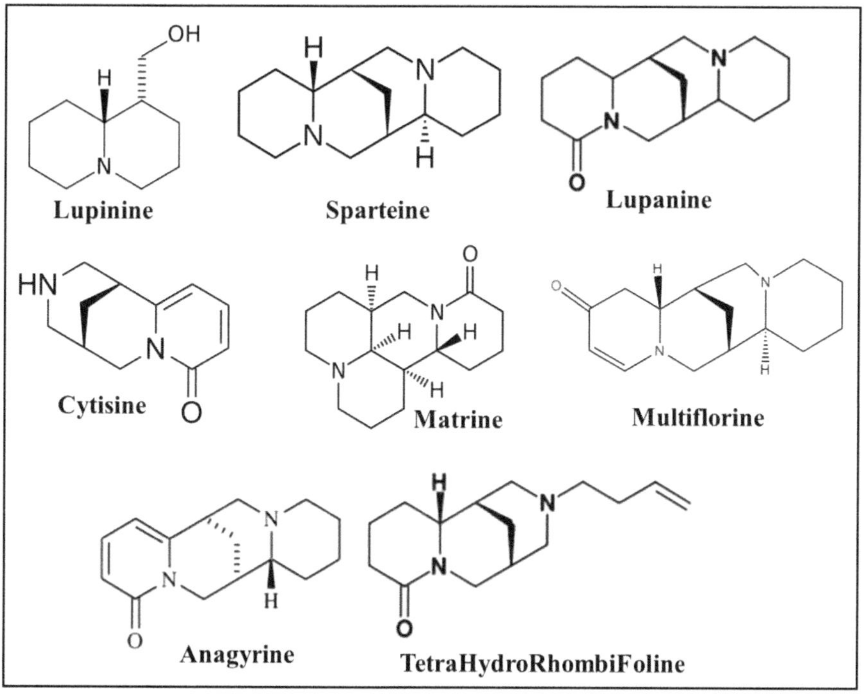

FIGURE 1.5   Structure of different types of quinolizidine alkaloids.

aqueous thermal treatment, and alkaline thermal treatment. Alkaline thermal treatment alone is very effective means of controlling QAs in legumes. NaHCO$_3$ solution (0.5%, pH 8.1) enhances the cooking ability and leaching out of the QAs. The cooking of *L. albus* seeds from Dembecha and from Debretabor in presence of NaHCO$_3$ reduced the level of QAs up to 99.56% and 99.62%, respectively (Shimelis and Rakshit, 2007). Similarly, Jimenez-Martinez et al. (2001) reported a reduction of QAs up to 99.9% in debittered lupin seeds (*L. campestris*) after alkaline (NaHCO$_3$) thermal treatment.

1.2.13.2   SIGNIFICANCE IN HUMAN HEALTH

The ingestion of QAs causes an acute toxicity, the symptoms of which include malaise, nausea, progressive weakness, respiratory arrest, and even coma in extreme case (Grande et al., 2004). A benzylisoquinoline alkaloid (papaverine) is reported to have a potent inhibitory effect on the replication of viruses like cytomegalovirus, human immunodeficiency virus, and measles (Turano et al., 1989). Besides this, it has other biological activities like inhibition of the viruses' multiplication (Wink, 1987), inhibits the growth of bacteria (Wink, 1984; Tyski et al., 1988; De la Vega et al., 1996), and certain fungi (Wink, 1984; Wippich and Wink, 1985). QAs like 13-tigloyloxylupanine, cytisine, lupanine, and sparteine have toxic effects against some Lepidoptera (Paolisso et al., 1985; Korcz et al., 1987; Wink, 1992, 1993).

1.2.14 SAPONINS

The chemical compound (Figure 1.2F) with a carbohydrate moiety (mono/oligosaccharide) in the structure of aglycone belong to the secondary group of plant metabolites id known as Saponins. They are found in the range of 0.05%–0.23% in the legumes like lupins (*L. campestris*) (Woldemichael et al., 2003), lentils (*L. culinaris*) (Morcos et al., 1976; Ruiz et al., 1996), and chickpeas (*C arietinum*) (El-Adawy, 2002), as well various beans, and peas (Shi et al., 2004). The variation in the saponins content (Table 1.7) depends on the type of cultivars (Khokhar and Chauhan, 1986), locations (Fenwick and Oakenfull, 1983; Price et al., 1987), irrigation condition, soil and climatic conditions.

TABLE 1.7   Saponin Presence Certain Leguminous Plants

Leguminous Plants	Saponin Yield (g/kg Dry Weight)
Bengal gram	56.0
Soybean	43.0
Navy beans	
Australia	21.0
Canada	6.7
USA	4.5
Green beans	13.0
Red kidney beans	16.0
Green gram	5.7
Lentil	3.7–4.6
Faba beans	4.3
Broad beans	3.5
Green peas	11.0
Lima beans	1.1
Haricot beans	19.0

Sources: Fenwick and Oakenfull (1983) [Reprinted from Fenwick, D. E.; Oakenfull, D. G. Saponin content of food plants and some prepared foods. *Journal of the Science of Food and Agriculture*, 1983, *34* (2), 186–191. © 1983 John Wiley & Sons with permission]

1.2.14.1   EFFECT OF COOKING AND PROCESSING METHODS

The treatments like soaking, germination, and cooking reduce the saponin contents of pulses. Soaking of pulses has been reported to reduce saponin by 5%–20% which is further reduces upon rising the soaking period (Kataria and Chauhan, 1988; Kataria et al., 1989). This decrease in saponin content during soaking is due to its leaching out into water (Kataria and Chauhan, 1988). Cooking reduces saponin content of chickpea (*C. arietinum*), mung bean (*V. radiata*), and urdbean (*V. mungo*) (Jood et al., 1987; Kataria et al., 1989), and losses are more in pressure cooking as compared to ordinary cooking (Kataria et al., 1989; Jain et al., 2009).

1.2.14.2   SIGNIFICANCE IN HUMAN HEALTH

Saponins are undesirable because of the toxicity and the hemolytic effect. However, there is enormous structural diversity, and only a few are toxic (Shi et al., 2004). They show promising effects for the hyperlipidemic (Shi et al., 2004) and heart patients (Geil and Anderson, 1994) besides the anticancer activity (Chang et al., 2006; Ellington et al., 2006; Shi et al., 2004). Chang et al. (2006) reported the decrease in the expression of R-2, 3-linked sialic acid on the cell surface due to soya-saponin I followed by the suppression of the metastatic potential of melanoma cells by the sialyltransferase inhibitory activity. Further evidences suggest for saponin regulation of the apoptosis pathway enzymes (AKT, Bcl, and ERK1/2), which cause a programmed cell death of cancerous cells (Ellington et al., 2006; Godlewski et al., 2006; Xiao et al., 2007; Zhu et al., 2005).

1.2.15   TANNINS

Tannins (Figure 1.2G) are secondary metabolites and phenolic in nature that are widely distributed through the plant kingdom, especially in legumes (MacRae and Ulyatt, 1974; Min et al., 2000). They exist primarily in condensed and hydrolyzable (HT) forms (Haslam, 1989). The HT molecule contains a carbohydrate (generally D-glucose) as a central core. They are present in pulses like pigeon pea, urdbean, and pea with the highest content. Their content differs based on the color of the seed coat. Light colored seeds contain less tannin than brown dark colored pulses. White varieties of *P. vulgaris* have negligible tannin contents (Jain et al., 2009). The complex of tannins—protein is responsible for decreased amino acid availability, increased fecal nitrogen, and low protein digestibility.

1.2.15.1 EFFECT OF COOKING AND PROCESSING METHODS

The various treatments like boiling and pressure cooking reduce tannins up to 93%. The decrease may be attributed to the heat labile and its water solubility nature. Khattab and Arntfield (2009) also reported reduction of tannins on boiling, autoclaving, and microwave cooking of legume. Dehulling eliminates about 68%–99% of tannins in beans (Alonso et al., 2000; Egounlety and Aworh, 2003; Ghavidel and Prakash, 2007). Soaking of seeds before cooking is usually followed in household practice in order to soften the texture and enhance the cooking process. The leaching out of tannins increases with the soaking time (Kataria and Chauhan, 1988). Overnight soaking in water and subsequent germination for 48 h have been reported to remove most of the tannins in pigeon pea, chickpea (*C. arietinum*), mung bean (*V. radiata*), and urdbean (Jood et al., 1987; Kataria et al., 1989). Cooking followed by discarding of cooking water reduces 37.5%–77% of tannin content (Reddy et al., 1985). Cooking reduces tannins in black grams (*V. mungo*), red kidney, white kidney beans, and in mung bean seeds (*V. radiata*) (Rehman and Shah, 2005; Wang et al., 2010).

1.2.15.2 SIGNIFICANCE IN HUMAN HEALTH

Tannic acid leads to hepatic necrosis in humans as well as in the grazing animals. A single subcutaneous injection of tannic acid at the rate of 700 mg/kg body weight caused a significant breakdown of polyribosomes in mouse liver. Tannins stick to and precipitate the epithelial proteins. They ultimately damage the liver by penetrating through the superficial cells (Chung et al., 1998). Dietary quercetin at 0.1% induces intestinal and bladder carcinomas in Norwegian rats. Similarly, other tannin-related compounds namely rutin, kaempferol, and catechin cause cancer (MacGregor, 1984). Tannins even cause tumors in experimental animals and, hence, are listed as Category I carcinogens by the Occupational Safety and Health Administration (OSHA). The carcinogenic activity of tannins is because of irritation and cellular damage rather than the DNA mutation.

1.2.16 TOXIC AMINO ACIDS (TAAS)

The TAAs are reported in a number of tropical legumes (D'Mello, 1982). These amino acids are antagonistic to certain amino acids which are nutritionally very important (Liener, 1980). According to Bell (1971), nonprotein amino acids act as storage metabolites and even defend plants by the attack of various animals and lower plants. The TAAs are djenkolic acids, mimosine, and canavanine. Mimosine is found in the legume (*Leucaena leucocephala*) (D'Mello and Acamovic, 1989; D'Mello, 2000). It inhibits DNA replication and protein synthesis and has been reported for defleecing sheep and goats (Jacquemet et al., 1990; Luo et al., 2000). Fowden (1971) reported that the metabolic pathways for the synthesis of certain nonprotein amino acids that alter the genome sequence responsible for the formation of some vital amino acids.

1.2.16.1   EFFECT OF COOKING AND PROCESSING METHODS

The TAAs are eliminated by traditional processing methods like as soaking, boiling, and fermentation (Hill, 2003). Over 90% of the 3-*N*-oxalyl-L-2,3-diaminopropanoic acid (ODPA) toxin has been removed by soaking the seeds overnight followed by steaming, roasting, or sun drying (Liener, 2003). Although low-ODPA lines of grass pea which have been developed through traditional breeding and selection, the removal of the neurotoxin from their need novel transgenic methods to remove them which are still under research and trial (Dixon and Sumner, 2003).

1.2.16.2   SIGNIFICANCE IN HUMAN HEALTH

In the legume family, the two toxic nonprotein amino acids having major negative effect on humans and animals are mimosine and ODPA (Hill, 2003; Liener, 2003; Michaels, 2004). These are highly toxic, and cause human toxicoses like lathyrism which is a nonprogressive motor neuron disease associated with high consumption of grass peas (*L. sativus*). Grass peas are common in arid regions, such as Ethiopia and the Indian subcontinent; they contain high levels of ODPA in their seeds. Their consumption causes neurological disorders and even effects on bone formation, especially in children. It is also reported that the consumption of *Lathyrus* is sex linked as it mainly affects young males (Hill, 2003; Dixon and Sumner, 2003).

1.3   SUMMARY AND CONCLUSION

There are various plant sources of nutrition on which humans depend for the livelihood. Among them legumes comprise one of the major sources for body building nutrition and vital ingredients since ancient times. Different researchers have reported their health beneficial artifacts. Despite these, some of the antinutritional factors present in certain legume varieties pose severe threat to the health of human as well as animals. In order to mitigate such adverse effects, the techniques like soaking, cooking, roasting, etc., are employed for better nutritional benefits and ensure consumers' safety at a priority level. Legumes are an important source antinutritional substances which affect normal metabolism and nutritional conditions adversely if used for consumption of both human and animal. The major antinutritional substances of legumes include: amylase inhibitors, chlorogenic acid, cyanogenic glycosides, goitrogens, gossypol, isoflavones, lectins (phytohemagglutinins), oligosaccharides, oxalates, phytic acid (phytates), protease inhibitors (trypsin inhibitors), pyrimidine glycosides, QA saponins, tannins, and TAAs. These substances are with a diverse array of potential nutritional and health benefits and could have beneficial health effects on some important human diseases, namely, cancers, cardiovascular, diabetes, and digestive diseases.

ACKNOWLEDGMENT

Author, Deepak Kumar Verma is highly thankful to Dipendra Kumar Mahato (Project Assistant, Agricultural and Food Engineering Department, Indian Institute of Technology Kharagpur, Kharagpur 721 302, West Bengal, India) and his colleagues Sheetal Devi (Technical, SABMiller India Ltd., Nagavara Village, Bangalore 560045, Karnataka, India) for their consistent support, cooperation, and timely suggestion on technical corrections of this chapter.

KEYWORDS

- **antinutritional phytochemical**
- **cyanogenic glycosides**
- **human health**
- **isoflavones**
- **legumes**
- **phytic acid**
- **polyphenolic compounds**
- **processing methods**
- **saponins**
- **trypsin inhibitors**

REFERENCES

Abd Allah, M. A.; Foda, Y. H.; Abu Salem, F.; Abd Allah, Z. Treatments for reducing total vicine in Egyptian faba bean (Giza 2 variety). *Plant Foods for Human Nutrition*, 1988, *38*, 201–210.

Abd El-Hady, E. A.; Habiba, R. A. Effect of soaking and extrusion conditions on antinutrients and protein digestibility of legume seeds. *LWT—Food Science and Technology*, 2003, *36*, 285–293.

Abdullaev, F. I.; Gonzalez de Mejia, E. Antitumor effect of plant lectins. *Natural Toxins*, 1997, *5*, 157–163.

Akande, K. E.; Doma, U. D.; Agu, H. Q.; Adamu, H. M. Major antinutrients found in plant protein sources: their effect on nutrition. *Pakistan Journal of Nutrition*, 2010, *9* (8): 827–832.

Akinyele, O. T. Effect of traditional methods of processing on nutrient content and some antinutritional factors in cowpea (*Vigna unguiculata*). *Food Chemistry*, 1989, *33*, 291–299.

Alford, B. B.; Liepa, G. U.; Vanbeber, A. D. Cottonseed protein, what does the future hold. *Plant Foods Human Nutrition*, 1996, *49*, 1–11.

Allen, L. H. Calcium bioavailability and absorption: a review. *The American Journal of Clinical Nutrition*, 1982, *35*, 783–808.

Allred, C. D.; Allred, K. F.; Ju, Y. H.; Virant, S. M.; Helferich, W. G. Soy diets containing varying amounts of genistein stimulate growth of estrogen-dependent (MCF-7) tumors in a dose-dependent manner. *Cancer Research*, 2001, *61*, 5045–5050.

Alonso, R.; Aguirre, A.; Marzo, F. Effects of extrusion and traditional processing methods on antinutrients and in vitro digestibility of protein and starch in faba and kidney beans. *Food Chemistry*, 2000, *68*, 159–165.

Alonso, R.; Oruae, E.; Marzo, F. Effects of extrusion and conventional processing methods on protein and antinutritional factor contents in pea seeds. *Food Chemistry*, 1998, *63*, 505–512.

Ambekar, S.; Patil, S. C.; Giri, A. P.; Kachole, M. S. Proteinaceous inhibitors of trypsin and amylases in developing and germinating seeds of pigeon pea (*Cajanus cajan* (L.) Millsp.). *Journal of the Science of Food and Agriculture*, 1996, *72*, 57–62.

Andriot, I.; Le Quéré, J.-L.; Guichard, E. Interactions between coffee melanoidins and flavor compounds: impact of freeze-drying (method and time) and roasting degree of coffee on melanoidins retention capacity. *Food Chemistry*, 2004, *85* (2), 289–294.

Anna, Y.; Medentsev, A. G.; Krupyanko, V. I. Gossypol inhibits electron transport and stimulates ROS generation in Yarrowia lipolytica mitochondria. *Open Biochemistry Journal*, 2012, *6*, 11–15.

Apata, D. F.; Ologhobo, A. D. Trypsin inhibitors and other antinutritional factors in tropical legume seeds. *Tropical Science*, 1997, *37*, 52–59.

Aumaitre, A.; Bourdon, D.; Peiniau, J.; Freire, J. B. Effect of graded levels of raw and processed rapeseed on feed digestibility and nutrient utilization in young pigs. *Animal Feed Science and Technology*, 1989, *24*, 275–287.

Badawy, S. Z. A.; Souid, A.-K.; Cuenca, V.; Montalto, N.; Shue, F. Gossypol inhibits proliferation of endometrioma cells in culture. *Asian Journal of Andrology*, 2007, *9* (3), 388–393.

Bailey, C. J. New approaches to the pharmacotherapy of diabetes. In: *Pickup, J. C.; William, G. (Eds.), Textbook of Diabetes*. Vol. 2, 3rd Ed., Blackwell Science Ltd., UK, 2003.

Bainbridge, Z.; Harding, S.; French, L.; Kapinga, R.; Westby, A. A study of the role of tissues disruption in the removal of cyanogens during cassava root processing. *Food Chemistry*, 1998, *62*, 291–297.

Balakrishnan, K.; Wierda, W. G.; Keating, M. J.; Gandhi, V. Gossypol, a BH3 mimetic, induces apoptosis in chronic lymphocytic leukemia cells. *Blood*, 2008, *112* (5), 1971–1980.

Barraza, M. L.; Coppock, C. E.; Brooks, K. N.; Wilks, D. L.; Saunders, R. G.; Latimer, G. W. Iron sulfate and feed pelleting to detoxify FG in cottonseed diets for dairy cattle. *Journal of Dairy Science*, 1991, *74* (10), 3457–3467.

Beck, V.; Rohr, U.; Jungbauer, A. Phytoestrogens derived from red clover: an alternative to estrogen replacement therapy. *Journal of Steroid Biochemistry and Molecular Biology,* 2005, *94*, 499–518.

Bell, E. A. Comparative biochemistry of nonprotein amino acids. In: *Harborne, J. B.; Boulter, B.; Turner, B. L. (Eds.), Chemotaxonomy of the Leguminosae.* Academic Press, New York, USA, 1971, pages 179–206.

Bell, E. A.; Charlwood, B. V. Secondary plant products. *Encyclopedia of Plant Physiology.* Vol. 8, Springer-Verlag, Berlin, Heidelberg, 1980, page 674.

Belmar, R.; Nava-Montero, R.; Sandoval-Castro, C.; McNab, J. M. Jack bean (*Canavalia ensiformis* L. DC.) in poultry diets: Antinutritional factors and detoxification studies—a review. *World's Poultry Science Journal*, 1999, *55*, 37–59.

Belsey, M. A. The epidemiology of favism. *Bulletin of the World Health Organisation,* 1973, *48* (1), 1–13.

Berardi, L. C.; Goldblatt, L. A. Gossypol. In: *Liener, I. E. (Ed.), Toxic Constituents of Plant Foodstuffs.* 2nd Ed., Academic Press, NY, USA, 1980, pages 183–237.

Bhat, R.; Karim, A. A. Exploring the nutritional potential of wild and underutilized legumes. *Comprehensive Reviews in Food Science and Food Safety,* 2009, *8* (4), 305–331.

Bisby, F. A.; Buckinham, J.; Harborne, J. B. *Phytochemical dictionary of the Leguminosae.* Vols. 1 and 2, Chapman and Hall, London, 1994.

Boerjan, W.; Ralph, J.; Baucher, M. Lignin biosynthesis. *Annual Review of Plant Biology*, 2003, *54*, 519–546.

Bowman, D. E. Some studies on the biochemical and nutritional aspects of selected edible legume seeds. PhD Thesis, University of Sri Jayewardenepura, Nugegoda, Sri Lanka, 1945.

Bunce, T. J.; Howard, M. D.; Allee, G. L.; Pace, L. W. Protective effects of fructooligosaccharide (FOS) in prevention of mortality and morbidity from infectious *E. coli* K: 88 challenge. *Journal of Animal Science*, 1995, *73* (Suppl. 1), 69.

Campos-Vega, R.; Raynoso-Camacho, R.; Pedraza-Aboytes, G.; Acosta-Gallegos, J. A.; Guzman-Maldonado, S. H.; Paredes-Lopez, O.; Oomah, B. D.; Loarca-Pina, G. Chemical composition and *in vitro* polysaccharide fermentation of different beans (*Phaseolus vulgaris* L.). *Journal of Food Science,* 2009, *74*, T59–T65.

Cappellini, M. D.; Fiorelli, G. Glucose-6-phosphate dehydrogenase deficiency. *Lancet*, 2008, *371*, 64–74.

Cardador-Martínez, A.; Maya-Ocaña, K.; Ortiz-Moreno, A.; Herrera-Cabrera, B. E.; Dávila-Ortiz, G.; Múzquiz, M.; Martín-Pedrosa, M.; Burbano, C.; Cuadrado, C.; Jiménez-Martínez, C. Effect of roasting and boiling on the content of vicine, convicine and 1-3,4 dihydroxyphenylalanine in *Vicia faba* L. *Journal of Food Quality*, 2012, *35* (6), 419–428.

Cardoso, A. P.; Mirione, E.; Ernesto, M.; Massaza, F.; Cliff, J.; Haque, R. M.; Bradbury, J. H. Processing of cassava roots to remove cyanogens. *Journal of Food Composition and Analysis*, 2005, *18*, 451–460.

Cassidy, A.; Bingham, S.; Setchell, K. D. R. Biological effects of a diet of soy protein rich in isoflavones on the menstrual cycle of premenopausal women. *American Journal of Clinical Nutrition,* 1994, *60*, 333–340.

Castelluccio, C.; Paganga, G.; Melikian, N.; Bolwell, G. P.; Pridham, J.; Sampson, J.; Rice, E. C. Antioxidant potential of intermediates in phenylpropanoid metabolism in higher plants. *FEBS Letters,* 1995, *368*, 188–192.

Chai, W.; Liebman, M. Oxalate content of legumes, nuts, and grain-based flours. *Journal of Food Composition and Analysis,* 2005, *53* (8): 723–729.

Champ, M. J. M. Non-nutrient bioactive substances of pulses. *British Journal of Nutrition,* 2002, *88* (Suppl. 3), S307–S319.

Chang, W. W.; Yu, C. Y.; Lin, T. W.; Wang, P. H.; Tsai, Y. C. Soyasaponin I decreases the expression of alpha 2,3-linked sialic acid on the cell surface and suppresses the metastatic potential of B16F10 melanoma cells. *Biochemical and Biophysical Research Communications,* 2006, *341*, 614–619.

Cheeke, P. R. *Toxicants of Plant Origin: Glycosides*. Vol. II, CRC Press, Boca Raton, FL, USA, 1989, pages 288.

Chien, C.-C.; Ko, C.-H.; Shen, S.-C.; Yang, L.-Y.; Chen, Y.-C. The role of COX-2/PGE2 in gossypol-induced apoptosis of colorectal carcinoma cells. *Journal of Cellular Physiology,* 2012, *227* (8), 3128–3137.

Choudhury, A.; Maeda, K.; Murayama, R.; Dimagno, E. P. Character of a wheat amylase inhibitor, preparation and effects on fasting human pancreaticobiliary secretions and hormones. *Gastroenterology,* 1996, *111*, 1313–1320.

Chung, K.-T.; Wong, T. Y.; Wei, C. I.; Huang, Y. W.; Lin, Y. Tannins and human health: a review. *Critical Review in Food Science and Nutrition,* 1998, *38* (6), 421–464.

Church, D. C. *Livestock Feeds and Feeding*. 3rd Ed., Prentice Hall Incorporation, New Jersy, USA, 1991, pages 546.

Cleveland, D. A.; Soleri, D. An ecological, nutritional and social approach to small scale households food production. *Food from Dry Land Gardens*, Centre for People, Food, and Environment (CPFE), USA. 1991, pages 26–29.

Clifford, M. N. Chlorogenic acids and other cinnamates—nature, occurrence and dietary burden. *Journal of the Science of Food and Agriculture,* 1999, *79*, 362–372.

Conn, E. E. Secondary plant products. In: *The Biochemistry of Plants*. Vol. 7, Academic Press, New York, USA, 1981.

Cowden, W.; Ramshaw, I.; Badenoch-Jones, P. Divicine-induced free radical killing of tumour cells. *Medical Science Research,* 1987, *15*, 997–998.

D'Mello, J. P. F. Toxic factors in some tropical legumes. *World Review of Animal Production,* 1982, *18*, 41–46.

D'Mello, J. P. F.; Acamovic, T. *Leucaena leucocephala* in poultry nutrition: a review. *Animal Feed Science and Technology,* 1989, *26*, 1–28.

D'Mello, J. P. F. Anti-nutritional factors and mycotoxins. In: *Farm Animal Metabolism and Nutrition*. CAB International Wallingford, UK, 2000, pages 383–403.

De la Vega, R.; Gutie´rrez, M. P.; Sanz, C.; Calvo, R.; Robredo, L. M.; de la Cuadra, C.; Muzquiz, M. Bactericide-like effect of Lupinus alkaloids. *Industrial Crops and Products,* 1996, *5*, 141–148.

Delzenne, N. M.; Kok, N.; Fiordaliso, M. F.; Deboyser, D. M.; Goethals, F. M.; Roberfroid, M. B. Dietary fructooligosaccharides modify lipid metabolism in rats. *American Journal of Clinical Nutrition,* 1993, *57* (Suppl.), 820S.

Dixon, R. A. Phytoestrogens. *Annual Review of Plant Biology,* 2004, **55**, 225–261.

Dixon, R. A.; Sumner, L. W. Legume natural products: understanding and manipulating complex pathways for human and animal health. *Plant Physiology*, 2003, *131*, 878–885.

Duhan, A.; Chauhan, B. M.; Punia, D.; Kapoor, A. C. Phytic acid content of chickpea (*Cicer arietinum*) and black gram (*Vigna mungo*): varietal differences and effect of domestic processing and cooking methods. *Journal of the Science of Food and Agriculture,* 1989, *49* (4), 449–455.

Duke, J. A. 1981. *Handbook of Legumes of World Economic Importance.* Springer, USA, pages 345.

Egounlety, M.; Aworh, O. C. Effect of soaking, dehulling, cooking and fermentation with *Rhizopus oligosporus* on the oligosaccharides, trypsin inhibitor, phytic acid and tannins of soybean (*G. max* Merr.), cowpea (*Vigna unguiculata* L. Walp) and groundbean (*Macrotyloma geocarpa* Harms). *Journal of Food Engineering*, 2003, *56*, 249–254.

El-Adawy, T. A. Nutritional composition and antinutritional factors of chickpeas (*Cicer arietinum* L.) undergoing different cooking methods and germination. *Plant Foods for Human Nutrition*, 2002, *57*, 83–97.

Ellington, A. A.; Berhow, M. A.; Singletary, K. W. Inhibition of Akt signaling and enhanced ERK1/2 activity are involved in induction of macroautophagy by triterpenoid B-group soyasaponins in colon cancer cells. *Carcinogenesis,* 2006, *27*, 289–306.

Enriori, P. J.; Evans, A. E.; Sinnayah, P.; Cowley, M. A. Leptin resistance and obesity. *Obesity*, 2012, *14*, 254S-258S.

Evans, R. C.; Fear, S.; Ashby, D.; Hackett, A.; Williams, E.; van der Vliet, M.; Dunstan, F. D. J.; Rhodes, J. M. Diet and colorectal cancer: an investigation of the lectin/galactose hypothesis. *Gastroenterology*, 2002, *122*, 1784–1792.

Farmakalidis, E.; Murphy, P. Isolation of 6-O-acetyldaidzein from toasted defatted soyflakes. *Journal of Agriculture and Food Chemistry,* 1985, *33*, 385–389.

Fenwick, D. E.; Oakenfull, D. Saponin content of food plants and some prepared foods. *Journal of the Science of Food and Agriculture*, 1983, *34*, 186–191.

Fenwick, G. R.; Spinks, E. A.; Wilkinson, A. P.; Heaney, R. K.; Legoy, M. A. Effect of processing on the antinutrient content of rapeseed. *Journal of the Science of Food and Agriculture*, 1986, *37*, 735–741.

Flo, G.; Abbott, T.; Vermout, S.; Boven, M. V.; Daenens, P.; Decuypere, E.; Pedersen, M.; Cokelaere, M. Growth performance of rats fed jojoba proteins: possible correlations with trypsin inhibitory activity in jojoba proteins. *Journal of Agricultural and Food Chemistry,* 1997, *45*: 4384–4387.

Folsch, U. R.; Winckler, K.; Wormsle, K. G. Effect of a soy bean diet on enzyme content and ultrastructure of the rat exocrine pancreas. *Digestion,* 1974, *11*, 161–171.

Fowden, L. Amino acid biosynthesis. In: *Pridham, J. B. and Swain, T. (Eds.), Biosynthetic Pathways in Higher Plants.* Academic Press, New York, USA, 1971, pages 73–99.

Francis, G.; Makkar, H. P. S.; Becker, K. Antinutritional factors present in plant-derived alternate fish feed ingredients and their effects in fish. *Aquaculture*, 2001, *199*, 197–227.

Franke, A.; Custer, L.; Cerna, C.; Narala, K. Rapid HPLC analysis of dietary phytoestrogens from legumes and from human urine. *Proceedings of the Society for Experimental Biology and Medicine*, 1995, *208*, 18–26.

Fukuba, H.; Igarashi, O.; Briones, C. M.; Mendoza, E. M. T. Determination anddetoxification of cyanide in cassava and cassava products. *Philippians Journal of Crop Science*, 1982, *7*, 170–175.

Gaitan, E.; Lindsay, R. H.; Cooksey, R. C. Millet and the thyroid. In: *Gaitan, E. (Ed), Environmental Goitrogenesis*, CRC Press, Boca Raton, Florida, 1989, pages 195–206.

Garcia-Olmedo, F.; Salcedo, G.; Sanchez-Monge, R.; Gomez, L.; Rexo, J.; Carbonero, P. Plant proteinaceous inhibitor of proteinases and *a*-amylases. *Oxford Surveys of Plant Molecular and Cell Biology*, 1987, *4*, 275.

Geil, P. B.; Anderson, J. W. Nutrition and health implications of dry beans: a review. *Journal of the American College of Nutrition*, 1994, *13*, 549–558.

Genovese, M. I.; Lajolo, F. M. Effect of bean (*Phaseolus vulgaris*) albumins on phaseolin *in vitro* digestibility, role of trypsin inhibitors. *Journal of Food Biochemistry*, 1996, *20*, 275–294.

Gepts, P.; Beavis, W. D.; Brummer, E. C.; Shoemaker, R. C.; Stalker, H. T.; Weeden, N. F.; Young, N. D. Legumes as a model plant family. Genomics for food and feed report of the cross-legume advances through genomics conference. *Plant Physiology*, 2005, **137** (4): 1228–1235.

Ghavidel, R. A.; Prakash, J. The impact of germination and dehulling on nutrients, anti-nutrients, *in vitro* iron and calcium bioavailability and *in vitro* starch and protein digestibility of some legume seeds. *LWT—Food Science and Technology*, 2007, *40*, 1292–1299.

Gibson, G. R.; Wang, X. Bifidogenic properties of different types of fructooligosaccharides. *Food Microbiology*, 1994, *11*, 491–498.

Giri, A. P. Role of proteinaceous inhibitors of pigeon pea in insect pest resistance. PhD Thesis. Dr Babasaheb Ambedkar Marathwada University, Aurangabad, India, 1964.

Giri, A. P.; Kachole, M. S. Amylase inhibitors of pigeon pea (*Cajanus cajan*) seeds. *Phytochemistry*, 1998, *47*, 197–202.

Godlewski, M. M.; Slazak, P.; Zabielski, R.; Piastowska, A.; Gralak, M. A. Quantitative study of soybean-induced changes in proliferation and programmed cell death in the intestinal mucosa of young rats. *Journal of Physiology and Pharmacology*, 2006, *57*, 125–133.

Golenser, J.; Miller, J.; Spira, D.; Navok, T.; Chevion, M. Inhibitory effect of a fava bean component on the in vitro development of *Plasmodium falciparum* in normal and glucose-6-phosphate dehydrogenase deficient erythrocytes. *Blood*, 1983, *61*, 507–510.

Gomes, J. C.; Koch, U.; Brunner, J. R. Isolation of a trypsin inhibitor from navy beans by affinity chromatography. *Cereal Chemistry*, 1979, *56* (6) 525–529.

Graf, E. Phytic acid: a natural antioxidant. *Journal of Biological Chemistry*, 1987, *262*, 11647–11650.

Graham, P. H.; Vance, C. P. Legumes. Importance and constraints to greater use. *Plant Physiology*, 2003, *131*, 872–877.

Grande, A. D.; Paradiso, R.; Amico, S.; Fulco, G.; Fantauzza, B.; Noto, P. Anticholinergic toxicity associated with lupin seed ingestion: case report. *European Journal of Emergency Medicine*, 2004, *11*, 119–120.

Grant, G.; Edwards, J. E.; Pusztai, A. α-Amylase inhibitor levels in seeds generally avail-able in Europe. *Journal of the Science of Food and Agriculture*, 1995, *67*, 235–238.

Guillon, F.; Champ, M. M.-J. Carbohydrate fractions of legumes: uses in human nutrition and potential for health. *British Journal of Nutrition*, 2002, *88*, S293–S306.

Gupta, Y. P. Anti-nutritional and toxic factors in food legumes: a review. *Plant Foods for Human Nutrition*, 1987, *37*, 201–228.

Habtie, T.; Admassu, S.; Asres, K. Effects of processing methods on some phytochemicals present in the seeds of *Lupinus albus* L. grown in Ethiopia. *Ethiopian Pharmaceutical Journal*, 2009, *27* (2), 91–102.

Han, I. H.; Baik, B. K. Oligosaccharide content and composition of legumes and their reduction by soaking, cooking, ultrasound, and high hydrostatic pressure. *Cereal Chemistry.* 2006, *83*, 428–433.

Han, M. L.; Wang, Y. F.; Tang, M. Y.; Ge, Q. S.; Zhou, L. F.; Zhu, P. D.; Sun, Y. T. Gossypol in the treatment of endometriosis and uterine myoma. *Contributions to Gynecology and Obstetrics*, 1987, *16*, 268–270.

Harland, B. F.; Morris, E. R. Phytate: a good or a bad food component. *Nutrition Research,* 1995, *15*, 733–754.

Haslam, E. *Plant Polyphenols. Vegetable Tannins Revisited.* Cambridge University Press, Cambridge, UK, 1989.

Herrmann, K. Flavonols and flavones in food plants: a review. *Journal of Food Technology,* 1976, *11*, 433–438.

Hidaka, H.; Eida, T.; Tokunaga, T.; Tashiro, Y. Effects of fructooligosaccharides on intestinal flora and human health. *Bifidobacteria and Microflora*, 1986, *5*, 37–50.

Hidaka, H.; Tashiro, Y.; Eida, T. Proliferation of bifidobacteria by oligosaccharides and their useful effect on human health. *Bifidobacteria and Microflora*, 1991, *10*, 65–79.

Hidayat, A.; Zuraida, N.; Hanarida, I. The cyanogenic potential of roots and leaves of ninety nine cassava cultivars. *Indonesian Journal of Agricultural Science*, 2002, *3*, 25–32.

Hill, G. D. *Plant Antinutritional Factors/Characteristics.* Elsevier Science Ltd.; Lincoln University, Canterbury, 2003, pages 4578–4586.

Honow, R.; Hesse, A. Comparison of extraction methods for the determination of soluble and total oxalate in foods by HPLC-enzyme-reactor. *Food Chemistry,* 2002, *78*, 511–521.

Howes, M. J. R.; Pery, N. S.L.; Houghton, P. J. Plants with traditional uses and activities, relevant to the management of Alzheimer's disease and other cognitive disorders. *Phytotherapy Research*, 2003, *17*, 1–18.

Hsiao, W.-T.; Tsai, M.-D.; Jow, G.-M.; Tien, L.-T.; Lee, Y. J. Involvement of Smac, p53, and caspase pathways in induction of apoptosis by gossypol in human retinoblastoma cells. *Molecular Vision*, 2012, *18*, 2033–2042.

Huang, S.; Liang, M.; Lardy, G.; Huff, H. E.; Kerley, M. S.; Hsieh, F. Extrusion process of rapeseed meal for reducing glucosinolates. *Animal Feed Science and Technology,* 1995, *56*, 1–9.

Ishizuki, Y.; Hirooka, Y.; Murata, Y.; Togashi, K. The effects on the thyroid gland of soybeans administered experimentally in healthy subjects. *Nippon Naibunpi Gakkai Zasshi*, 1991, *67*, 622–629.

Jackson, C. J. C.; Dini, J. P.; Lie, L.; Kingsmill, C.; Faulkner, H.; De Grandis, S. The influence of variety, location and growth year on phytoestrogen levels in Ontario soybeans and processed food products. *Journal of Medicinal Food*, 1999, *2*, 3–4.

Jacquemet, N.; Fernandez, J. M.; Sahlu, T.; Lu, C. D. Mohair quality and metabolic profile of Angoragoats during acute mimosine toxicity. *Journal of Animal Science,* 1990, *75* (1), 69–79.

Jain, A. K.; Sudhir Kumar, S.; Panwar, J. D. S. Antinutritional factors and their detoxification in Pulses—a review. *Agricultural Reviews,* 2009, *30* (1), 64–70.

Jamalian, J. Favism-inducing toxins in broad beans (*Vicia faba*). Determination of vicine content and investigation of other non-protein nitrogenous compounds in different broad bean cultivars. *Journal of the Science of Food and Agriculture*, 1978, *29*, 136–140.

Jansz, E. R.; Uluwaduge, D. I. Biochemical aspects of cassava (manihotesculentacrantz) with special emphasis on cyanogenic glucosides—a review. *Journal of the National Science Council of Sri Lanka*, 1997, *25*, 1–24.

Jiang, J.; Slivova, V.; Jedinak, A.; Sliva, D. Gossypol inhibits growth, invasiveness, and angiogenesis in human prostate cancer cells by modulating NF-κB/AP-1 dependent and independent-signaling. *Clinical and Experimental Metastasis*, 2012, *29* (2), 165–178.

Jimenez-Martinez, C.; Hernandez-Sánchez, H.; Alvarez-Manilla, G.; Robledo-Quintos, N.; Martınez-Herrera, J.; Dávila-Ortiz, G. Effect of aqueous and alkaline thermal treatments on chemical composition and oligosaccharide, alkaloid and tannin contents of *L. campestris* seeds. *Journal of the Science of Food and Agriculture*, 2001, *81*, 421–428.

Johnson, P. W. M. New targets for lymphoma treatment. *Annals of Oncology*, 2008, *19* (4), iv56–iv59.

Jönsson, T.; Olsson, S.; Ahrén, B.; Bøg-Hansen, T. C.; Dole, A.; Lindeberg, S. Agrarian diet and diseases of affluence—Do evolutionary novel dietary lectins cause leptin resistance? *BMC Endocrine Disorders*, 2005, *5* (10), 1–7.

Jood, S.; Chauhan, B. M.; Kapoor, A. C. Polyphenols of chickpea and blackgram as affected by domestic processing and cooking methods. *Journal of the Science of Food and Agriculture*, 1987, *39*, 145–149.

Ju, Y. H.; Allred, C. D.; Allred, K. F.; Karko, K. L.; Doerge, D. R.; Helferich, W. G. Physiological concentrations of dietary genistein dose-dependently stimulate growth of estrogen-dependent human breast cancer (MCF-7) tumors implanted in athymic nude mice. *Journal of Nutrition*, 2001, *131*, 2957–2962.

Ju, Y. H.; Fultz, J.; Allred, K. F.; Doerge, D. R.; Helferich, W. G. Effects of dietary daidzein and its metabolite, equol, at physiological concentrations on the growth of estrogen-dependent human breast cancer (MCF-7) tumors implanted in ovariectomizedathymic mice. *Carcinogenesis*, 2006, *27*, 856–863.

Kalogeropoulos, N.; Chiou, A.; Ioannou, M.; Karathanos, V. T.; Hassapidou, M.; Andrikopoulos, N. K. Nutritional evaluation and bioactive microconstituents (phytosterols, tocopherols, polyphenols, triterpenic acids) in cooked dry legumes usually consumed in the Mediterranean countries. *Food Chemistry*, 2010, *121*, 682–690.

Kasai, H.; Fukada, S.; Yamaizumi, Z.; Sugie, S.; Mori, H. Action of chlorogenic acid in vegetables and fruits as an inhibitor of 8-hydroxydeoxyguanosine formation in vitro and in a rat carcinogenesis model. *Food and Chemical Toxicology*, 2000, *38*, 467–471.

Kataria, A.; Chauhan, B. M. Contents and digestibility of carbohydrates of mung beans (*Vigna radiata* L.) as affected by domestic processing and cooking. *Plant Foods for Human Nutrition*, 1988, *38*, 51–59.

Kataria, A.; Chauhan, B. M.; Punia, D. Antinutrients and protein digestibility (in vitro) of mung bean as affected by domestic processing. *Food Chemistry*, 1989, *32* (1), 9–17.

Khalil, A. H.; Mansour, E. H. The effect of cooking, autoclaving and germination on the nutritional quality of faba beans. *Food Chemistry*, 1995, *54*, 177–182.

Khattab, R. Y.; Arntfield, S. D.; Nyachoti, C. M. Nutritional quality of legume seeds as affected by some physical treatments, Part 1: Protein quality evaluation. *LWT—Food Science and Technology*, 2009, *42*, 1107–111.

Khattab, R.Y.; Arntfield, S. D. Nutritional quality of legume seeds as affected by some physical treatments 2. Antinutritional factors, *LWT—Food Science and Technology*, 2009, *42*, 1113–1118.

Khokhar, S.; Chauhan, B. M. Antinutritional factors in moth bean: varietal differences and effects of methods of domestic processing and cooking. *Journal of Food Science*, 1986, *51*, 591–594.

Kilpatrick, P. C.; Pusztai, A.; Grant, G.; Graham, C.; Ewen, S. W. B. Tomato lectin resists digestion in the mammalian alimentary canal and binds to intestinal villi without deleterious effects. *FEBS Letters*, 1985, *185* (2), 299–305.

Kim, M.; Shin, H. K. The water soluble extract of chicory influences serum and liver lipid concentrations, cecal short-chain fatty acid concentrations and fecal lipid excretion in rats. *Journal of Nutrition,* 1998, *128*, 1731–1736.

Kinghorn, D. A.; Balandrin, M. F. Quinolizidine alkaloids of the Leguminosae: structural types, analysis, chemotaxonomy, and biological activities. In: *Pelletier, W. S. (Ed.), Alkaloids: Chemical and Biological Perspectives*, 2nd Ed., John Wiley and Sons, New York, 1984, pages 105–148.

Korcz, A.; Markiewicz, M.; Pulikowska, J.; Twardowski, T. Species-specific inhibitory effects of lupine alkaloids on translation in plants. *Journal of Plant Physiology*, 1987, *128*, 433–438.

Kuhnau, J. The flavonoids. A class of semi-essential food components: their role in human nutrition. *World Review of Nutrition and Dietetics,* 1976, *24*, 117–191.

Kwon, S. H.; Lee, H. K.; Kim, J. A.; Hong, S. I.; Kim, H. C. Jo, T. H.; Park, Y. I.; Lee, C. K.; Kim, Y. B.; Lee, S. Y.; Jang, C. G. Neuroprotective effects of chlorogenic acid on scopolamine-induced amnesia via anti-acetyl cholinesterase and anti-oxidative activities in mice. *European Journal of Pharmacology,* 2010, *649*, 210–217.

Laranjinha, J. A.; Almeida, L. M.; Madeira, V. M. Reactivity of dietary phenolic acids with peroxyl radicals: antioxidant activity upon low density lipoprotein peroxidation. *Biochemical Pharmacology,* 1994, *48*, 487–494.

Lee, C. W.; Won, T. J.; Kim, H. R.; Lee, D.; Hwang, K. W.; Park, S. Y. Protective effect of chlorogenic acid against Ab-induced neurotoxicity. *Biomolecules and Therapeutics,* 2011, *19*, 181–186.

Lewis, G. P.; Schrire, B. D.; Mackinder, B. A.; Lock, M. In: *Lewis, G. P.; Schrire, B. D.; Mackinder, B. A.; Lock, M. (Eds.*), *Legumes of the World* Royal Botanic Garden, Kew, UK, 2005.

Liener, I. E. Heat labile antinutritional factors. In: *Summerfield, R. J.; Bunting, A. H. (Eds.), Advances in Legume Science.* Royal Botanic Gardens, Kew, London, 1980, pages 157–170.

Liener, I.. E.. Antitryptic and other anti-nutritional factors in legumes. In: *Milner, M. (Ed.), Nutritional Improvement of Food Legumes by Breeding.* Wiley Interscience Publication, John Wiley and Sons, New York, 1975, pages 239–258.

Liener, I. E. *Plant Antinutritional Factors/Detoxification.* Elsevier Science Ltd.; University of Minnesota, St. Paul, MN, USA, 2003, pages 4587–4593.

Luo, J.; Litherland, A. J.; Sahlu, T.; Puchala, R.; Lachicaand, M.; Goetsch, A. L. Effects of mimosine on fiber shedding, follicle activity and fiber regrowth in Spanish goats. *Journal of Animal Science,* 2000, *78*, 1551–1555.

Luzzatto, L.; Sydney, B.; Jeffrey, H. M. Favism. In: *Reeve, E. C. R. (Ed.), Encyclopedia of Genetics.* Taylor and Francis Ltd., Oxford, 2001, pages 683–683.

MacGregor, J. T. Genetic and carcinogenic effects of plant flavonoids: an overview. In: *Friedman, M. (Ed.), Nutritional and Toxicological Aspects of Food Safety. Advances in Experimental Medicine and Biology,* Springer , Boston, MA, USA, Vol. 177, 1984, pages 497–526.

MacRae, J. C.; Ulyatt, M. J. Quantitative digestion of fresh herbage by sheep: II. The sites of digestion of some nitrogenous constituents. *Journal of Agricultural Science, Cambridge*, 1974, *82* (2), 309–319.

Mager, J.; Chevion, M.; Glaser, G. Favism. In: *Liener, I. E. (Ed.), Toxic Constituents of Plant Foodstuffs*. 2nd Ed., Academic Press, NY, USA, 1980, pages 265–294.

Maheshwari, P. N.; Stanley, D. W.; Van de Van, F. R. Microwave treatment of dehulled rapeseed meal to inactivate myrosinase and its effect on oil meal quality. *Journal of the American Oil Chemists' Society,* 1980, *57*, 194–199.

Marshall, J. J.; Lauda, C. M. Purification and properties of Phaseolanin, an inhibitor of α-amylase from the kidney bean, *Phaseolus vulgaris. Journal of Biological Chemistry*, 1975, *250*, 8031–8037.

Massey, L. K. Dietary influences on urinary oxalate and risk of kidney stones. *Frontiers in Biosciences,* 2003, *8*, s584–s594.

Massey, L. K.; Palmer, R. G.; Horner, H. T. Oxalate content of soybean seeds (*Glycine max*: Leguminosae), soyfoods, and other edible legumes. *Journal of Agricultural and Food Chemistry*, 2001, *49*, 4262–4266.

McDonald, P.; Edwards, R. A.; Greenhalgh, J. F. D.; Morgan, C. A. *Animal Nutrition*. 5th Ed., Longman Group Ltd., UK, 1995, pages 607.

Mckay, A. Hydrolysis of vicine and convicine from faba beans by microbial b-glucosidase enzymes. *Journal of Applied Microbiology,* 1992, *72*, 475–478.

Melmed, R. N.; Boucher, I. A. D. A further physiological role for naturally occurring trypsin inhibitors: the evidence for a throphic stimulant of the pancreatic acinar cells. *Gut,* 1969, *10*, 973–979.

Menezes, E. W.; Laljo, F. M. Inhibition of starch digestion by a black bean amylase inhibitor in normal and diabetic rats. *Nutrition Reports International,* 1987, *36*, 1185.

Michaels, T. E. *Pulses, Overview*. Elsevier Ltd, University of Minnesota, St. Paul, MN, USA, 2004, pages 494–501.

Min, B. R.; McNabb, W. C.; Barry, T. N.; Peters, J. S. Solubilization and degradation of ribulose-1,5-*bis*phosphate carboxylase/oxygenase (EC 4.1.1.39; Rubisco) protein from white clover (*Trifolium repens*) and *Lotus corniculatus* by rumen microorganisms and the effect of condensed tannins on these processes. *Journal of Agricultural Science, Cambridge*, 2000, *134*, 305–317.

Morcos, S. R.; Gabriel, G. N.; El-Hafez, M. A. Nutritive studies on some raw and prepared leguminous seeds commonly used in the Arab Republic of Syria. *Zeitschrift fuer Ernaehrungswissenchaft*, 1976, *15*, 378–386.

Murphy, P. A. Separation of genistin, daidzin and their aglycones and coumesterol by gradient high-performance liquid chromatography. *Journal of Chromatography,* 1981, *211*, 166–169.

Nagabhushana Rao, G.; Shrivastava, S. K. Toxic and antinutritional factors of new varieties of pea seeds. *Research Journal of Pharmaceutical, Biological and Chemical Sciences,* 2011, *2* (2), 512–523.

Nagalakshmi, D.; Sastry, V. R. B.; Agrawal, D. K. Detoxification of undecorticated cottonseed meal by various physical and chemical methods. *Animal Feed Science and Technology,* 2002, *2* (2), 117–126.

Nagalakshmi, D.; Sastry, V. R. B.; Pawde, A. Rumen fermentation patterns and nutrient digestion in lambs fed cottonseed meal supplemental diets. *Animal Feed Science and Technology,* 2003, *103*: 1–4.

Nambisan, B. Evaluation of the effect of various processing techniques on the cyanogens reduction in cassava. *Acta Horticulture*, 1994, *375*: 193–202.

Nardini, M.; D'Aquino, M.; Tomassi, G.; Gentili, V.; Di-Felice, M.; Scaccini, C. Inhibition of human low-density lipoprotein oxidation by caffeic acid and other hydroxycinnamic acid derivatives. *Free Radical Biology and Medicine,* 1995, *19*, 541–552.

Ngudi, D. D.; Kuo, Y. H.; Lambein, F. Cassava cyanogens and free amino acids in raw and cooked leaves. *Food and Chemical Toxicology*, 2003, *41*, 1193–1197.

Nicoli, M. C.; Anese, M.; Parpinel, M. T. Influence of processing on the antioxidant properties of fruit and vegetables. *Trends Food Science Technological*, 1999, *10*, 94–100.

Nikmarama, N.; Leong, S. Y.; Koubaa, M.; Zhu, Z.; Barba, F. J.; Greiner, R.; Oey, I.; Roohinejad, S. Effect of extrusion on the anti-nutritional factors of food products: an overview. *Food Control*, 2017, *79*, 62–73.

Noonan, S. C.; Savage, G. P. Oxalate content of foods and its effect on humans. *Asia Pacific Journal of Clinical Nutrition*, 1999, *8*, 64–74.

Noratto, G.; Porter, W.; Byrne, D.; Cisneros-Zevallos, L.; Identifying peach and plum polyphenols with chemopreventive potential against estrogen-independent breast cancer cells. *Journal of Agricultural and Food Chemistry.* 2009, *57*, 5219–5226.

Nwinuka, N. M.; Abbe, B. W.; Ayalogu, E. O. Effect of processing on flatus producing oligosaccharides in cowpea (*Vigna unguiculata*) and the tropical African yam bean (*Sphenostylis stenocarpa*). *Plant Foods for Human Nutrition,* 1997, *51*, 209–218.

Oberleas, D. Phytates. In: *Strong, F. M. (Ed.), Toxicants Occurring Naturally in foods*. 2nd Ed., National Academy of Sciences, Washington, DC, USA, 1973, pages 363–371.

Oberleas, D.; Prasad, A. S. Growth as affected by zine and protein nutrition. *American Journal of Clinical Nutrition,* 1969, *22*, 1304–1314.

Okubo, K.; Kobayzshi, Y.; Takahashi, K. Improvement of soymilk and tofu process on the behavior of undesirable taste component such as glycosides. *Up to Date Food Processing,* 1983, *18*, 16–22.

Oliveira, A. C.; Vidal, B. C.; Sgarbieri, V. C. Lesions of intestinal epithelium by ingestion of bean lectins in rats. *Journal of Nutritional Science and Vitaminology (Japan)*, 1989, *35*, 315–322.

Onigbinde, A. O.; Akinyele, I. O. Oligosaccharide content of 20 varieties of cowpeas in Nigeria. *Journal of Food Science,* 1983, *48*, 1250–1254.

Orhan, I.; Kartal, M.; Tosun, F.; Sener, B. Screening of various phenolic acids and flavonoid derivatives for their anticholinesterase potential. *Zeitschrift für Naturforschung C*, 2007, *62*, 829–832.

Oyenuga, V. A.; Fetuga, B. L. Dietary importance of fruits and vegetables. *Proceeding of First National Seminar on Fruits and Vegetables*, Ibadan, 1975, pages 122–129.

Pan, W.; Ikeda, K.; Takebe, M.; Yamori, Y. Genistein, daidzein and glycitein inhibit growth and DNA synthesis of aortic smooth muscle cells from strokeprone spontaneously hypertensive rats. *Journal of Nutrition*, 2001, *131* (4), 1154–1158.

Paolisso, G.; Nenquin, M.; Schmeer, W.; Mathot, F.; Meissner, H. P.; Henquin, J. C. Sparteine increases insulin release by decreasing the K+ permeability of the B-cell membrane. *Biochemical Pharmacology*, 1985, *34* (13), 2355–2361.

Pedrosa, M. M.; Cuadrado, C.; Burbano, C.; Allaf, K.; Haddad, J.; Gelencsér, E.; Takács, K.; Guillamón, E.; Muzquiz, M. Effect of instant controlled pressure drop on the oligosaccharides, inositol phosphates, trypsin inhibitors and lectins contents of different legume. *Food Chemistry* 2012, *131,* 862–868.

Polsky B.; Segal, S. J.; Baron, P. A.; Gold, J. W. M.; Ueno, H.; Armstrong, D. Inactivation of human immunodeficiency virus in vitro by gossypol. *Contraception*, 1989, *39* (6), 579–587.

Price, K. R.; Johnson, I. T.; Fenwick, G. R. The chemistry and biological significance of saponins in food and feeding stuffs. *Critical Review in Food Science and Nutrition*, 1987, *26*, 27–135.

Puls, W.; Keup, N. Influence of an α-amylase inhibitor in blood glucose, serum insulin and NEFA in starch loading tests in rats, dogs and man. *Diabetologia*, 1973, *9*, 97–101.

Purseglove, J. W. *Tropical Crops: Dicotyledons.* Longman Scientific and Technical Co., John Wiley and Sons Inc.,United States, New York, USA, 1991.

Pusztai, A. Biological effects of dietary lectins. In: *Recent Advances of Research in Antinutritional Factors in Legume Seeds: Animal Nutrition, Feed Technology and Analytical Methods.* Pudoc, Wageningen (Netherlands), 1989, pages 17–29.

Pusztai, A.; Watt, W. B.; Stewart, J. C. A comprehensive scheme for the isolation of trypsin inhibitors and agglutinins from soybean seeds. *Journal of the Science of Food and Agriculture*, 1991, *39*, 862–866.

Ramadoss, B. R.; Shunmugam, A. S. K. Anti-dietetic factors in legumes—local methods to reduce them. *International Journal of Food and Nutritional Sciences*, 2014, *3* (2), 84–89.

Randel, R. D.; Chase Jr, C. C.; Wyse, S. J. Effect of gossypol and cottonseed products on reproduction in mammals. *Journal of Animal Science,* 1992, *70*, 1628–1638.

Randhir, R.; Kwon, Y. I.; Shetty, K. Effect of thermal processing on phenolics, antioxidant activity and health-relevant functionality of select grain sprouts and seedlings. *Innovative Food Science and Emerging Technologies,* 2008, *9*, 355–364.

Randhir, R.; Kwon, Y. I.; Shetty, K. Improved health-relevant functionality in dark germinated Mucuna pruriens sprouts by elicitation with peptide and phytochemical elicitors. *Bioresource Technology,* 2009, *100*, 4507–4514.

Reddy, N. R.; Pierson, M. D.; Sathe, S. K.; Salunkhe, D. K. Dry bean tannins: a review of nutritional implications. *Journal of the American Oil Chemists' Society,* 1985, *62*, 541–549.

Rehman, Z.; Shah, W. H. Thermal heat processing effects on anti-nutrients, protein and starch digestibility of food legumes. *Food Chemistry,* 2005, *91*, 327–331.

Rice-Evans, C. A.; Miller, N. J.; Paganga, G. Structure-antioxidant activity relationships of flavonoids and phenolic acids. *Free Radical Biology and Medicine,* 1996, *20*, 933–956.

Roberfroid, M. B.; Vanloo, J. A. E.; Gibson, G. R. The bifidogenic nature of chicory inulin and its hydrolysis products. *Journal of Nutrition,* 1998, *128*, 11–19.

Robinson, E. H. Improvement of cottonseed meal protein with supplemental lysine in feeds for channel catfish. *Journal of Applied Aquaculture*, 1991, *1*, 1–14.

Robinson, P. H.; Getachew, G.; De Peters, E. J.; Calhoun, M. C. Influence of variety and storage for up to 22days on nutrient composition and gossypol level of Pima cottonseed (*Gossypium* spp.). *Animal Feed Science and Technology,* 2001, *91*, 149–156.

Roth, E. F.; Raventos-Suarez, C.; Rinaldi, A.; Nagel, R. L. Glucose-6-phosphate dehydrogenase deficiency inhibits in vitro growth of *Plasmodium falciparum. Proceedings of the National Academy of Sciences of the USA,* 1983, *80*, 298–299.

Ruiz, R. G.; Price, K. R.; Arthur, A. E.; Rose, M. E.; Rhodes, M. J. C.; Fenwick, R. G. Effect of soaking and cooking on the saponin content and composition of chickpeas (*Cicer arietinum*) and lentils (*Lens culinaris*). *Journal of Agricultural and Food Chemistry*, 1996, *44*, 1526–1530.

Santos, M. D.; Almeida, M. C.; Lopes, N. P.; Souza, G. E. Evaluation of the antiinflammatory, analgesic and antipyretic activities of the natural polyphenol chlorogenic acid. *Biological and Pharmaceutical Bulletin,* 2006, *29,* 2236–2240.

Schuurman, M.; Van Waardenburg, D.; Costa, J.; Niemarkt, H.; Leroy, P. Severe hemolysis and methemoglobinemia following fava beans ingestion in glucose-6-phosphatase dehydrogenase deficiency: case report and literature review. *European Journal of Pediatrics,* 2009, *168,* 779–782.

Sharpley, A. N.; Charpa, S. C.; Wedepohl, R.; Sims, J. Y.; Daniel, T. C.; Reddy, K. R. Managing agricultural phosphorus for protection of surface waters: issues and options. *Journal of Environmental Quality,* 1994, *23,* 437–451.

Sheehan, D. M. Isoflavone content of breast milk and soy formulas: benefits and risks [Editorial]. *Clinical Chemistry,* 1997, *43,* 850.

Sheehan, D. M. Herbal medicines, phytoestrogens, and toxicity: risk/benefit considerations. *Proceedings of the Society for Experimental Biology and Medicine,* 1998, *217,* 379–385.

Shepard, T. H.; Pyne, G. E.; Kirschvink, J. F.; McLean, C. M. Soybean goiter. *New England Journal of Medicine,* 1960, *262,* 1099–1103.

Shi, J.; Arunasalam, K.; Yeung, D.; Kakuda, Y.; Mittal, G.; Jiang, Y. Saponins from edible legumes: chemistry, processing, and health benefits. *Journal of Medicinal Food,* 2004, *7,* 67–78.

Shi, A. H.; Zhang, Y.; Qu, P.; Yan, J. G.; Xiao, H. J. Screening and breeding of highly-effected degrading cotton-phenol strains and study on detoxification technology and conditions. *Acta Microbiologica Sinica,* 1998, *38* (4), 318–320.

Shibata, H.; Sakamoto, Y.; Oka, M.; Kono, Y. Natural antioxidant, chlorogenic acid, protects against DNA breakage caused by monochloramine. *Bioscience, Biotechnology, and Biochemistry,* 1999, *63,* 1295–1297.

Shimelis, A. E.; Rakshit, S. K. Effect of processing on antinutrients and *in vitro* protein digestibility of kidney bean (*Phaseolus vulgaris* L.) varieties grown in East Africa. *Food Chemistry,* 2007, *103,* 161–172.

Sievwright, C. A.; Shipe, W. F. Effect of storage conditions and chemical treatments on firmness, in vitro protein digestibility, condensed tannins, phytic acid and divalent cations of cooked black beans (*Phaseolus vulgaris*). *Journal of Food Science,* 1986, *51, 982–987.*

Simpson, T. S.; Savage, G. P.; Sherlock, R.; Vanhanen, L. Oxalate content of silver beet leaves at different stages of maturation and the effect of cooking with different milk sources. *Journal of Agricultural and Food Science,* 2009, *57,* 10804–10808.

Smithard, R. R.; Eyre, M. D. The effect of dry extrusion of rapeseed with other feedstuffs upon its nutritional value and anti-thyroid activity. *Journal of the Science of Food and Agriculture,* 1986, *37,* 136–140.

Spreadbury, I. Comparison with ancestral diets suggests dense acellular carbohydrates promote an inflammatory microbiota, and may be the primary dietary cause of leptin resistance and obesity. *Diabetes, Metabolic Syndrome and Obesity: Targets and Therapy,* 2012, *5,* 175–189.

Stacewicz-Sapuntzakis, M.; Bowen, P. E.; Hussain, E. A.; Damayanti-Wood, B. I.; Farnsworth, N. R. Chemical composition and potential health effects of prunes: a functional food? *Critical Reviews in Food Science and Nutrition,* 2001, *41* (4), 251–286.

Strumeyer, D. H. Protein amylase inhibitors of the gliadin fraction of wheat, rye flour and possible factors in coeliac disease. *Nutrition Reports International,* 1972, *6,* 45–49.

Tabatabai, F.; Golian, A.; Salarmoeini, M. Determination and detoxification methods of cottonseed meal gossypol for broiler chicken rations. *Journal of Agricultural Science and Technology* 2002, *16* (1), 3–15.

Tabekhia, M. M.; Luh, B. S. Effect of germination, cooking, and canning on phosphorus and phytate retention in dry beans. *Journal of Food Science,* 1980, *45,* 406–408.

Tarling, C. A.; Woods, K.; Zhang, R.; Brastianos, H. C.; Brayer, G. D.; Andersen, R. J.; Withers, S. G. The search for novel human pancreatic-amylase inhibitors: high-throughput screening of terrestrial and marine natural product extracts. *ChemBioChem,* 2008, *9,* 433–438.

Tikkanen, M. J.; Adlercreutz, H. Dietary soy-derived isoflavone phytoestrogens: could they have a role in coronary heart disease prevention? *Biochemical Pharmacology,* 2000, *60,* 1–5.

Tikkanen, M. J.; Wahala, K.; Ojala, S.; Vihma, V.; Adlercreutz, H. Effect of soybean phytoestrogen intake on low density lipoprotein oxidation resistance. *Proceedings of the National Academy of Sciences of the USA,* 1998, *95,* 3106–3110.

Tokunaga, T.; Oku, T; Hosoya, N. Utilization and excretion of a new sweetener, fructooligosaccharide in rats. *Journal of Nutrition,* 1989, *119,* 553–559.

Trugo, L. C.; Ramos, L. A.; Trugo, N. M. F.; Souza, M. C. P. Oligosaccharide composition and trypsin inhibitor activity *of Phaseolus vulgaris* and the effect of germination on the alpha-galactoside composition and fermentation in the human colon. *Food Chem*istry, 1990, *36,* 53–61.

Tucker, S. C. Floral development in legumes. *Plant Physiology,* 2003, *131,* 911–926.

Turano, A.; Scura, G.; Caruso, A.; Bonfanti, C.; Luzzati, R.; Basetti, D.; Manca, N. Inhibitory effect of papaverine on HIV replication *in vitro. AIDS Research and Human Retroviruses,* 1989, *5,* 183–191.

Turco, E.; Vizzuso, C.; Franceschini, S.; Ragazzi, A.; Stefanini, F. M. The *in vitro* effect of gossypol and its interaction with salts on conidial germination and viability of *Fusarium oxysporum* sp. vasinfectum isolates. *Journal of Applied Microbiology,* 2007, *103* (6): 2370–2381.

Tyski, S.; Markiewicz, M.; Gulewicz, K.; Twardowski, T. The effect of lupin alkaloids and ethanol extracts from seeds of *L. angustofolius* and selected bacterial strains. *Journal of Plant Physiology,* 1988, *133* (2), 240–242.

Uzogara, S. G.; Morton, I. D.; Daniel, J. W. Changes in some antinutrients of cowpeas (*Vigna unguiculata*) processed with 'kanwa' alkaline salt. *Plant Foods Human Nutrition,* 1996, *40,* 249–258.

van der Schouw, Y. T.; Pijpe, A.; Lebrun, C. E. I.; Bots, M. L.; Peeters, P. H. M.; van Staveren, W. A.; Lamberts, S. W. J.; Grobbee, D. E. Higher than usual dietary intake of phytoestrogens is associated with lower aortic stiffness in postmenopausal women. *Arteriosclerosis, Thrombosis, and Vascular Biology,* 2002, *22,* 1316–1322.

Van Poznak, C.; Seidman, A. D.; Reidenberg, M. M.; Moasser, M. M.; Sklarin, N.; Van Zee, K.; Borgen, P.; Gollub, M.; Bacotti, D.; Yao, T. J.; Bloch, R.; Ligueros, M.; Sonenberg, M.; Norton, L.; Hudis, C. Oral gossypol in the treatment of patients with refractory metastatic breast cancer: a phase I/II clinical trial. *Breast Cancer Research and Treatment,* 2001, *66* (3), 239–248.

Vijayakumari, K.; Siddhuraju, P.; Janardhanan, K. Chemical composition and nutritional potential of the tribal pulse (Bauhinia malabarica Roxb). *Plant Foods for Human Nutrition,* 1993, *44,* 291–298.

Walsh, P. N.; Ahmad, S. S. Proteases in blood clotting. *Essays in Biochemistry,* 2002, *38,* 95–111.

Wang, H. J.; Murphy, P. A. Isoflavone content in commercial soybean foods. *Journal of Agriculture and Food Chemistry,* 1994, *42,* 1666–1673.

Wang, H. J.; Murphy, P. A. Mass balance study of isoflavones during soybean processing. *Journal of Agriculture and Food Chemistry,* 1996, *44,* 2377–2383.

Wang, N.; Hatcher, D. W.; Tyler, R. T.; Toews, R.; Gawalko, E. J. Effect of cooking on the composition of beans (*Phaseolus vulgaris* L.) and chickpeas (*Cicer arietinum* L.). Food Research International, 2010, *43,* 589–594.

Wang, X.; Wang, J.; Wong, S. C.; Chow, L. S.; Nicholls, J. M.; Wong, Y. C.; Liu, Y.; Kwong, D. L.; Sham, J. S.; Tsa, S. W. Cytotoxic effect of gossypol on colon carcinoma cells. *Life Sciences,* 2000, *67* (22), 2663–2671.

Weiping, Y.; Hsiang-Lin, C.; Li-Shu, W.; Yi-Wen, H.; Sherry, S.; Yasuro, S.; Michael, K. D.; Peter, J. W.; Young C. L. Modulation ofmultidrug resistance gene expression in human breast cancer cells by (−)-gossypol-enriched cottonseed oil. *Anticancer Research,* 2007, *27* (1), 107–116.

Wilson, R. P.; Robinson, E. H.; Poe, W. E. Apparent and true availability of amino acids from *Nutrition,* 1981, *111,* 923–929.

Wink, M. Chemical defense of Leguminosae. Are quinolizidine alkaloids part of the antimicrobial defense system of lupins? *Zeitschrift für Naturforschung,* 1984, *39,* 548–552.

Wink, M. Interference of alkaloids with neuroreceptors and ion channels. In: *Atta-Ur-Rahman (Ed.), Bioactive Natural Products.* Vol. 11, Elsevier, Amsterdam, 2000, pages 3–129.

Wink, M. Quinolizidine alkaloids: biochemistry, metabolism, and function in plants and cell suspension cultures. *Planta Medica,* 1987, *53,* 509–514.

Wink, M. The role of quinolizidine alkaloids in plant-insect interactions. In: *Bernays, E. A. (Ed.), Insect-Plant Interactions.* Vol. IV, CRC Press, Boca Raton, FL, 1992, pages 131–166.

Wink, M. Quinolizidine alkaloids. In: *Waterman, P. (Ed.), Methods in Plant Biochemistry.* Vol. 8, Academic Press, London, 1993, pages 197–239.

Wink, M.; Witte, L. Quinolizidine alkaloids as nitrogen source for lupin seedlings and cell suspension cultures. *Zeitschrift für Naturforschung,* 1985, *40,* 767–775.

Wippich, C.; Wink, M. Biological properties of alkaloids. Influence of quinolizidine alkaloids and gramine on the germination and development of powdery mildew, Erysiphe graminist f. sp. hordei. *Experientia,* 1985, *41,* 1477–1479.

Woldemichael, G. M.; Montenegro, G.; Timmermann, B. N. Triterpenoidal lupin saponins from the Chilean legume *Lupinus oreophilus* Phil. *Phytochemistry,* 2003, *63,* 853–857.

Wood, J. A.; Grusak, M. A. Nutritional value of chickpea. In: *Yadav, S. S.; Redden, R.; Chen, W. and Sharma, B. (Eds.), Chickpea Breeding and Management.* CAB International, Wallingford, UK, 2007, pages 101–142.

Wood, C. E.; Register, T. C.; Franke, A. A.; Anthony, M. S.; Cline, J. M. Dietary soy isoflavones inhibit estrogen effects in the postmenopausal breast. *Cancer Research,* 2006, *66,* 1241–1249.

Wu, X. Y.; Chen, J. X. The utilization of microbes to break down FG in cottonseed meal. *Scientia Agricultura Sinica,* 1989, *22* (2), 82–86.

Xiao, J. X.; Huang, G. Q.; Zhu, C. P.; Ren, D. D.; Zhang, S. H. Morphological study on apoptosis HeLa cells induced by soyasaponins. *Toxicology in Vitro,* 2007, *21,* 820–826.

Yang, J.; Chen, G.; Li, L.; Pan, W.; Zhang, F.; Yang, J.; Wu, S.; Tien, P. Synthesis and anti-H5N1 activity of chiral gossypol derivatives and its analogs implicated by a viral entry blocking mechanism. *Bioorganic* and *Medicinal Chemistry Letters,* 2013, *23* (9), 2619–2623.

Yang, J.; Zhang, F.; Li, J.; Chen, G.; Wu, S.; Ouyang, W.; Pan, W.; Yu, R.; Yang, J.; Tien, P. Synthesis and antiviral activities of novel gossypol derivatives. *Bioorganic and Medicinal Chemistry Letters*, 2012, *22* (3), 1415–1420.

Yildirim-Aksoy, P.; Lim, C.; Dowd, M. K.; Wan, P. J.; Klesius, P. H.; Shoemaker, C. *In vitro* inhibitory effect of gossypol from gossypol-acetic acid, and (+)- and (−)-isomers of gossypol on the growth of *Edwardsiella ictaluri*. *Journal of Applied Microbiology*, 2004, *97* (1): 87–92.

Zhang, J.; Shi, J.; Ilic, S.; Jun, X. S.; Kakuda, Y. Biological properties and characterization of lectin from red kidney bean (*Phaseolus vulgaris*). *Food Reviews International*, 2009, *25*, 12–27.

Zhu, J.; Xiong, L.; Yu, B.; Wu, J. Apoptosis induced by a new member of saponin family is mediated through caspase-8-dependent cleavage of Bcl-2. *Molecular Pharmacology*, 2005, *68*, 1831–1838.

CHAPTER 2

Sorghum Phytochemicals: Extraction, Processing, Application, and Health Benefits

SMITA SINGH[1], DEEPAK KUMAR VERMA[2], MAMTA THAKUR,
SOUBHAGYA TRIPATHY, SANKHADIP BOSE, PREM PRAKASH SRIVASTAV,
MÓNICA L. CHÁVEZ-GONZÁLEZ, and CRISTOBAL NOE AGUILAR

[1]*Department of Life Sciences (Food Technology), Graphic Era
(Deemed to be) University, Dehradun, Uttarakhand 248002, India
E-mail: sweetsmita1004@gmail.com*

[2]*Agricultural and Food Engineering Department, Indian Institute of
Technology Kharagpur, Kharagpur 721302, West Bengal, India.
E-mail: deepak.verma@agfe.iitkgp.ernet.in*

ABSTRACT

Sorghum, popularly known as milo, is a versatile crop which can easily grow in drought-prone areas. It has high nutritional value and is a good source of phytochemicals, that is, tannins, flavonoids, phytosterols, and policosanols. These phytochemicals have high antioxidant activity as compared with other cereals and also exhibit positive health benefits. Processing conditions result in the reduction of antioxidant properties. Consumption of sorghum in the regular diet has shown anticancerous properties and prevents cardiovascular diseases, esophageal cancer, and many more. This chapter reviews and discusses the information on sorghum phytochemicals, their processing, and development of food products as well as human health application.

2.1 INTRODUCTION

Cereals are consumed by millions of people all over the world as a staple food. Grains are important sources of dietary fiber, energy, minerals, protein, vitamins, and phytochemicals (such as lignans, phenolic acid, phytic acids, and phytoestrogens). Cereals are known to be the richest source of soluble dietary fiber (SDF) (Plaami, 1997). The major components of SDF are arabinoxylans, with some amount of β-D-glucans (Rao and Muralikrishna, 2004). Crops other than wheat and rice are referred to as coarse cereals. These coarse cereal crops (Figure 2.1) are widely grown in semiarid regions which are also known as poor man's crop (Rai et al., 2008)

Sorghum (*Sorghum bicolor* (L.) Moench) is a member of the family "*Poaceae*" and grows up to a height of 6 feet (Figure 2.2). It is popularly used as food and feed worldwide. Sorghum contains higher contents of fat and protein than other cereals making it suitable as feed for livestock. Table 2.1 shows the proximate composition of sorghum grain (SG). Tables 2.2 and

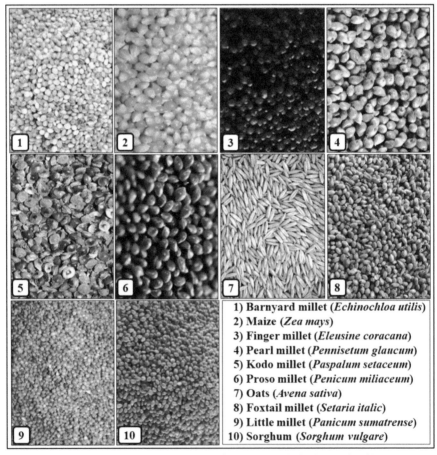

1) Barnyard millet (*Echinochloa utilis*)
2) Maize (*Zea mays*)
3) Finger millet (*Eleusine coracana*)
4) Pearl millet (*Pennisetum glaucum*)
5) Kodo millet (*Paspalum setaceum*)
6) Proso millet (*Penicum miliaceum*)
7) Oats (*Avena sativa*)
8) Foxtail millet (*Setaria italic*)
9) Little millet (*Panicum sumatrense*)
10) Sorghum (*Sorghum vulgare*)

FIGURE 2.1   List of some important grains of course cereals for human health.

2.3 compare the nutrient component of sorghum with other cereal crops. Due to low nutritional value and other reasons like poor digestibility and limited diversification of its product, sorghum is considered as poor food which limits its utilization in human food (Mella, 2011; Raihanatu et al., 2011). Figure 2.3 shows the factors for poor digestibility of sorghum protein stated by Doudou et al. (2003).

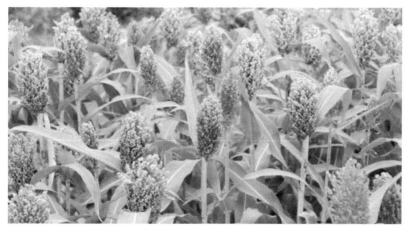

FIGURE 2.2   Standing field crop of *Sorghum vulgare* with the grains.

TABLE 2.1   Nutritional Value of Sorghum Grain

Nutrients Components	Value per 100 g (3.5 oz)	Nutrients Components	Value per 100 g (3.5 oz)
Proximate		Vitamin B$_6$	0.443 mg
Energy	1377 kJ (329 kcal)	Niacin (B$_3$)	3.688 mg
Carbohydrates	72.09 g	Folate (B$_9$)	20 μg
Dietary fiber	6.7 g	Vitamin E (α-tocopherol)	0.50 mg
Fat	3.46 g	**Minerals**	
Saturated	0.610 g	Calcium (Ca)	13 mg
Monounsaturated	1.131 g	Iron (Fe)	3.36 mg
Polyunsaturated	1.558 g	Magnesium (Mg)	165 mg
Protein	10.62 g	Phosphorus (P)	289 mg
Vitamins		Potassium (K)	363 mg
Thiamine (B$_1$)	0.332 mg	Sodium (Na)	2 mg
Riboflavin (B$_2$)	0.096 mg	Zinc (Zn)	1.67 mg

Source: Adapted from USDA (2017).

TABLE 2.2 Composition of Nutrient of Sorghum Grain With Comparison to Various Other Cereal Crops

Cereals and Millets Crop	Protein (g)	Fat (g)	Fiber (g)	Minerals (g)	Iron (mg)	Calcium (mg)	Calories (kcal)
Sorghum	10.4	3.1	2	1.6	5.4	25	329
Rice	6.8	2.7	0.2	0.6	0.7	10	362
Wheat	11.8	2	1.2	1.5	5.3	41	348
Corn	9.4	4.7	–	–	2.71	7	365.0
Barnyard millet	11.2	3.9	10.1	4.4	15.2	11	342
Finger millet	7.3	1.5	3.6	2.7	3.9	344	336
Foxtail millet	12.3	4	8	3.3	2.8	31	473
Kodo millet	8.3	3.6	9	2.6	0.5	27	309
Little millet	7.7	5.2	7.6	1.5	9.3	17	207
Pearl millet	10.6	4.8	1.3	2.3	16.9	38	378
Proso millet	12.5	2.9	2.2	1.9	0.8	14	356

Source: Modified from Kapri et al. (2017); USDA (2017).

TABLE 2.3 Composition of Essential Amino Acids of Sorghum Grain With Comparison to Various Other Cereal Crops (in mg/g)

Amino Acids	Sorghum and Other Cereal Crops							
	Sorghum	Barnyard Millet	Common Millet	Finger Millet	Foxtail Millet	Kodo Millet	Little Millet	Pearl Millet
Cystine	94	175	–	163	–	–	–	148
Leucine	832	725	762	594	1044	419	679	598
Isoleucine	245	288	405	275	475	188	416	256
Lysine	126	106	189	181	138	188	114	214
Methionine	87	133	160	194	175	94	142	154
Phenylalanine	306	362	307	325	419	375	297	301
Threonine	189	231	147	263	194	194	212	241
Tryptophan	63	63	49	191	61	38	35	122
Tyrosine	167	150	–	–	–	213	–	203

Source: Adapted from FAOUN (1970); Indira and Naik (1971).

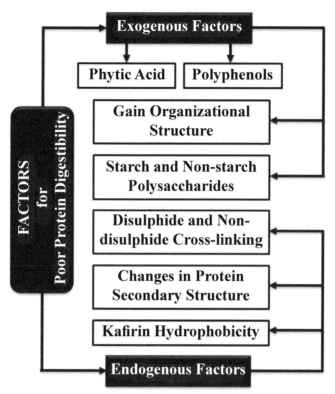

FIGURE 2.3   Factors for poor digestibility of sorghum protein (Doudou et al., 2003).

Sorghum is known with different names such as *Durra, Egyptian millet, Guinea corn, Jowar, Milo, Shallu,* and *Sudan grass* depending on the geographical area. The major sorghum producing country is the United States with about 10.25 million ton per annum, followed by Mexico, Nigeria, and India with 7.0, 6.3, and 5.0 million ton, respectively (FAOUN, 2016). A region of China, that is, Shaanxi province was reported to be the largest consumer of sorghum with 1.4–3.2 lesser amount of mortality from esophageal cancer (Chen et al., 1993). It has also been reviewed that biofortified sorghum and millets are being developed through conventional breeding and recombinant DNA technology to combat malnutrition in developing countries (Taylor et al., 2014).

Sorghum is a rich source of phytochemicals beneficial for human health and a source of natural colorants (Awika and Rooney, 2004; Etuk et al., 2012). The people of Africa and India consume 35% of sorghum directly, whereas the rest is used for animal feed and production of bioethanol. The consumption of sorghum comes at fifth place, after wheat, rice, maize, and barley all over the world (Klopfesntein and Hoseney, 1995; Mohammed et al., 2011; Paiva et al., 2015). Processing is done to increase the consumption of this grain. More recently, dry and wet heat have been used for the processing of SG. Dry heat (oven/milling, milling/oven, and popped grains/ milling) did not affect the content of 3-deoxyanthocyanidins, total phenolics compounds, and antioxidant activity. It increased vitamin E content but decreased carotenoid content in sorghum flour (BRS 301 genotype). Wet heat (cooking in water/drying/milling) was less efficient as compared to dry heat, as it decreased 3-deoxyanthocyanidins and all the other compounds, whereas carotenoid got increased in the flour (Cardoso et al., 2014).

Therefore, this chapter is framed to focus on sorghum phytochemicals, their chemistry, processing, and development of food products as well as potential human health application and their role in chronic disease.

2.2 PHYTOCHEMICALS

Phytochemicals are known as phytonutrients. There are thousands different types of phytochemicals are found in different fruits and vegetables (Xin et al., 2006; De la Rosa et al., 2010), whole grains (Okarter and Liu, 2010; Koistinen and Hanhineva, 2017), legumes (Rochfort and Panozzo, 2007; Admassu, 2009), beans (Abu-Reidah et al., 2013; Seidu et al., 2014), herbs (Kennedy and Wightman, 2011), spices (Kadam et al., 2015), and nuts (Oliver Chen and Blumberg, 2008; Bolling et al., 2010). Some of these phytochemical compounds are glucosinolates, lectins monoterpenes, phytoestrogens, phytosterols, polyphenols, protease inhibitors, salicylates, saponins, sulfides, terpenes, and so on. The general classification of these phytochemical compounds is given based on chemical structures and their functional properties.

These bioactive phytochemicals are not uniformly distributed in grains because some part like bran and germ reported in the literature to have higher concentrations. The main examples of such grains are sorghum, barley, rice, wheat, corn, oats, rye, triticale, millet, amaranth, and teff in which bioactive phytochemicals are found in the majority.

Recent research indicates that the beneficial effect of whole grain may arise from the combined action of several components such as fiber, vitamins, phenolics, carotenoids, alkylresorcinols, and other phytochemicals (Okarter and Liu, 2010; Liu, 2007; Koistinen and Hanhineva, 2017). In cereal grains, the most diversified and complex group of phytochemicals found dominantly are known as phenolic compounds (Ragaee et al., 2014; Wanga et al., 2014; Van Hung, 2016). They contain various derivatives of benzoic and cinnamic acids as well as alkylresorcinols, anthocyanidins, avenanthramides, flavones and flavonols, flavonoids, and lignans.

Many reports state that the phenolic acids of the most cereal grains are found in the bran and embryo of the cell walls (Stevenson et al., 2012; Belobrajdic and Bird, 2013; Goufo and Trindade, 2014) and exist mostly being minor entities in different forms such as free form, insoluble bound form, and soluble-conjugated form (Fardet, 2010; Jonnalagadda et al., 2011). The insoluble bound form of most of the phenolic acids are found in cereal grains, these form of phenolic acids in wheat are reported about 80% of the total phenolic acids (Liyana-Pathirana and Shahidi, 2006; Li et al., 2008; Fernandez-Orozco et al., 2010). It is considered that the total antioxidant capacity of whole grains mainly contributed by the content of these phenolic acids (Jonnalagadda et al., 2011). Notwithstanding this, these minor grains have some most useful quality characteristics. Notably, they are character-ized by being rich in many "health-promoting" phytochemicals, which exhibit antioxidant and free-radical scavenging activity (Przbylski et al., 1998; Dykes and Rooney, 2006). Black rice has gained increasing popularity today as a staple food and is replacing white rice, due to its high potential health-promoting and chronic-disease-preventing properties (Chiang et al., 2006; Wang et al., 2007; Norkaew et al., 2017). The health benefits of black rice are attributed to the bioactive pigments located in the bran layer of the rice (Norkaew et al., 2017). Two major anthocyanins found in black rice are cyanidin-3-O-glucoside and peonidin-3-O-glucoside (Hou et al., 2013). The phytochemicals found in sorghum and their potential health benefit when people consume it as a part of their diet are subject of great concern that has been described in the following sections.

2.2.1 SORGHUM PHYTOCHEMICALS

In the world, Sorghum is the fifth leading crop among the cereal (Dlamini et al., 2007; Raihanatu et al., 2011) which has noted to have the highest content of polyphenols when compare with other cereals such as barley, millet, wheat, or rye (Ragaee et al., 2006). However, the phenolic compounds of sorghum are found in the outer layers (pericarp and testa) of the grain (Beta et al., 2000) while the whole SG contain higher amounts of dietary fiber and biologically active phytochemicals, viz. 3-deoxyanthocyanins, phenolic acids, phytosterols, policosanols, and procyanidins (Awika et al., 2005; Dykes et al., 2011).

The phytochemicals have extended increased interest because of their many possible health benefits viz. antioxidant activity, cancer prevention, cardiovascular disease, cholesterol-lowering properties, diabetes, and obesity (Awika and Rooney, 2004; Liu, 2007; Awika et al., 2009; Okarter and Liu, 2010; Belobrajdic and Bird, 2013; Proietti et al., 2015; Stefoska-Needham et al., 2015; de Morais Cardoso et al., 2017). Phenolic acids and flavonoids are two major classes of sorghums phenols, in which phenolic acids are described as the derivatives of benzoic or cinnamic acid (Hahn et al., 1983; Waniska et al., 1989), while anthocyanins and tannins describe to the flavonoids class as the most important components extracted from sorghum to date (Gupta and Haslam, 1978; Gujer et al., 1986; Gous, 1989; Krueger et al., 2003).

Sorghum phytosterols have mostly free sterols or stanols and their fatty acid/ferulate esters which are reported in corn with structural similarity (Avato et al., 1990; Singh et al., 2003). Sorghums have been classified into two types due to their phytochemical specification (Figure 2.4); one of them is on the basis of extraction of their tannin content, and another is on the basis both appearance and the extraction of their total phenols content (Cummings and Axtel, 1973; Price et al., 1978; Awika and Rooney, 2004).

The phytochemicals commonly present in sorghum are tannins, anthocyanin, phenolic acids, phytosterols, and policosanols. Along with SG, bran, and leaves, SG cuticle has also been reported to be rich in phytochemicals viz. flavonoids, tannins, and anthocyanins (Kaluza et al., 1988; Rey et al., 1993). The presence of these phytochemicals in sorghum foods and beverages show various functional and health-promoting effects. They may also impart probiotic effects due to the action of their lactic acid bacteria-fermented products (Taylor and Duodu, 2014).

2.2.1.1 FLAVONOIDS AND ANTHOCYANIN

Flavonoids are a group of polyphenolic compounds. They are ubiquitous and are classified according to their chemical structure into different classes such as entities anthocyanidins catechins, chalcones flavanones, flavones, flavonols, and isoflavones. The structure of major sorghum flavonoids is depicted in Figure 2.5. Rooney and coworkers developed black, red, and lemon-yellow sorghums in 2013, which have high flavonoids with or without condensed tannins (Rooney et al., 2013a, b) and best natural colorants source

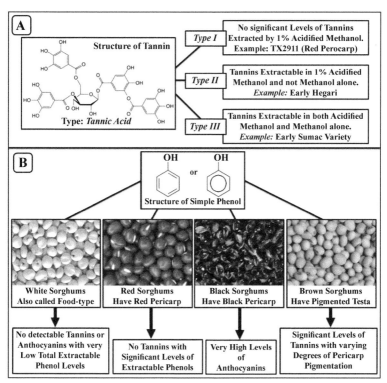

FIGURE 2.4 Classification of sorghums based on (A) tannin content extraction (Cummings and Axtel, 1973; Price et al., 1978) and (B) appearance and total phenols content extraction (Awika and Rooney, 2004).

with known health beneficial effects on human (Shih et al., 2007; Bralley et al., 2008; Burdette et al., 2010; Devi et al., 2011). Genotypic and environmental conditions of sorghum are responsible to regulate the flavonoids metabolism (Boddu et al., 2005; Shih et al., 2006).

Sorghum flavonoids are divided into three groups reported by Dykes et al. (2009, 2011) in high amounts in different genotypes of SGs such as 3-deoxyanthocyanidins (32–680 mg/g), flavones (60–386 mg/g), and flavanones (134–1780 mg/g). The group of flavonoids "3-deoxyanthocyanidins" is predominantly fond in black sorghum genotypes which are known as potential natural sources of colorants for low pH foods and also reported for their anti-cancer and anti-inflammatory activities (Shih et al., 2007; Yang et al., 2009; Burdette et al., 2010). The 3-deoxyanthocyanidin sorghum flavonoids (Figure 2.6) are of two types; (1) methoxylated and (2) nonmethoxylated (Dykes et al., 2009; Taleon et al., 2012). The methoxylated forms of 3-deoxyanthocyanidins

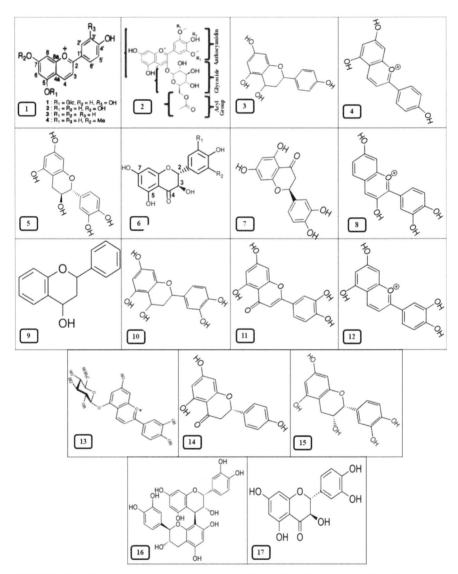

FIGURE 2.5 Structure of sorghum flavonoid. (A) 7-*O*-methyl apigeninidin (Pale et al., 1997); (B) anthocyanins and anthocyanidins (R$_1$, R$_2$, and R$_3$ are each independently –H, –OH, or –OCH$_3$; and R$_4$ is a sugar either a galactose, glucose, arabinose, xylose, or rhamnose) (Barnes et al., 2009); (C) apiforol; (D) apigeninidin; (E) catechin; (F) dihydroflavonol (R$_1$ = H and R$_2$ = H; R$_1$ = H and R$_2$ = OH; R$_1$ = OH and R$_2$ = OH) (Trabelsi et al., 2011); (G) eriodictoyl; (H) fisetinidin; (I) flavan-4-ols; (J) luteoforol; (K) luteolin; (L) luteolinidin; (M) luteolinidin-5-glucoside; (N) naringenin; (O) proanthocyanidin; (P) procyanidin B$_1$; and (Q) taxifolin.

sorghum flavonoids show stronger anticarcinogenic activity and was confirmed by Yang et al. (2009), whereas flavanones show anticancer activity was confirmed by Ko et al. (2002) and Lee et al. (2008). These flavanones with high concentrations were reported by Dykes et al. (2009, 2011) in red and lemon-yellow genotypes of sorghum with tan secondary plant color. These groups of phenolic compounds are associated to human health with beneficial effects (Hahn et al., 1983, 1984; Dykes et al., 2005, 2006, 2009, 2011, 2013; Luthria and Liu, 2013; Taylor et al., 2014) since reports of many researchers point out that the consumption of high levels of flavonoids in foods of daily routine may have potential to solve many chronical diseases like some cancers such as breast, colon, and pancreatic cancers (Slavin et al., 1997; Awika and Rooney, 2004, 2005; Shih et al., 2007; Rai et al., 2008; Yang et al., 2009, 2012; Devi et al., 2011; Carbonneau et al., 2014; de Morais Cardoso et al., 2017).

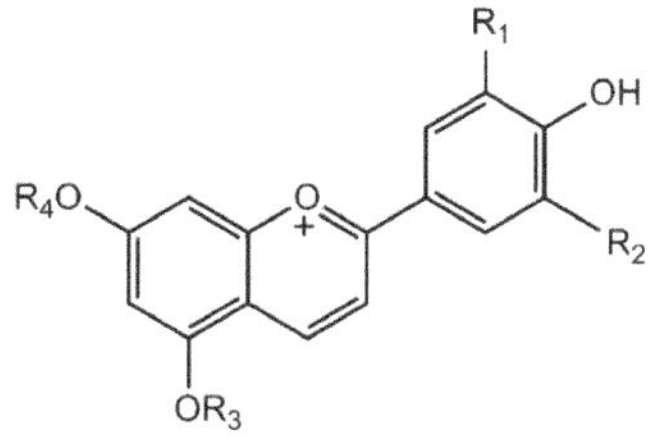

FIGURE 2.6   Structure of 3-deoxyanthocyanidin sorghum flavonoid.

Anthocyanins are a group of pigments that are widely distributed among plant species. They may be provided in the diet by a variety of fruits, vegetables, and grains. Anthocyanins are of interest in foods because they exhibit various bioactive properties and function as a natural food colorant, providing red-blue-purple hues (Wrolstad, 2004). However, the use of these pigments is limited by their stability under processing conditions such as pH and temperature (Wrolstad, 2004). Chemically, anthocyanin is glycosides of anthocyanidins, the basic chemical structure of which is shown in Figure 2.5. They have been reported as the major class of flavonoids in sorghum. Cyanidin, malvidin, petunidin, delphinidin, pelargonidin, and peonidin are the common anthocyanins found in cereals.

Table 2.4 shows the flavonoid compounds present in sorghum (Figure 2.5). Sorghum anthocyanins have a unique character as they lack the hydroxyl group in the 3-position of C-ring. This unique anthocyanin is named as 3-deoxyanthocyanin (Dykes and Rooney, 2006). The absence of hydroxyl group makes it stable at high pH (Sweeny and Iacobucci, 1981; Awika et al., 2004a, b). This property makes flavonoids perfect food colorants.

Luteolinidin, apigeninidin, and their derivatives (Figure 2.5) are the most prevalent sorghum 3-deoxyanthocyanins. Apigeninidin and luteolinidin in yellow and orange color respectively are two common 3-deoxyanthocyanins which found in SGs. The 3-deoxyanthocyanins have been shown to exhibit greater stability to pH change as compared to anthocyanins (Awika et al., 2004a); therefore, sorghum may be of interest as a source to supply natural food colorants. Sorghum 3-deoxyanthocyanins have also been shown to have a protective effect against the proliferation of cancer cells (Yang et al., 2009). Some sorghum varieties are unique in their anthocyanin composition in that they contain high levels of 3-deoxyanthocyanins, a group of anthocyanins less common than those found in fruits and vegetables (Awika et al., 2004a, b). The high-performance liquid chromatography (HPLC) analysis has shown that black (Tx430 Black) and brown (Hi Tannin) sorghum brans contained 36%–50% of luteolinidin and apigeninidin (Awika et al., 2004a, b). The highest level of 3-deoxyanthocyanin is found in sorghum with black pericarp located in the bran (Awika et al., 2004a, b; Dykes et al., 2005). Specialty sorghums have also been developed which have unique colors and high flavonoid content (Taleon et al., 2012).

2.2.1.2   PHENOLIC ACID

A phenolic acid is a type of phytochemical called a polyphenol. Phenolic compounds have a benzene ring in their structure with one or add more than one hydroxyl groups (Figure 2.7) and could be negative in terms of reducing sugar (i.e., starch), macromolecule (i.e., protein), and minerals digestibility (Stefoska-Needham et al., 2015; Wu et al., 2016). However, these compounds are receiving more importance and attention in food and health research (Awika and Rooney, 2004; Dicko et al., 2005; Crozier et al., 2009; Fraga, 2010; Visioli et al., 2011; Luthria et al., 2013; Taylor et al., 2013, 2014; Carbonneau et al., 2014) due to their antioxidant activity (Table 2.5). Many reports describe the potential health benefits of these phenolic compounds and their role in chronic diseases, which are consumed in the daily routine of human diets. For instances, these compounds are aging, cancer, diabetes, reducing oxidative stress, cardiovascular diseases, asthma, and providing anti-inflammatory and anticarcinogenic properties (Kondratyuk and Pezzuto, 2004; Dykes et al., 2005, 2013; Graf et al., 2005; Foti, 2007; Pandey and Rizvi, 2009; Del Rio et al., 2010, 2012; Fraga et al., 2010; Vauzour et al., 2010; Gyllinga et al., 2014; Stefoska-Needham et al., 2015; de Morais Cardoso et al., 2017).

TABLE 2.4 Flavonoids Compounds Detected in Sorghum Grain

Flavonoids Compounds of Sorghum		
7-O-methyl apigeninidin[a–e]	Eriodictyol[a, b, f]	Naringenin[g]
7-O-methyl luteolin[h]	Fisetinidin[i]	Polyflavan-3-ol[j, k]
Anthocyanidins[i, l, m, n, e]	Flavan-4-ols[o, p]	Proanthocyanidins[q, j, k, r, s]
Anthocyanins[m, n]	Flavanones[g, k, f]	Proapigeninidin[k, s]
Apiforol [p]	Flavones[h, t]	Procyanidin B$_1$[r]
Apigeninidin[u, a, b, l, n]	Luteoforol[o]	Prodelphinidin[q, s]
Apigeninidin-5-glucoside[m, n, e]	Luteolin[a, b, d, n]	Proluteolinidin[k, s]
Catechin [k, r]	Luteolinidin[u, l, n]	Taxifolin[k]
Dihydroflavonol [k]	Luteolinidin-5-glucoside[m, n, e]	Taxifolin 7-O-β-glucoside[k]

Sources: [a]Dykes et al. (2013), [b]Dykes et al. (2009), [c]Pale et al. (1997), [d]Seitz (2005), [e]Wu and Prior (2005), [f]Kambal and Bate-Smith (1976), [g]Awika et al. (2003), [h]Misra and Seshadri (1967), [i]Blessin et al. (1963), [j]Gu et al. (2002), [k]Gujer et al. (1986), [l]Gous (1989), [m]Nip and Burns (1969), [n]Nip and Burns (1971), [o]Bate-Smith and Luteoforol (1969), [p]Watterson and Butler (1983), [q]Brandon et al. (1982), [r]Gupta and Haslam (1978), [s]Krueger et al. (2003), [t]Stafford (1965), and [u]Carbonneau et al. (2014).

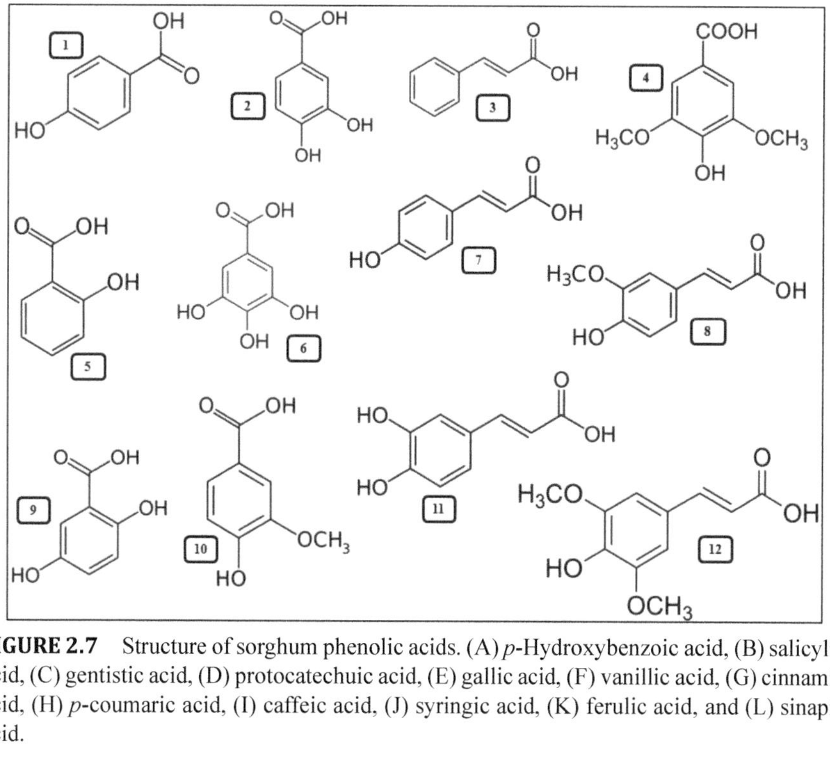

FIGURE 2.7 Structure of sorghum phenolic acids. (A) *p*-Hydroxybenzoic acid, (B) salicylic acid, (C) gentistic acid, (D) protocatechuic acid, (E) gallic acid, (F) vanillic acid, (G) cinnamic acid, (H) *p*-coumaric acid, (I) caffeic acid, (J) syringic acid, (K) ferulic acid, and (L) sinapic acid.

TABLE 2.5 In-vitro Antioxidant Activities of Sorghum and Sorghum Commodities Measured by Different Methods

Sorghum and Commodity	In-vitro Antioxidant Activity	Reference
DPPH (2,2-diphenyl-1-picrylhydrazyl) Radical Scavenging Activity		
Black PI Tall	177.2 ± 2.3 µmol TE/g	Dykes et al. (2013)
Hi-Tannin	44.7 ± 1.6 µmol TE/g	Awika et al. (2009)
Nontannin whole grain	15.3–22.2 µmol TE/g	Awika et al. (2009)
Shawaya Black	45.1 ± 1.7 µmol TE/g	Dykes et al. (2013)
Sumac	41.5 ± 0.6 µmol TE/g	Awika et al. (2009)
T×3362	32.4 ± 0.2 µmol TE/g	Dykes et al. (2013)
T×430	15.3 ± 1.1 µmol TE/g	Awika et al. (2009)
Tannin whole grain	17.7–44.7 µmol TE/g	Awika et al. (2009)
ABTS (2,2′-azino-bis(3-ethylbenzothiazoline-6-sulphonic acid)) Radical Scavenging Activity		
Black PI Tall	334.2 ± 8.1 µmol TE/g	Dykes et al. (2013)
Black sorghum bran	190–400 µmol TE/g	Awika et al. (2004a)
Black sorghum grain	52–112 µmol TE/g	Awika et al. (2004a)
Hi-Tannin	108 ± 4.6 µmol TE/g	Awika et al. (2009)
Leaf-sheaths of dye sorghum	1026.2 (mg /g DM)	Kayodéa et al. (2012)
Non-tannin whole grain	63.9–78.9 µmol TE/g	Awika et al. (2009)
Red sorghum grain	30–80 µmol TE/g	Dicko et al. (2005)
Shawaya Black	110.4 ± 2.0 µmol TE/g	Dykes et al. (2013)
Sumac	125 ± 3.1 µmol TE/g	Awika et al. (2009)
T×3362	80.0 ± 2.5 µmol TE/g	Dykes et al. (2013)
T×430	78.9 ± 4.3 µmol TE/g	Awika et al. (2009)
Tannin whole grain	61.6–125 µmol TE/g	Awika et al. (2009)
White sorghum grain	16–62 µmol TE/g	Dicko et al. (2005)
ORAC (Oxygen Radical Absorbance Capacity) Scavenging Activity		
Black sorghum bran	3.7 µmol TE/mg	González-Montilla et al. (2012)
Hi-Tannin	2630 ± 190 µmol TE/g	Awika et al. (2009)
Non-tannin whole grain	81.6–126 µmol TE/g	Awika et al. (2009)
Sumac	5180 ± 530 µmol TE/g	Awika et al. (2009)
T×430	2910 ± 210 µmol TE/g	Awika et al. (2009)
Tannin whole grain	72.4–236 µmol TE/g	Awika et al. (2009)
FRAP (Ferric Reducing Ability of Plasma) Assay		
Leaf-sheaths of dye sorghum	49.7 mg/g DM	Kayodéa et al. (2012)

DM, dry matter; *TE*, Trolox equivalent.

Notes: *Sample = dry weight basis.

In sorghum grains, a wide ranging of phenolic compounds have been reported including condensed tannins, flavonoids, and phenolic acids (Figure 2.7) (Stefoska-Needham et al., 2015). A wide natural variation found among the sorghum varieties which contribute to the diverse polyphenolic composition. In SG, phenolic acids (Hahn et al., 1983), 3-deoxyanthocyanins (pigments) (Awika et al., 2004b), and proanthocyanidins (tannins) (Strumeyer and Malin, 1975) have been identified and quantified. Because of these characteristics, sorghum has been proposed as a functional ingredient to increase the phenolic content of bread, pasta, and flatbreads, as an alternative grain for use in gluten-free bread, and a natural antioxidant to retard lipid oxidation in ground beef products (Schober et al., 2005, 2007; Hemphill, 2006; Boswell, 2010; Yousif et al., 2012; Khan et al., 2013). Like other cereal grains, phenolic acids in sorghum may be bound to the cell wall components (Hahn et al., 1983); however, new evidence suggests that glycerol ester derivatives of phenolic acids are predominant in sorghum (Yang et al., 2012). Phenolic acids and their antioxidant properties are believed to contribute to the protective effects of whole grains against chronic diseases (Slavin et al., 1997). The highest level of phenolic content and antioxidant activity were reported by Dykes et al. (2005) in a study on sorghum genotypes with pigmented testa. Whereas lower content of phenolic and simpler phenolic profiles was found by Wu et al. (2016) in white-grained sorghum genotypes as compare to colored one's genotypes of sorghum.

All varieties of sorghum are rich in phenolic acids present in testa, aleurone layer, endosperm, and pericarp (Hahn et al., 1984; McDonough et al., 1986). Ferulic acid is the most common phenolic acid of sorghum (Hahn et al., 1983). Some of the other phenolic acids are found very abundantly in sorghum, they are caffeic, *p*-coumaric, protocatechuic, sinapic, and syringic (Waniska et al., 1989). Table 2.6 enlists the major phenolic acids present in SG and bran. Sorghum marrow stem and leaf sheath contain four times more phenolic acid than SG (Pascal et al., 2012). It has been reported that gallic acid is present only in bound form (12.9–46.0 µg/g, d/w), whereas cinnamic acid in free form (2.0–10.7 µg/g, d/w) (Hahn et al., 1984).

2.2.1.3 PHYTOSTEROLS

Phytosterols are a large family of chemical compounds that are found mainly in the cell walls and membranes of plants (Figure 2.8). Structurally, considered as to closely associate with cholesterol but have a big difference with

TABLE 2.6 Detected Major Phenolic Acids From Sorghum

Phenolic Compounds	Chemical Formula	Detected Amounts* (µg/g [d/w])	Reference
Ferulic acid	$[C_{10}H_{10}O_4]$	100–500 (Grain)	Hahn et al. (1984); Hahn and Rooney (1986)
		1400–2170 (Bran)	Hahn et al. (1984)
p-Coumaric acid	$[C_9H_8O_3]$	70–230 (Grain)	Hahn et al. (1983)
		0–970 (Bran)	Hahn et al. (1984)
Sinapic acid	$[C_{11}H_{12}O_5]$	50–140 (Grain)	Hahn et al. (1983)
		100–630 (Bran)	Hahn et al. (1984)

Notes: *Total (free and bound) measured by HPLC.

d/w: Dry weight.

the side chain found in the structure of cholesterol depicted very clearly in Figure 2.9 (Gyllinga et al., 2014). A steroid skeleton is contained in their structure with a hydroxyl (−OH) group linked to the C-3 atom of the A-ring while aliphatic side chain in structure linked to the C-17 atom of the D-ring. A double bond is found in sterol moiety, typically between C-5 and C-6 atoms. In human and animal studies, dietary phytosterols have been well documented which can help to lower serum low-density lipoprotein and total cholesterol concentrations with the help of reduction in intestinal cholesterol absorption (Jones et al., 1999; Sierksma et al., 1999). Phytosterols are hypocholesterolemic.

In SG, phytosterols and its wet-milled fractions were evaluated by Singh et al. (2003). The findings state that significantly two classes of phytosterol can be distinguished from sorghum kernels, one of them was *free phytosterols* (St) while the second was *fatty acyl phytosterol esters* (St:E) (Table 2.7). Wet-milled fiber fraction was noticed in their study to have a high concentration of these phytosterols followed by the germ fraction (Table 2.7). Singh et al. (2003) observed an average of total phytosterol ~48.4 mg/100 g two hybrids sorghum grain viz. Cargill 737 (Hybrid A) and Cargill 888Y (Hybrid B). In addition to phytosterols, their findings reported that the kernels of SG have 72%–93% fewer phytosterols than corn kernels on compression.

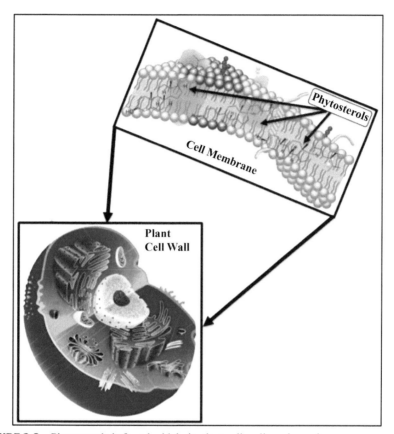

FIGURE 2.8 Phytosterols is found widely in plant cell walls and membranes.

TABLE 2.7 Concentration of Two Classes of Phytosterol in Sorghum Kernels (Mean ± SD, $n = 2$)

Sample	Phytosterol in Hybrid Sorghum Kernels					
	Free Phytosterols (St) (in %)		Fatty Acyl Phytosterol Esters (St:E) (in %)		Total Phytosterol (mg/100 g)	
	Cargill 737 (Hybrid A)	Cargill 888Y (Hybrid B)	Cargill 737 (Hybrid A)	Cargill 888Y (Hybrid B)	Cargill 737 (Hybrid A)	Cargill 888Y (Hybrid B)
Kernels	0.96 ± 0.07	0.59 ± 0.07	0.61 ± 0.05	0.63 ± 0.08	51.10	45.68
Fiber	1.32 ± 0.10	1.11 ± 0.29	1.36 ± 0.37	1.08 ± 0.18	11.43	14.18
Germ	0.52 ± 0.09	0.56 ± 0.00	0.32 ± 0.03	0.27 ± 0.02	8.62	10.08
Protein	1.99 ± 0.66	1.50 ± 0.03	0.83 ± 0.42	0.62 ± 0.11	1.74	1.56
Starch	2.63 ± 0.52	1.67 ± 0.33	0.00 ± 0.00	0.00 ± 0.00	5.74	7.52

Sources: Singh et al. (2003). (Reprinted from Singh, V.; Moreau, R. A. and Hicks, K. B. Yield and phytosterol composition of oil extracted from grain sorghum and its wet-milled fractions. *Cereal Chem,* 2003, *80*(2), 126–129. © 2003 John Wiley & Sons with permission).

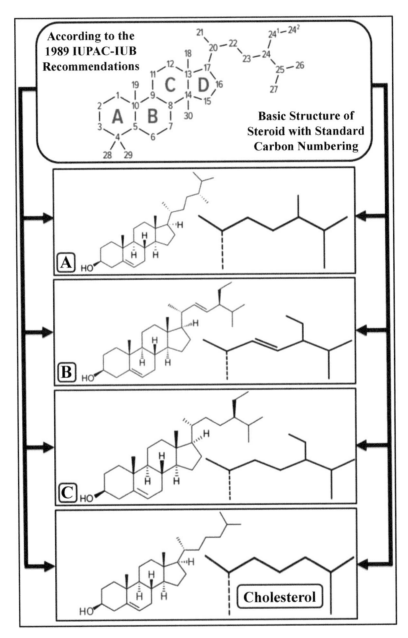

FIGURE 2.9 Basic structure of steroid (Moss, 1989), structure of commonly present phytosterols in sorghum (A) Campesterol, (B) Stigmasterol, and (C) Sitosterol (Avato et al., 1990; Awika and Rooney, 2004) and their structural compression with cholesterol (Gyllinga et al., 2014).

In 2007, whole kernel, stalks, and leaves of different nine parent lines of sorghum were studied by Christiansen et al. (2007) who reported stigmasterol as predominant phytosterols extracted from the whole kernel in SGs while sitosterol and campesterol were with higher amounts in sorghum stalks and leaves. Leguizamón et al. (2009) studied SGs for characterization of phytosterol using two extraction methods viz. soxhlet and reflux extraction (Table 2.8). Sitosterol was the major phytosterol among the whole kernel, ground kernel, and dried distillers grains with solubles sorghum samples.

TABLE 2.8 Soxtec and Reflux Extraction Method for Phytosterols From Sorghum Grains (Mean ± SD, $n = 3$)

Samples	Extracted Phytosterols Composition (mg/g of Lipids)					
	Campesterol		Stigmasterol		Sitosterol	
	Soxtec	Reflux	Soxtec	Reflux	Soxtec	Reflux
Whole Kernel	1.04 ± 0.04	0.97 ± 0.37	1.02 ± 0.04	1.08 ± 0.30	1.92 ± 0.09	0.93 ± 0.33
Ground Kernel	2.86 ± 0.28	2.69 ± 0.18	1.73 ± 0.18	1.74 ± 0.06	5.66 ± 0.57	5.07 ± 0.29
DDGS	2.54 ± 0.24	2.52 ± 0.20	1.21 ± 0.11	1.18 ± 0.10	6.04 ± 0.57	6.04 ± 0.52

DDGS: dried distillers grains with solubles.

Source: Leguizamón et al. (2009). (Partially adapted from Leguizamón, C.; Weller, C. L.; Schlegel, V. L.; and Carr, T. P. Plant sterol and policosanol characterization of hexane extracts from grain sorghum, corn and their DDGS. *J Am Oil Chem Soc*, 2009, *86*(7), 707–716. © 2009 John Wiley & Sons with permission).

2.2.1.4 POLICOSANOLS

Policosanols are classified as the group of high molecular weight biologically active long chains of aliphatic primary alcohols between the carbon atoms 22 to 38 (Hwang et al., 2002a, b, 2005; Vali et al., 2005; Pham et al., 2018), according to their sources of occurrence such as beeswax (Irmak et al., 2005), sugarcane (Irmak et al., 2005), perilla seeds (Adhikari et al., 2006), and cereals (Hwang et al., 2005) like rice (Wang et al., 2007; Pham et al., 2018), wheat (Irmak et al., 2005; Dunford et al., 2010; Pham et al., 2018), sorghum (Hwang et al., 2004; Leguizamón et al., 2009; Pham et al., 2018) as described in the literature.

These policosanols phytochemicals are very unique in sorghum grain due to their presence in nonesterified forms (Althwab et al., 2015). Although in another source of plants, these compounds are found in esterified forms (Adhikari et al., 2006). Policosanols phytochemical is with high amounts especially in sorghum and their most commercial form are docosanol (C_{22}), hexacosanol (C_{26}). Octacosanol (C_{28}), triacontanol (C_{30}), and dotriacontanol

(C_{32}) which are available and sold in the markets as nutritional supplements (Hwang et al., 2002b, 2005; Irmak et al., 2005; Vali et al., 2005). Structure of major policosanols reported in sorghum grain is depicted in Figure 2.10. Octacosanol (C_{28}) and triacontanol (C_{30}) in sorghum grain do the representation of most predominant policosanols when compare with hexacosanol (C_{26}) and dotriacontanol (C_{32}) (Hwang et al., 2004; Leguizamón et al., 2009).

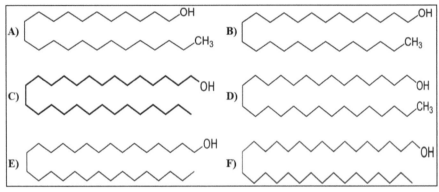

FIGURE 2.10   Structure of major sorghum policosanols. (A) Lignoceryl alcohol, (B) hexacosanol, (C) octacosanol, (D) nonacosanol, (E) triacontanol, and (F) dotriacontanol.

These phytochemicals are gaining more popularity due to their physiological function and beneficial health effects (Figure 2.11) which have been documented in many reports worldwide (Arruzazabala et al., 1994, 1996; Kabir and Kimura, 1995; Kato et al., 1995; Sttisser et al., 1998; Mas et al., 1999; Castano et al., 2001; Gouni-Berthold and Berthold, 2002; Carr et al., 2005; Vali et al., 2005; Lee et al 2014). Therefore, researchers and scientists are giving more emphasis on its uses in pharmaceutical industries because of the significant presence of policosanols phytochemicals in sorghum grain (Irmak et al., 2005; Wang et al., 2007; Dunford et al., 2010). The common policosanols of SG kernels are given in Table 2.9, which reported by many workers.

2.3   HIGH-PERFORMANCE LIQUID CHROMATOGRAPHY: METHODS FOR EXTRACTION AND QUANTIFICATION OF SORGHUM PHYTOCHEMICALS

An HPLC instrument is known as the most important and useful analytical tool for analysis in food and other allied fields (Figure 2.12) (Gupta et al., 2012) because of its many characteristics features (Charde et al., 2014) which

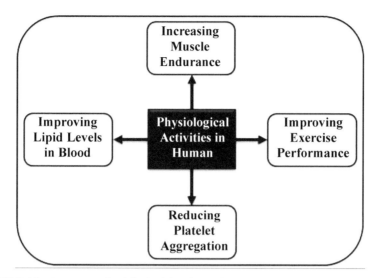

FIGURE 2.11   Important physiological functions of policosanols in human body.

TABLE 2.9   Policosanols of Sorghum Grain Kernels

Common Policosanols	IUPAC Name	Chemical Formula	Amounts (%, w/w)[a]
Docosanol	Docosan-1-ol	$C_{22}H_{46}O$	0.4–0.5
Lignoceryl alcohol	Tetracosan-1-ol	$C_{24}H_{50}O$	0.4–3.1
Pentacosanol	Pentacosan-1-ol	$C_{25}H_{52}O$	0.1
Hexacosanol	Hexacosan-1-ol	$C_{26}H_{54}O$	6.1–8.2
Heptacosanol	Heptacosan-1-ol	$C_{27}H_{56}O$	0.8
Octacosanol	Octacosan-1-ol	$C_{28}H_{58}O$	43.0–47.2
Nonacosanol	Nonacosan-1-ol	$C_{29}H_{60}O$	1.3–1.5
Triacontanol	Triacontan-1-ol	$C_{30}H_{62}O$	40.9–42.8
Dotriacontanol	Dotriacontan-1-ol	$C_{32}H_{66}O$	1.4–3.5

Source: Avato et al. (1990), Hwang et al. (2002b, 2004), and Awika and Rooney (2004).
[a]Hwang et al. (2004).

are as follows; (1) high resolution, (2) small diameter, (3) stainless steel, glass column, rapid analysis, (4) relatively higher mobile phase pressure, and (5) controlled flow rate of mobile phase.

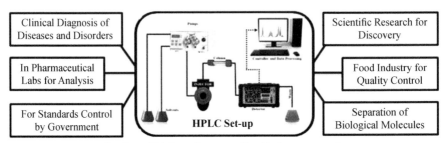

FIGURE 2.12   Application of high-performance liquid chromatography.

Today, this instrument has been widely used in cereals for extraction, identification, and quantification of each phytochemical's component from the sample matrix. Instrumentation of HPLC depends upon pumps which help to pass the sample matrix in the form of pressurized liquid solvents via column which contains solid adsorbent material (Figure 2.13). Each phytochemical component in sample matrix interacts together slight differently with the solid adsorbent material; resulting different flow rates according to the phytochemical components and further proceeds to the extraction of those components as they flow out in HPLC column. Extracted and quantified sorghum phytochemicals are shown in Table 2.10. One of the studies has suggested that sorghum brans are a rich source of anthocyanin (4.0–9.8 mg luteolinidin equivalents/g) than pigmented fruits and vegetables (0.2–10 mg/g). Samples of sorghum variety (T*430) were analyzed by using spectrophotometric detection and HPLC method, for anthocyanins. The extracting solvents used were 1% HCl in methanol and 70% aqueous acetone. The result showed that the methanol solution gave higher values for total anthocyanins than aqueous acetone. Moreover, sorghum brans contain three to four times more anthocyanins than contained in the whole grain (Awika et al., 2004a, b).

A study detected the presence of bioactive amines using quantification by ion-pair HPLC along with fluorimetric detection. Sorghum particle size was reduced to 420 μm and then extraction was done using 5% of trichloroacetic acid. The result showed 100% presence of spermine and spermidine, 77% putrescine, and 14% cadaverine. It was also observed that sorghum without tannin contained higher levels of the amine as compared to sorghum with tannin (Paiva et al., 2015).

Phenolic acids and flavonoids such as anthocyanins are separated by reverse phase chromatography using C18 columns (Chen et al., 2001; Lopez et al., 2001). The detector used is ultraviolet-visible photodiode array set at 280 and 360 nm, and identification is done by matching retention time and

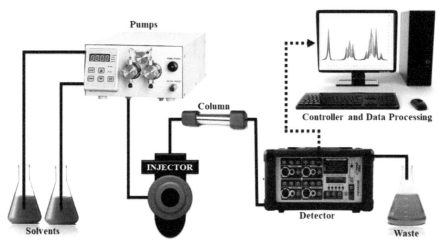

FIGURE 2.13 Diagrammatic presentation of high-performance liquid chromatography for phytochemicals extraction and quantification.

TABLE 2.10   Methods of Extraction and Quantification of Sorghum Phytochemicals

Method of Extraction and Quantification	Extracted and Quantified Compounds	References
Et/H$_2$O	Apigeninidin, Luteolinidin, Anthocyanins (AU/g)	Kayodéa et al. (2012)
HPLC	5-Methoxy-luteolinidin, 7-Methoxy-apigeninidin Apigeninidin, Luteolinidin,	Dykes et al. (2009, 2013)
HPLC with PDA (photodiode array) and mass spectral detection method	Caffeic acid, *p*-Coumaric acid, Ferulic acid, Sinapic acid, Ferulic acid isomer	Luthria and Liu (2013)

spectral characteristics of the flavonoids and phenolic compounds with those of standards (Chen et al., 2001). For quantification, standard calibration curves are prepared by plotting the area of peaks against different concentrations of phenolic compound standards (Lopez et al., 2001). Condensed tannins or procyanidin profile in tannin sorghum is determined on normal phase Luna silica columns, after the sample extract has been cleaned of sugars and phenols, using aqueous methanol, on Sephadex LH-20 columns (Awika et al., 2003). The initial separation of procyanidins from the rest of the phenolic compounds is based on the finding that, in alcohol (95% ethanol), tannins were adsorbed on Sephadex LH-20, after which they could be eluted with aqueous acetone (Strumeyer and Malin, 1975).

2.4   EFFECT OF PROCESSING ON NUTRITIONAL AND PHYTOCHEMICAL COMPOSITION OF SORGHUM

2.4.1   EFFECT OF CLEANING

Cleaning is the first step in the processing of cereals. It usually removes debris and germs from the grain. The organic impurities, ferromagnetic components, and mineral matter are separated from the grains. Cleaning is especially done for removal of bran from endosperm of the grain. The main function of cleaning is to moisturize the grains to reduce the adhesion between bran and endosperm. Cleaning is a prerequisite step before milling to provide optimum moisture content to grains.

2.4.2   EFFECT OF DECORTICATION AND MILLING

Milling converts cereals into a more-palatable and desirable form. Milling results in the recovery of the starchy endosperm and removal of the bran. It increases the palatability of the product but decreases its nutritional value. While, decortication is a process involved in the removal of the outer layers with the help of de-huller or mortar and pestle, resulting reduction in the losses of fat, fiber, and ash contents. This reduction is in the levels of fat, fiber, and ash content due to decrease decortication. Arginine, histidine, and lysine contents from the composition of amino acid of decorticated grains are found decreased during laboratory analysis. Reduction in grain weight and lysine content of sorghum after decortication is depicted in Table 2.11.

TABLE 2.11   Reduction in Sorghum Grain After Decortication

Weight Loss From Initial Weight (%)	Lysine Content (%)	Reference
20–25	40	Eggum et al. (1983)
14	10	Serna-Saldivar et al. (1987, 1988)

2.4.3   EFFECT OF FERMENTATION

Fermentation is a method which involves the metabolic process and employed to converts carbohydrate to acids, gases, or alcohol. It takes place in yeast and bacteria. This process also takes place in lactic acid fermentation in oxygen-starved muscle cells. Fermentation is described widely as bulk microbial growth on a growth medium to produce a specific chemical in food products. These food products are known as *"Fermented foods"* and subjected to the microbial or enzymatic action for desirable changes in biochemical reactions to give significant modification in the food. Products produced from various cereal substrates fermented by lactic acid bacteria, yeast, and/or fungi are included (Murooka and Yamshita, 2008). Numerous traditional fermented foods have been studied and demonstrated their health effects on metabolisms and immune systems in vitro and in vivo models. New bioactive metabolites reported by Poutanen et al. (2009) in cereals which are produced from raw materials due to the presence of starters during the fermentation process. The bioaccessibility of these bioactive compounds is increased during fermentation because of the modification in the cereal matrix. The traditional cereal-fermented products can enhance their properties of nutritional companions through increasing their nutrient and energy densities while mineral status with the help of combine mineral fortification and dephytinization (Nout, 2009).

Several processing parameters viz. cooking, decortication, soaking, germination including fermentation are reported to reduce the amounts of phytochemicals in sorghum (Elmaki et al., 1999; Mahgoub and Elhag, 1998; Youssef, 1998). Kayodéa et al. (2006) studied processing methods on sorghum phytochemicals with simultaneous effects in which they found degradation of phytate because of increases phytase activities during germination and lactic acid fermentation. Iron (Fe) bioavailability improves in sorghum flours during fermentation (Kayodéa et al., 2006). Microbial enzymes are responsible for tannins degradation during fermentation process (Towo et al., 2006) which is accountable to reduce the levels of tannin content in food products prepare from sorghum and also involve to improve in vitro protein and starch digestibility (Kazanas and Fields, 1981; Taylor, 1983; Hassan and El Tinay, 1995, Dewar et al, 1997; Bvochora et al., 1999; Doudou et al., 2003; Osman, 2004). The improved digestibility of protein means improvement in the nutritional values of sorghum such as proximate composition, essential amino acids composition, and minerals content viz. calcium (Ca), iron (Fe), magnesium (Mn), potassium (K), and zinc (Zn) (Au and Fields, 1981; Taylor, 1983; Chavan et al., 1988; Dewar et al, 1997). Dlamini et al. (2007) suggested that the antioxidant properties of sorghum flour may be contributed by tannins. However, Beta et al. (2000) reported that the reason behind the reduction of extracted phenolic compounds from sorghum is because of the self-polymerization and/or interaction with proteins macromolecules.

2.5   USES OF SORGHUM IN FOOD AND NONFOOD INDUSTRY

2.5.1   FOOD INDUSTRY

Sorghum is a cheap cereal grain and forage crop which is used to produce a variety of consumable and nonconsumable food products. Drought resistance and efficient energy conversion make sorghum a viable alternative crop (Rosenow et al., 1983). These agronomic advantages in combination with the composition of sorghum, such as the presence of high levels of polyphenolic compounds and the absence of gluten proteins, contribute to sorghum's potential as a food ingredient (Taylor et al., 2013). In many food products, sorghum is used instead of wheat and maize. Sorghum is widely used to develop starch-based sweeteners (Udachan et al., 2012) as it contains 68%–75% starch (Subramanian et al., 1994; Shinde, 2005; Singh et al., 2009). Ferreira et al. (2016) studied through their research that a mixed proportion of sorghum flour, rice, and potato flour (in combination; 40:20:40) used for the preparation of gluten-free pasta. It has shown its importance in the case of patients suffering from celiac disease. Table 2.12 enlists the products obtained from sorghum and its commodities.

TABLE 2.12   Different Products Obtained From Sorghum and Their Properties

Sorghum Products	Properties	Reference
Beer	Properties of sorghum starch and its beta-amylase activity are utilized	Ezeogu and Okolo (1994, 1995)
Bioethanol	Higher yield is given by decorticated grain, sweet sorghum juice	Almodares and Hadi (2009), Alvarez et al. (2010)
Biopolymer film	Made by sorghum flour, darker in color due to kafirin, high tensile strength	Duodu et al. (2003), Emmambux et al. (2004)
Bread	Gluten-free, flat-shaped, light-colored product	Murty and Kumar (1995), Nout (2009)
Flour	White-colored, tanned product with high gelatinizing property	Waniska and Rooney (2002), Yousif et al. (2012)
Muffins	Dark-colored, especially made of bran	Brannan et al. (2001)
Porridge	Fermented product of sorghum flour, thick or thin in appearance	Akingbala et al. (1981a, b)
Tortilla	Unleavened product, made in combination with maize flour	Choto et al. (1985)

2.5.2 NONFOOD INDUSTRY

2.5.2.1 BIOETHANOL

Ethanol as an alternative fuel is being used increasingly worldwide. The reason behind this is the depletion of oil reserves on a larger scale (Sheoran et al., 1998). Agronomic data have suggested that more than 1300 gallons of ethanol per hectare could be obtained from sorghum (CRADA, 2001). According to the study done by Khalil et al. (2015) stalks of varieties Mn-1054, Ramada, and SS-301 had a higher content of fibers, so their bagasse was used for bioethanol production. Bagasse was pretreated and hydrolyzed thermo-chemically with 2% (v/v) sulfuric acid (98%) at 120 °C for 60 min and filtered, and the sugar-rich filtrate was neutralized and supplemented with nutrients for bioethanol production.

Fermentation of sweet sorghum sugars or acid-hydrolyzed neutralized bagasse into bioethanol was conducted by *Saccharomyces cerevisiae*, *Zymomonas mobilis*, or mixed-culture of both organisms at 1:1 ratio. The highest production of bioethanol was obtained from juice and bagasse of variety SS-301, by the mixed-culture treatment. From the juice, bioethanol concentration was 50.26 mL/L, whereas, from bagasse, bioethanol concentration was 10.5 mL/L. Finally, it could be estimated that 160 mL of bioethanol can be produced out of each 1 kg of variety SS-301, when using both juice and bagasse. Lignocellulosic biomass of sorghum was converted into ethanol by using three unit operations: pretreatment, hydrolysis, and fermentation. The yield of ethanol obtained was 91.94 g per kg sorghum. The process of conversion was carried out without any detoxification and washing of pretreated biomass; whereas mild acidic treatment was done which was followed by enzymatic hydrolysis and fermentation.

2.5.2.2 BIOPOLYMER FILM

Sorghum flour is also used for making biobased coatings and films. It has been reported that sorghum prolamine protein, that is, kafirin is most suitable for making bioplastics (Duodu et al., 2003). The color of the film is due to the presence of the phenolic compound. Properties of kafirin film can be enhanced by cross-linking with condensed tannins (Emmambux et al., 2004). Tannin addition in kafirin increases the tensile strength by 50%–100%.

2.6 SORGHUM PHYTOCHEMICALS AND HUMAN HEALTH

Health-promoting properties of SG have been shown in Table 2.13. It has been reported by Yang et al. (2009) that a stronger anticarcinogenic activity is shown by methoxylated 3-deoxyanthocyanidins than nonmethoxylated

TABLE 2.13   Health Benefits of Sorghum Grain Consumptions

Beneficial Properties	Sample	Findings	Reference
Anticancer properties	Acidified aqueous acetone extracts of tannin and non-tannin sorghums	Extracts from black sorghum had highest phase II enzyme inductor activity compared to white sorghum	Awika et al. (2009)
	Acidified aqueous acetone extracts of black, red and white sorghum	Black sorghum extracts with high levels of methoxylated 3-deoxyanthocyanins induced quinone reductase activity strongly	
Antidiabetic properties	Ethanolic extracts from sorghum	Oral administration of sorghum extract significantly reduced blood glucose concentration by inhibition of hepatic gluconeogenesis	Kim and Park (2012)
Anti-inflammatory properties	Ethanolic extracts from sorghum bran	Ethanolic extract of black sorghum significantly inhibited secretion of IL-1beta and TNF-alpha. Also, reduced edema inflamed mouse ears	Burdette et al. (2010)
	Experimental diets enriched with tannin and non-tannin sorghum flour	Lower expression of TNF-alpha in epididymal adipose of adult male rats	Moraes et al. (2012)
Oxidative stress	Sorghum flour mixed with cowpea (sorghum-cowpea porridge)	Reduction in production of ROS/RNS	Apea-Bah et al. (2014)
Hypercholesterolemia	Extract of sorghum policosanol	In connection with the treatment of atherosclerosis seen a positive response	Mas (2000)

3-deoxyanthocyanidins. The anticancerous activity has also been demonstrated in flavanones and flavones (Kuntz et al., 1999; Ko et al., 2002; Lee et al., 2008). It has been demonstrated that consumption of sorghum as a regular diet helps in reducing obesity (Awika and Rooney, 2004). Sorghum proves to be the best substitute for people having a wheat-gluten allergy since it does not contain gluten. Sorghum provides phytosterols and unsaturated fatty acids that helps in lowering of blood cholesterol (Bernardo-Gil et al., 2002). Recently policosanol has been used in more than 25 countries for the treatment of hypercholesterolemia (Mas, 2000). Sorghum and cowpea when combined in food preparation, they showed a reduction in oxidative stress and inflammation resulting from overproduction of ROS/RNS (Apea-Bah et al., 2014). The sorghum–cowpea porridge has been reported to be more effective than maize–soybean composite porridge.

2.7 FINAL REMARKS

Sorghum is rich in a variety of antioxidants which prevent human health deterioration with positive effects. It has an anticarcinogenic property and can be used in the treatment of cardiovascular diseases. Sorghum tannin imparts positive action against obesity. Processing of SGs eliminates the toxicity of antinutrients and retains the nutritional value. It is not easy to utilize the antioxidants directly from grain; therefore various methods have been adopted for their extraction with maximum yield. Sorghum is used as a substitute for wheat and rice in many developing countries, especially in Africa. Products of sorghum flour are highly accepted by consumers. As the sorghum phytochemicals have high nutritional value, they are widely used for making food products like bread, cookies, pasta, and so on. Moreover, it is widely used as a food colorant, because sorghum anthocyanins are more stable than fruit anthocyanin. It is also being used for the production of alcoholic and nonalcoholic products. Care should be given that tannin, phenol, and phytate contents should not be in high amount. These highly affect the color of the product. Rather than food products, sorghum is also used to produce ethanol, gums resins, and so on. Production of bio-based products is also taking on a large scale, but certain investments are needed to enhance it. Much more demonstration is needed to utilize the under-effects of sorghum.

KEYWORDS

- antioxidant activity
- extraction method
- flavonoids
- health-promoting properties
- nutritional value
- phenolic compounds
- physiological functions
- phytochemicals
- phytosterols
- policosanols
- polyphenol
- processing
- proximate composition
- sorghum grain

REFERENCES

Abu-Reidah, I. M.; Arráez-Román, D.; Lozano-Sánchez, J.; Segura-Carretero, A.; and Fernández-Gutiérrez, A. Phytochemical characterisation of green beans (*Phaseolus vulgaris* L.) by using high-performance liquid chromatography coupled with time-of-flight mass spectrometry. *Phytochem Anal,* **2013**, *24*(2): 105–116.

Adhikari, P.; Hwang, K. T.; Park, J. N.; and Kim, C. K. Policosanol content and composition in Perilla seeds. *J Agric Food Chem,* **2006**, *54*, 5359–5362.

Admassu, S. Potential health benefits and problems associated with phytochemicals in food legumes. *East African J Sci,* **2009**, *3*(2), 116–133.

Akingbala, J. O.; Faubion, J. M.; and Rooney, L. W. A laboratory procedure for the preparation of Ogi, a Nigerian fermented food. *J Food Sci,* **1981a**, *46*(5), 1523–1526.

Akingbala, J. O.; Faubion, J. M.; and Rooney, L. W. Physical, chemical and organoleptic evaluation of Ogi from sorghum of differing kernel characteristics. *J Food Sci,* **1981b**, *46*(5), 1532–1536.

Almodares, A.; Hadi, M. R. Production of bioethanol from sweet sorghum: a review. *Afr J Agric Res,* **2009**, *4*, 772–780.

Althwab, S.; Carr, T. P.; Weller, C. L.; Dweikat, I. M.; and Schlegel, V. Advances in grain sorghum and its co-products as a human health promoting dietary system. *Food Res Int,* **2015**, *77*, 349–359.

Alvarez, M.; Perez-Carrillo, E.; and Serna-Saldivar, S. O. Effect of decortication and protease treatment on the kinetics of liquefaction, saccharification and ethanol production from sorghum. *J Chem Technol Biotechnol*, **2010**, *885*(8), 1122–1129.

Apea-Bah, B. F.; Minnaar, A.; Bester, J. M.; and Duodu, G. K. Does a sorghum-cowpea composite porridge hold promise for contributing to alleviating oxidative stress? *Food Chem*, **2014**, *157*, 157–166.

Arruzazabala. M. L.; Carbajal, D.; Mas, R.; Molina, V.; Valdes, S.; and Laguna. A. Cholesterol-lowering effects of policosanol in rabbits. *Biol Res*, **1994**, *27*, 205–208.

Arruzazabala, M. L.; Valdes, S.; Mas. R.; Fernandez, L.; and Carbajal, D. Effect of policosanol successive dose increases on platelet aggregation in healthy volunteers. *Pharmacol Res*, **1996**, *34*, 181–185.

Au, P. M.; Fields, M. L. Nutritive quality of fermented sorghum. *J Food Sci*, **1981**, *46*, 652–654.

Avato, P.; Bianchi, G.; and Murelli, C. Aliphatic and cyclic lipid components of Sorghum plant organs. *Phytochemistry*, **1990**, *29*, 1073–1078.

Awika, J. M.; Dykes, L.; Gu, L.; Rooney, L. W.; Prior, L. R. Processing of sorghum (*Sorghum bicolor*) and sorghum products alters procyanidin oligomer and polymer distribution and content. *J Agric Food Chem*, **2003**, *51*, 5516–5521.

Awika, J. M.; McDonough, C. M.; and Rooney, L. W. Decorticating sorghum to concentrate healthy phytochemicals. *J Agric Food Chem*, **2005**, *53*, 6230–6234.

Awika, J. M.; Rooney, L. W. Sorghum phytochemicals and their potential impact on human health. *Phytochemistry*, **2004**, *65*, 1199–1221.

Awika, J. M.; Rooney, L. W.; and Waniska, R. D. Anthoycanins from black sorghum and their antioxidant properties. *Food Chem*, **2004a**, *90*, 293–301.

Awika, J. M.; Rooney, L. W.; and Waniska, R. D. Properties of 3- deoxyanthocyanins from sorghum. *J Agric Food Chem*, **2004b**, *52*, 4388–4394.

Awika, J. M.; Yang, L.; Browning, J. D.; and Faraj, A. Comparative antioxidant, antiproliferative and phase II enzyme inducing potential of sorghum (*Sorghum bicolor*) varieties. *LWT—Food Sci Technol*, **2009**, *42*, 1041–1046.

Barnes, J. S.; Nguyen, H. P.; Shen, S.; and Schug, K. A. General method for extraction of blueberry anthocyanins and identification using high performance liquid chromatography–electrospray ionization-ion trap-time of flight-mass spectrometry. *J Chromatogr A*, **2009**, *1216*, 4728–4735.

Bate-Smith, E. C. Luteoforol (30,4,40,5,7-pentahydroxyflavan) in *Sorghum vulgare* L. *Phytochemistry*, **1969**, *8*, 1803–1810.

Belobrajdic, D. P.; Bird, A. R. The potential role of phytochemicals in wholegrain cereals for the prevention of type-2 diabetes. *Nutr J*, **2013**, *12*(62), 1–12.

Bernardo-Gil, M. G.; Grenha, J.; Santos, J.; and Cardoso, P. Supercritical fluid extraction and characterization of oil from hazelnut. *Eur J Lipid Sci Technol*, **2002**, *104*, 402–409.

Beta, T.; Rooney, L. W.; Marovatsanga, L. T.; and Taylor, J. R. N. Effect of chemical treatments on polyphenols and malt quality in sorghum. *J Cereal Sci*, **2000**, *31*, 295–302.

Blessin, C. W.; Vanetten, C. H.; and Dimler, R. J. An examination of anthocyanogens in grain sorghums. *Cereal Chem*, 1963, 40, 241–250.

Boddu, J.; Svabek, C.; Ibraheem, F.; Jones, D.; and Chopra, S. Characterization of a deletion allele of a sorghum Myb gene yellow seed1 showing loss of 3-deoxy-flavonoids. *Plant Sci*, **2005**, *169*, 542–552.

Bolling, B. W.; McKay, D. L.; and Blumberg, B. J. The phytochemical composition and antioxidant actions of tree nuts. *Asia Pac J Clin Nutr*, **2010**, *19*(1), 117–123.

Boswell, S. E. *Development of gluten-free baking methods utilizing sorghum flour*. MSc Dissertation, Texas A&M University: College Station, TX, 2010.

Bralley, E.; Greenspan, P.; Hargrove, J. L.; and Hartle, D. K. Inhibition of hyaluronidase activity by select sorghum brans. *J Med Food*, **2008**, *11*, 307–312.

Brandon, M. J.; Foo, L. Y.; Porter, L. J.; and Meredith, P. Proanthocyanidins of barley and sorghum composition as a function of maturity of barley ears. *Phytochemistry*, **1982**, *21*, 2953–2957.

Brannan, G. L.; Setser, C. S.; Kemp, K. E.; Seib, P. A.; and Roozeboom, K. Sensory characteristics of grain sorghum hybrids with potential for use in human food. *Cereal Chem*, **2001**, *78*, 693–700.

Burdette, A.; Garner, P. L.; Mayer, E. P.; Hargrove, J. L.; Hartle, D. K.; and Greenspan, P. Anti-inflammatory activity of select sorghum (*Sorghum bicolor*) brans. *J Med Food*, **2010**, *13*, 879–887.

Bvochora, J. M.; Reed, J. D.; Read, J. S. and Zvauya, R. Effect of fermentation processes on proanthocyanidins in sorghum during preparation of Mahewu, a non-alcoholic beverage. *Process Biochem*, **1999**, *35*, 21–25.

Carbonneau, M.-A.; Cisse, M.; Mora-Soumille, N.; Dairi, S.; Rosa, M.; Michel, F.; Lauret, C.; Cristol, J.-P.; and Dangles, O. Antioxidant properties of 3-deoxyanthocyanidins and polyphenolic extracts from Côte d'Ivoire's red and white sorghums assessed by ORAC and *in vitro* LDL oxidisability tests. *Food Chem*, **2014**, *145*, 701–709.

Cardoso, M. L.; Montini, A. T.; Pinheiro, S. S.; Ana, P. M. H.; Martino, D. S. H.; and Moreira, B. V. A. Effects of processing with dry heat and wet heat on the antioxidant profile of sorghum. *Food Chem*, **2014**, *152*, 210–217.

Carr, P. T.; Weller, L. C.; Schlegel, L. V.; Cuppett, L. S.; Guderian, M. D.; and Johnson, R. K. Grain sorghum lipid extract reduces cholesterol absorption and plasma non-HDL cholesterol concentration in hamsters. *J Nutr*, **2005**, *135*, 2236–2240.

Castano, G.; Mas, R.; Fernandez, J. C.; Illnait, J.; Fernandez, L.; and Alvarez, E. Effects of policosanol in older patients with type II hypercholesterolemia and high coronary risk. *J Gerontology: A Biol Sci Med Sci*, **2001**, *56*, M186–M192.

Charde, M. S.; Welankiwar, A. S. and Kumar, J. Method development by liquid chromatography with validation. *Int J Pharm Chem*, **2014**, *4*(2), 57–61.

Chavan, U. D.; Chavan, J. K.; and Kadam, S. S. Effects of fermentation on soluble proteins and in vitro digestibility of sorghum, green grain and sorghum green gram blends. *J Food Sci*, **1988**, *53*: 1574–1575.

Chen, F.; Cole, P.; Mi, Z.; and Xing, L. Y. Corn and wheat-flour consumption and mortality from esophageal cancer in Shanxi, *Chin J Cancer*, **1993**, *53*, 902–906.

Chen, H.; Zuo, Y. and Deng, Y. Separation and determination of flavonoids and other phenolic compounds in cranberry juice by high-performance liquid chromatography. *J Chromatogr A*, **2001**, *913*, 387–395.

Chiang, A.-N.; Wu, H.-L.; Yeh, H.-I.; Chu, C.-S.; Lin, H.-C.; and Lee, W.-C. Antioxidant effects of black rice extract through the induction of superoxide dismutase and catalase activities. *Lipids*, **2006**, *41*, 797–803.

Choto, C. E.; Morad, M. M.; and Rooney, L. W. The quality of tortillas containing whole sorghum and pearled sorghum alone and blended with yellow maize. *Cereal Chem*, **1985**, *62*, 51–55.

Christiansen, K. L.; Weller, C. L.; Schlegel, V. L.; Cuppett, S. L.; and Carr, T. P. Extraction and characterization of lipids from the kernels, leaves, and stalks of nine grain sorghum parent lines. *Cereal Chem*, **2007**, *84*, 463–470.

Christiansen, K. L.; Weller, C. L.; Schegel, V. L.; and Dweikat, I. M. Comparison of lipid extraction methods of food-grade sorghum (*Sorghum bicolor*) using hexane. *Biol Eng*, **2008**, *1*(1), 51–63.

CRADA (Cooperative Research and Development Agreement). (2011). Sorghum to Ethanol Research Initiative Cooperative Research and Development Final Report CRADA Number: CRD-08e291 CRADA Report NREL/TP- 7A10–52695, October 2011. URL: Accessed on August 17, 2018.

Crozier, A. A.; Jaganath, I. B.; and Clifford, M. N. Dietary phenolics: chemistry, bioavailability and effects on health. *Nat Prod Rep*, **2009**, *26*, 1001–1043.

Cummings, D. P.; Axtel, J. D. Relationships of pigmented testa to nutritional quality of sorghum grain in inheritance and improvement of protein quality in sorghum. Research Progress Report, Purdue University: West Lafayette, IN, 1973, p. 112.

De la Rosa, L. A.; Alvarez-Parrilla, E.; and González-Aguilar, G. A. *Fruit and Vegetable Phytochemicals Chemistry, Nutritional Value, and Stability*. 1st ed., Wiley-Blackwell Publishing: Singapore, 2010, pages 131–155.

de Morais Cardoso, L.; Pinheiro, S. S.; Martino, H. S. D.; and Pinheiro-Sant'Ana, H. M. Sorghum (*Sorghum bicolor* L.): nutrients, bioactive compounds, and potential impact on human health. *Crit Rev Food Sci Nutr*, **2017**, *57*(2), 372–390.

Del Rio, D.; Costa, L. G.; Lean, M. E.; and Crozier, A. Polyphenols and health: what compounds are involved?. *Nutr Metab Cardiovasc Dis*, **2010**, *20*(1), 1–6.

Del Rio, D.; Rodriguez-Mateos, A.; Spencer, J. P. E.; Tognolini, M.; Borges, G.; and Crozier, A. dietary (poly)phenolics in human health: structures, bioavailability, and evidence of protective effects against chronic diseases. *Antioxid Redox Signal*, **2012**, *18*, 1–73.

Devi, P. S.; Kumar, M. S.; and Das, S. M. Evaluation of antiproliferative activity of red sorghum bran anthocyanin on a human breast cancer cell Line (McF-7). *Int J Breast Cancer*, **2011**, *2011*, 1–6. http://dx.doi.org/10.4061/2011/891481

Dewar, J.; Taylor, J. R. N.; and Berjak, P. Effects of germination conditions with optimized steeping on sorghum malt quality with particular reference to free amino nitrogen. *J Inst Brew*, **1997**, *103*, 171–175.

Dicko, M. H.; Gruppen, H.; Traore, A. S.; van Berkel, W. J.; and Voragen, A. G. Evaluation of the effect of germination on phenolic compounds and antioxidant activities in sorghum varieties. *J Agric Food Chem*, **2005**, *53*(7), 2581–2588.

Dlamini, N. R.; Taylor, J. R. N.; and Rooney, L. W. The effect of sorghum type and processing on the antioxidant properties of African sorghum-based foods. *Food Chem*, **2007**, *105*, 1412−1419.

Doudou, K. G., Taylor, J. R. N., Belton, P. S.; and Hamaker, B. B. Factors affecting sorghum protein digestibility (Mini Review). *J Cereal Sci*, **2003**, *38*, 117–131.

Dunford, N. T.; Irmak, S.; and Jonnala, R. Pressurised solvent extraction of policosanol from wheat straw, germ and bran. *Food Chem*, **2010**, *119*(3), 1246–1249.

Duodu, K. G.; Taylor, J. R. N.; Belton, P. S.; and Hamaker, B. R. Factors affecting sorghum protein digestibility. *J Cereal Sci*, **2003**, *38*(2), 117–131.

Dykes, L.; Peterson, G. C.; Rooney, W. L.; and Rooney, L. W. Flavonoid composition of lemon-yellow sorghum genotypes. *Food Chem*, 2011, 128, 173–179.

Dykes, L.; Rooney, L. W. Sorghum and millet phenols and antioxidants. *J Cereal Sci,* **2006**, *44*(3), 236–251.

Dykes, L.; Rooney, W. L.; and Rooney, L. W. Evaluation of phenolics and antioxidant activity of black sorghum hybrids. *J Cereal Sci,* **2013**, *58*, 278–283.

Dykes, L.; Rooney, L. W.; Waniska, R. D.; and Rooney, W. L. Phenolic compounds and antioxidant activity of sorghum grains of varying genotypes. *J Agric Food Chem,* 2005, 53, 6813–6818.

Dykes, L.; Seiz, L. M.; Rooney, W. L.; and Rooney, L. W. Flavonoid composition of red sorghum genotypes. *Food Chem,* **2009**, *116*, 313–317.

Eggum, B. O.; Monowar, L.; Bach Knudsen, K. E.; Munck, L.; and Axtell, J. Nutritional quality of sorghum and sorghum foods from Sudan. *J Cereal Sci,* **1983**, *1*(2), 127–137.

Elmaki, H. B.; Babiker, E. E.; and El Tinay, A. H. Changes in chemical composition, grain malting, starch and tannin contents and protein digestibility during germination of sorghum cultivars. *Food Chem,* **1999**, *64*(3), 331–336.

Emmambux, M. N.; Stading, M.; and Taylor, J. R. N. Sorghum film property modification with hydrolysable and condensed tannins. *J Cereal Sci,* **2004**, *40*, 127–135.

Etuk, E. B.; Okeudo, N. J.; Esonu, B. O.; and Udedibie, A. B. I. Antinutritional factors in sorghum: chemistry, mode of action and effects on livestock and poultry. *Online J Animal Feed Res,* **2012**, *2,* 113–119

Ezeogu, L. I.; Okolo, B. N. Effect of final warm water steep and air rest cycles on malt properties of three improved Nigerian sorghum cultivars. *J Inst Brew,* **1994**, *100*, 335–338.

Ezeogu, L. I.; Okolo, B. N. Effects of air rest periods on malting sorghum response to final warm water steep. *J Inst Brew,* **1995**, *101*, 39–45.

FAOUN (Food and Agriculture Organization of the United Nations). *Amino-acid Content of Foods and Biological Data on Proteins.* FAO Nutrition Studies No. 24, Food and Agriculture Organization of the United Nations, Rome, Italy, 1970, pages 1–285.

FAOUN (Food and Agriculture Organization of the United Nations). *Food Outlook: Biannual Report on Global Food Markets,* 2016. URL: http://www.fao.org/3/a-I5703E.pdf. Accessed on July 17, 2017.

Fardet, A. New hypotheses for the health-protective mechanisms of whole-grain cereals: what is beyond fibre? *Nutr Res Rev,* **2010**, *23*, 65–134.

Fernandez-Orozco, R.; Li, L.; Harflett, C.; Shewry, P. R.; and Ward, J. L. Effects of environment and genotype on phenolic acids in wheat in the HEALTHGRAIN diversity screen. *J Agric Food Chem,* **2010**, *58*, 9341–9352.

Ferreira, S. M. R.; de Mello, A. P.; dos Anjos, R. C. M.; Krüger, H. C. C.; Azoubel, M. P.; and Márcia Aurelina de Oliveira Alves, A. M. Utilization of sorghum, rice, corn flours with potato starch for the preparation of gluten-free pasta. *Food Chem,* **2016**. *191*, 147–151.

Foti, M. C. Antioxidant properties of phenols. *J Pharm Pharmacol,* 2007, *59*(12), 1673–1685.

Fraga, C. G. (Eds.). *Plant Phenolics and Human Health: Biochemistry, Nutrition and Pharmacology.* John Wiley: New Jersey, 2010. ISBN 978–0–470–28721–7.

Fraga, C. G.; Galleano, M.; Verstraeten, S. V.; and Oteiza, P. I. Basic biochemical mechanisms behind the health benefits of polyphenols. *Mol Aspects Med,* **2010**, *31*(6), 435–445.

Giner, L. M.; Rodrigo, J. V.; Navarro, A. C. F.; and Burillo, V. L. C. Improved extraction procedures for coal products based on the Soxtec apparatus. *Energy Fuels,* **1996**, *10* (4), 1005–1011.

González-Montilla, F. M.; Chávez-Santoscoy, R. A.; Gutiérrez-Uribe, J. A.; and Serna-Saldivar, S. O. Isolation and identification of phase II enzyme inductors obtained from black Shawaya sorghum [*Sorghum bicolor* (L.) Moench] bran. *J Cereal Sci, 2012, 55*, 126–131.

Goufo, P.; Trindade, H. Rice antioxidants: phenolic acids, flavonoids, anthocyanins, proanthocyanidins, tocopherols, tocotrienols, γ-oryzanol, and phytic acid. *Food Sci Nutr, 2014, 2* (2): 75–104.

Gouni-Berthold, I.; Berthold, H. K. Policosanol: clinical pharmacology and therapeutic significance of a new lipid-lowering agent. *Am Heart J, 2002, 143*, 356–365.

Gous, F. *Tannins and phenols in black sorghum.* PhD Dissertation, Texas A&M University, College Station, TX, USA, 1989.

Graf, B. A.; Milbury, P. E.; and Blumberg, J. B. Flavonols, flavonones, flavanones and human health: epidemiological evidence. *J Med Food, 2005, 8*, 281–290.

Gu, L.; Kelm, M.; Hammerstone, J. F.; Beecher, G.; Cunnigham, D.; Vannozzi, S.; and Prior, L. Fractionation of polymeric procyanidins from lowbush blueberry and quantification of procyanidins in selected foods with an optimized normal-phase HPLC-MS fluorescent detection method. *J Agric Food Chem, 2002, 50*, 4852–4860.

Gujer, R.; Magnolato, D.; and Self, R. Glucosylated flavonoids and other phenolic compounds from sorghum. *Phytochemistry, 1986, 25*, 1431–1436.

Gupta, R. K.; Haslam, E. Plant proanthocyanidins. Part 5. Sorghum polyphenols. *J Chem Soc, Perkin Trans 1, 1978, 14* (8), 892–896.

Gupta, V.; Jain, A. D. K.; Gill, N. S.; and Gupta, K. Development and validation of HPLC method—a review. *Int Res J Pharm Appl Sci, 2012, 2*(4), 17–25.

Gyllinga, H.; Plat, J.; Turley, S.; Ginsberg, H. N.; Ellegård, L.; Jessup, W.; Jones, P. J.; Lütjohann, D.; Maerz, W.; Masana, L.; Silbernagel, G.; Staels, B.; Borén, J.; Catapano, A. L.; Backer, G. D.; Deanfield, J.; Descamps, O. S.; Kovanen, P. T.; and Chapman, M. J. Plant sterols and plant stanols in the management of dyslipidaemia and prevention of cardiovascular disease. *Atherosclerosis, 2014, 232*(2), 346–360.

Hahn, D. H.; Rooney, L. W.; and Earp, C. F. Tannins and phenols of sorghum. *Cereal Food World, 1984, 29*, 776–779.

Hahn, D. H.; Rooney, L. W.; and Faubion, J. M. Sorghum phenolic acids, their HPLC separation and their relation to fungal resistance. *Cereal Chem, 1983, 60*, 255–259.

Hassan, I. A. G.; El Tinay, A. H. Effect of fermentation on tannin content and in-vitro protein and starch digestibilities of two sorghum cultivars. *Food Chem, 1995, 53*, 149–151.

Hemphill, S. P. *Effect of sorghum bran addition on lipid oxidation and sensory properties of ground beef patties differing in fat levels.* MSc Dessertation, Texas A&M University: College Station, TX, 2006.

Hou, Z.; Qin, P.; Zhang, Y.; Cui, S.; and Ren, G. Identification of anthocyanins isolated from black rice (*Oryza sativa* L.) and their degradation kinetics. *Food Res Int, 2013, 50*, 691–697.

Hwang, K. T.; Cuppett, S. L.; Weller, C. L.; and Hanna, M. A. HPLC of grain sorghum wax classes highlighting separation of aldehydes from wax esters and steryl esters. *J Sep Sci, 2002a, 25*(9), 619–623.

Hwang, K. T.; Cuppett, S. L.; Weller, C. L.; and Hanna, M. A. Properties, composition, and analysis of grain sorghum wax. *J Am Oil Chem Soc, 2002b, 79*(6), 521–527.

Hwang, K. T.; Kim, J. E.; and Weller, C. L. Policosanol contents and compositions in wax-like materials extracted from selected cereals of Korean origin. *Cereal Chem, 2005, 82*(3), 242–245.

Hwang, K. T.; Weller, C. L.; Cuppett, S. L.; and Hanna, M. A. Policosanol contents and composition of grain sorghum kernels and dried distillers grains. *Cereal Chem,* **2004,** *831*(3), 345–349.

Indira, R.; Naik, M. S. Nutrient composition and protein quality of some minor millets. *Indian J Agric Sci,* **1971,** *41,* 795–797.

Irmak, S.; Dunford, N. T.; and Milligan, J. Policosanol contents of beeswax, sugar cane and wheat extracts. *Food Chem,* **2005,** *95,* 312–318.

Jones, P. J. H.; Ntanios, F. Y.; Raeini-Sarjaz, M.; and Vanstone, C. A. Cholesterol-lowering efficacy of a sitostanol-containing phytosterol mixture with a prudent diet in hyperlipidemic men, *Am J Clin Nutr,* **1999,** *69,* 1140–1150.

Jonnalagadda, S. S.; Harnack, L.; Liu, R. H.; McKeown, N.; Seal, C.; Liu, S.; and Fahey, G. C. Putting the whole grain puzzle together: health benefits associated with whole grains– summary of American Society for Nutrition 2010 Satellite Symposium. *Br J Nutr,* **2011,** *141,* 1011S–1022S.

Kabir, Y.; Kimura, S. Tissue distribution of (8–14C)-octacosanol in liver and muscle of rats after serial administration. *Ann Nutr Metab,* **1995,** *39,* 279–284.

Kadam, D. D.; Mane, P. C.; and Chaudhari, R. D. Phytochemical screening and pharmacological applications of some selected Indian spices. *Int J Sci Res,* **2015,** *4* (3), 704–706.

Kaluza, W. Z.; McGrath, R. M.; Roberts, T. C.; and Schroeder, H. H. Separation of phenolics of *Sorghum bicolor* (L.) Moench grain. *J Agric Food Chem,* **1988,** *28,* 1191–1196.

Kambal, A. E.; Bate-Smith, E. C. A genetic and biochemical study on pericarp pigments in a cross between two cultivars of grain sorghum, *Sorghum bicolor. Heredity,* **1976,** *37,* 413–416.

Kapri, M.; Verma, D. K.; Ajesh Kumar, V.; Billoria, S.; Mahato, D. K.; Yadav, B. S.; and Srivastav, P. P. Modified pearl millet starch: a review on chemical modification, characterization, and functional properties. In: Goyal, M. R. and Verma, D. K. (Eds.), *Engineering Interventions in Agricultural Processing.* Volume 8, as part of book series on Innovations in Agricultural and Biological Engineering. Apple Academic Press: USA, 2017.

Kaufmann, B.; Christen, P. Recent extraction techniques from natural products: microwave- assisted extraction and pressurized solvent extraction. *Phytochem Anal,* **2002,** *13* (2), 105–113.

Kayode, A. P. P.; Nout, M. J. R.; Bakker, E. J.; and Van Boekel, M. A.´ J. S. Evaluation of the simultaneous effects of processing parameters on the iron, and zinc solubility of infant sorghum porridge by response surface methodology. *J Agric Food Chem,* **2006,** *54,* 4253–4259.

Kayodéa A. P. P.; Bara, C. A.; Dalodé-Vieira, G.; Linnemann. A. R.; and Nout, M. J. R. Extraction of antioxidant pigments from dye sorghum leaf sheaths. *LWT—Food Sci Technol,* **2012,** *46,* 49–55.

Kazanas, N.; Fields, M. L. Nutritional improvement of sorghum by fermentation. *J Food Sci,* **1981,** *46,* 81–821.

Kennedy, D. O.; Wightman, E. L. Herbal extracts and phytochemicals: plant secondary metabolites and the enhancement of human brain function. *Adv Nutr,* **2011,** *2,* 32–50.

Khalil, R. A. S.; Abdelhafez, A. A.; and Amer, E. A. M. Evaluation of bioethanol production from juice and bagasse of some sweet sorghum varieties. *Ann Agric Sci,* **2015,** *60* (2), 317–324.

Khan, I.; Yousif, A.; Johnson, S. K.; and Gamlath, S. Effect of sorghum flour addition on resistant starch content, phenolic profile and antioxidant capacity of durum wheat pasta. *Food Res Int,* **2013**, *54*, 578–586.

Kim, J.; Park, Y. Anti-diabetic effect of sorghum extract on hepatic gluconeogenesis of streptozotocin-induced diabetic rats. *Nutr Metabol,* **2012**, *9*(1), 106. http:// dx.doi.org/10.1186/1743–7075-9–106

Klopfesntein, C. F.; Hoseney, R. C. Nutritional properties of sorghum and millets. In: Dendy, D. A. V. (Eds.), *Sorghum and Millets: Chemistry, Technology.* American Association of Cereal Chemists: St Paul, MN, 1995, pages 125–168.

Ko, C.; Shen, S.; Lin, H.; Hou, W.; Lee, W.; Yang, L.; and Chen, Y. Flavanones structure-related inhibition on TPA-induced tumor promotion through suppression of extracellular signal-regulated protein kinases: involvement of prostaglandin E2 in anti-promotive process. *J Cell Physiol,* **2002**, *193*, 93–102.

Koistinen, V. M.; Hanhineva, K. Mass spectrometry-based analysis of whole grain phytochemicals. *Crit Rev Food Sci Nutr,* **2017**, *57*(8), 1688–1709.

Kondratyuk, T. P.; Pezzuto, J. M. Natural product polyphenols of relevance to human health. *Pharm Biol,* **2004**, *42*, 46–63.

Krueger, C. G.; Vestling, M. A.; and Reed, J. D. Matrix-assisted laser desorption/ionization time-of-flight mass spectrometry of heteropolyflavan-3-ols and glucosylated heteropolyflavans in sorghum (*Sorghum bicolor* (L.) Moench). *J Agric Food Chem,* **2003**, *51*, 538–543.

Kuntz, S.; Wenzel, U.; and Daniel, H. Comparative analysis of the effects of flavonoids on proliferation, cytotoxicity, and apoptosis in human colon cancer cell lines. *Euro Br J Nutr,* **1999**, *38*, 133–142.

Lee, B. H.; Carr, T. P.; Weller, C. L.; Cuppett, S.; Dweikat, I. M.; and Schlegel, V. GS whole kernel oil lowers plasma and liver cholesterol in male hamsters with minimal wax involvement. *J Funct Foods,* **2014**, *7*, 709–718.

Lee, E. R.; Kang, Y. J.; Kim, H. J.; Choi, H. Y.; Kang, G. H.; Kim, J. H.; Kim, B. W.; Jeong, H. S.; Park, Y. S.; and Cho, S. G. Regulation of apoptosis by modified naringenin derivatives in human colorectal carcinoma RKO cells. *J Cell Biochem,* **2008**, *104*, 259–279.

Leguizamón, C.; Weller, C. L.; Schlegel, V. L.; and Carr, T. P. Plant sterol and policosanol characterization of hexane extracts from grain sorghum, corn and their DDGS. *J Am Oil Chem Soc,* **2009**, *86* (7), 707–716.

Li, L.; Shewry, P. R.; and Ward, J. L. Phenolic acids in wheat varieties in the HEALTHGRAIN diversity screen. *J Agric Food Chem,* **2008**, *56*, 9732–9739.

Liu, R. H. Whole grain phytochemicals and health. *J Cereal Sci,* **2007**, *46*, 207–219.

Liyana-Pathirana, C. M.; Shahidi, F. Importance of insoluble-bound phenolics to antioxidant properties of wheat. *J Agric Food Chem,* **2006**, *54*, 1256–1264.

Lopez, M.; Martinez, F.; Del Valle, C.; Orte, C. and Miro, M. Analysis of phenolic constituents of biological interest in red wines by high performance liquid chromatography. *J Chromatogr A,* **2001**, *922*, 395–363.

Luque de Castro, M. D.; Garcia-Ayuso, L. E. Soxhlet extraction of solid materials: An outdated technique with a promising innovative future. *Anal Chim Acta,* **1998**, *369*(1–2), 1–10.

Luthria, D. L.; Liu, K. Localization of phenolic acids and antioxidant activity in sorghum karnels. *J Food Sci.* **2013**, *5*, 1751–1760.

Mahgoub, S. E. O.; Elhag, S. A. Effect of milling, soaking, malting, heat-treatment and fermentation on phytate level of four Sudanese sorghum cultivars. *Food Chem,* **1998**, *61,* 77–80.

Mas, R. Policosanol—hypolipidemic antioxidant treatment of atherosclerosis. *Drugs Future,* **2000**, *25,* 569–586.

Mas, R.; Rivas, P.; Izquierdo, J. E.; Hernandez, R.; Fernandez, J.; Orta, S. D.; Illnait, J.; and Ricardo, Y. Pharmacoepidemiologic study of polycosanol. *Curr Ther Res,* **1999**, *60,* 458–467.

McDonough, C. M.; Rooney, L. W.; and Earp, C. F. Structural characteristics of *Eleusine coracana* (finger millet) using scanning electron and fluorescence microscopy. *Food Microstruct,* **1986**, *5,* 247–256.

Mella, O. N. O. *Effects of malting and fermentation on the composition and functionality of sorghum flour.* MSc Dissertation, University of Nebraska, USA, 2011.

Misra, K.; Seshadri, T. R. Chemical components of sorghum durra glumes. *Indian J Chem,* **1967**, *5,* 409.

Mohammed, N. A.; Mohammed, I. A.; and Barbiker, E. E. Nutritional evaluation of sorghum flour (*Sorghum bicolor* L. Moench) during processing of injera. *Int J Biolog Biomol Agril, Food Biotech Eng,* **2011**, 5, 99–103.

Moraes, E.A.; Natal, D. I. G.; Quieroz, V. A. V.; Schaffert, R. E.; Cecon, P. R.; de Paula, S. O.; dos Anjos Benjamin, L.; Ribeiro, S. M. R.; and Martino, H. S. D. Sorghum genotype may reduce low-grade inflammatory response and oxidative stress and maintains jejunum morphology of rats fed a hyperlipidic diet. *Food Res Int,* **2012**, *49,* 553–559.

Moss, G. P. The nomenclature of steroids: recommendations by the IUPAC–IUB joint commission on biochemical nomenclature. *Eur J Biochem,* **1989**, *186,* 429–458.

Murooka, Y.; Yamshita, M. Traditional healthful fermented products of Japan. *J Ind Microbiol Biotechnol,* **2008**, *35,* 791–798.

Murty, D. S.; Kumar, K. A. Traditional uses of sorghum and millets In: Dendy, D. A. V. (Ed.), *Sorghum and Millets: Chemistry and Technology.* American Association of Cereal Chemists: St. Paul, MN, 1995, pp. 185–221.

Nip, W. K.; Burns, E. E. Pigment characterization in grain sorghum. I. Red varieties. *Cereal Chem,* **1969**, *46,* 490–495.

Nip, W. K.; Burns, E. E. Pigment characterization in grain sorghum. II. White varieties. *Cereal Chem,* **1971**, *48,* 74–80.

Norkaew, O.; Boontakham, P.; Dumri, K. and Noenplab, L. N. A. Effect of post-harvest treatment on bioactive phytochemicals of Thai black rice. *Food Chem,* **2017**, *217,* 98–105.

Nout, M. J. Rich nutrition from the poorest—cereal fermentations in Africa and Asia. *Food Microbiol,* **2009**, *26*(7), 685–692.

Okarter, N.; Liu, R. H: Health benefits of whole grain phytochemicals. *Crit Rev Food Sci Nutr,* **2010**, *50,* 193–208.

Oliver Chen, C.-Y.; Blumberg, J. B. Phytochemical composition of nuts. *Asia Pac J Clin Nutr,* **2008**, *17* (S1), 329–332.

Osman, M. A. Changes in sorghum enzyme inhibitors, phytic acid, tannins and in vitro protein digestibility occurring during Khamir (local bread) fermentation. *Food Chem,* **2004**, *88,* 129–134.

Paiva, C. L.; Evangelista, W. P.; Queiroz, V. A. V.; and Glória, M. B. A. Bioactive amines in sorghum: Method optimisation and influence of line, tannin and hydric stress. *Food Chem,* **2015**, *173,* 224–230.

Pale, E.; Kouda-Bonafos, M.; Nacro, M.; Vanhaelex, M.; Vanhaelen-Fastreta, R.; and Ottinger, R. 7-*O*-Methylapigeninidin, an anthocyanidin from *Sorghum caudatum*. *Phytochemistry*, **1997**, *45*(5), 1091–1092.

Pandey, K. B.; Rizvi, S. I. Plant polyphenols as dietary antioxidants in human health and disease. *Oxidative Med Cell Longev*, **2009**, *2*(5), 270–278.

Pascal, D. C. A.; Tachon, C.; Bonin, H.; Chrostowka, A.; Fouquet, E.; and Sohounhloue, C. K. D. Phytochemical study of a tinctorial plant of benin traditional pharmacopoeia: the red sorghum (*Sorghum caudatum*) of benin. *Sci Study Res, Chem Eng Biotechnol Food Ind*, **2012**, *13* (2), 121–135.

Pham, T. -C. -T.; Angers, P.; and Ratti, C. Extraction of wax-like materials from cereals. *Can J Chem Eng*, **2018**, *96*(10), 2273–2281.

Piironen, V.; Toivo, J.; and Lampi, A.-M. Plant sterols in cereals and cereal products. *Cereal Chem*, **2002**, *79*, 148–154.

Plaami, S. P. Content of dietary fiber in foods and its physiological effects. *Food Rev Int*, **1997**, *13*(1), 29–76.

Poutanen, K.; Flander, L.; and Katina, K. Sourdough and cereal fermentation in a nutritional perspective, *Food Microbiol*, **2009**, *26*, 693–699.

Price, M. L.; Van Scoyoc, S.; and Butler, L. G. A critical evaluation of vanillin reaction as an assay for tannin in sorghum. *J Agric Food Chem*, **1978**, *26*, 1214–1218.

Proietti, I.; Frazzoli, C.; and Mantovani, A. Exploiting nutritional value of staple foods in the world's semi-arid areas: risks, benefits, challenges and opportunities of sorghum. *Healthcare*, **2015**, *3*(2), 172–193.

Przbylski, R.; Lee, Y. C.; and Eskin, N. A. M. Antioxidant and radical-scavenging activities in buckwheat seeds. *J Am Oil Chem Soc*, **1998**, *75*, 1595–1601.

Ragaee, S.; Abdel-Aal, E. M.; and Noaman, M. Antioxidant activity and nutrient composition of selected cereals for food use. *Food Chem*, **2006**, *98*, 32–38.

Ragaee, S.; Seetharaman, K.; and Abdel-Aal el-SM. The impact of milling and thermal processing on phenolic compounds in cereal grains. *Crit Rev Food Sci Nutr*, **2014**, *54*(7), 837–849.

Rai, K. N.; Gowda, C. L. L.; Reddy, B. V. S.; and Sehgal, S. The potential of sorghum and pearl millet in alternative and health food uses. *Compr Rev Food Sci Food Saf*, **2008**, *7*, 340–352.

Raihanatu, M. B.; Modu, S.; Falmata, A. S.; Shettima, Y. A.; and Heman, M. Effect of processing (sprouting and fermentation) of five local varieties of sorghum on some biochemical parameters. *Biokemistri*, **2011**, *23*, 91–96.

Rao, M. V. S. S. T. S.; Muralikrishna G. Structural analysis of arabionoxylans isolated from native and malted finger millet (*Eleusine coracana*, ragi). *Carbohydr Res*, **2004**, *339*, 2457–2463.

Rey, J. P.; Pousset, J. L.; Levesque, J.; and Wanty, P. Isolation and composition of a natural dye from the stems of *Sorghum bicolor* (L.) Moench subsp. Americanum caudatum. *Cereal Chem*, **1993**, *70*, 759–760.

Rooney, W. L.; Portillo, O. R.; and Hayes, C. Registration of A/BTx3363 black sorghum germplasm. *J Plant Regist*, **2013a**, *7*, 342–346.

Rooney, W. L.; Rooney, L. W.; Awika, J. A.; and Dykes, L. Registration of Tx3362 sorghum germplasm. *J Plant Regist*, **2013b**. *7*, 104–107.

Rosenow, D. T.; Quisenberry, J. E.; Wendt, C. W.; and Clark, L. E. Drought tolerant sorghum and cotton germplasm. *Agric Water Manag*, **1983**, 7, 207–222.

Schober, T. J.; Messerschmidt, M.; Bean, S. R.; Park, S. H.; and Arendt, E. K. Gluten-free bread from sorghum: quality differences among hybrids. *Cereal Chem,* **2005**, *82,* 394–404.

Seidu, K. K.; Osundahunsi, O. F.; Olaleye, M. T.; and Oluwalana, I. B. Chemical composition, phytochemical constituents and antioxidant potentials of lima bean seeds coat. *Ann Food Sci Technol,* **2014**, *15*(2), 288–298.

Seitz, L. M. *3-Deoxyanthocyanidins and other phenolic compounds in grain from sorghum sister lines with white, red, and yellow pericarp.* AACC Annual Meeting Program Book, USA, 2005, pages 153.

Serna-Saldivar, S. O.; Knabe, D. A.; Rooney, L. W.; Tanksley Jr, T. D.; and Sproule, A. M. Nutritional value of sorghum and maize tortillas. *J Cereal Sci,* **1988**, *7*(2), 83–94.

Serna-Saldivar, S. O.; Tellez-Giron, A.; and Rooney, L. W. Production of tortilla chips from sorghum and maize. *J Cereal Sci,* **1987**, *8*(3), 275–284.

Sheoran, A.; Yadav, B. S.; Nigam, P.; and Singh, D. Continuous ethanol production from sugarcane molasses using a common reactor of immobilised *Saccharomyces cereviaceae* HAV -1. *J Basic Microbiol,* **1998**, *38,* 123–128.

Shih, C. H.; Chu, I. K.; Yip, W. K.; and Lo, C. Differential expression of two flavonoid 30—hydroxylase cDNAs involved in biosynthesis of anthocyanin pigments and 3-deoxyanthocyanidin phytoalexins in sorghum. *Plant Cell Physiol,* **2006**, *47,* 1412–1419.

Shih, C. H.; Siu, S. O.; Ng, R.; Wong, E.; Chiu, L. C.; Chu, I. K.; and Lo, C. Quantitative analysis of anticancer 3-deoxyanthocyanidins in infected sorghum seedlings. *J Agric Food Chem,* **2007**, *55,* 254–259.

Shinde, V. V. Production kinetics and functional properties of carboxymethyl sorghum starch. *Indian J Nat Prod Res,* **2005**, *4*(6), 466–470

Sierksma, A.; Weststrate, J. A.; and Meijer, G. W. Spreads enriched with plant sterols, either esterified 4,4-dimethylsterols or free 4-desmethylsterols, and plasma total- and LDL-cholesterol concentrations. *Br J Nutr,* **1999**, *82,* 273–282.

Singh, H.; Singh, S. N.; and Singh, N. Structure and functional properties of acid thinned sorghum starch. *Int J Food Prop,* **2009**, *12,* 713–725.

Singh, V.; Moreau, R. A.; and Hicks, K. B. Yield and phytosterol composition of oil extracted from grain sorghum and its wet-milled fractions. *Cereal Chem,* **2003**, *80*(2), 126–129.

Slavin, J.; Jacobs, D.; and Marquart, L. Whole-grain consumption and chronic disease: protective mechanisms. *Nutr Cancer,* **1997**, *27,* 14–21.

Stafford, H. A. Flavonoids and related phenolic compounds produced in the first internode of *Sorghum vulgare* preserved in darkness and in light. *Plant Physiol,* **1965**, *40,* 130–139.

Stefoska-Needham, A.; Beck, E. J.; Johnson, S. K.; and Tapsell, L. C. Sorghum: an underutilized cereal whole grain with the potential to assist in the prevention of chronic disease. *Food Rev Int,* **2015**, *31,* 401–437.

Stevenson, L.; Phillips, F.; O'sullivan, K.; and Walton, J. Wheat bran: its composition and benefits to health, a European perspective. *Int J Food Sci Nutr,* **2012**, *63*(8), 1001–1013.

Strumeyer, D. H.; Malin, M. J. Condensed tannins in grain sorghum: isolation, fractionation, and characterization. *J Agric Food Chem,* **1975**, *23,* 909–914.

Subramanian, V.; Hoseney, R. C.; and Bramel-Cox, P. Factors affecting the colour and appearance of Sorghum starch. *Cereal Chem,* **1994**, *71,* 275–278.

Sweeny, J. G.; Iacobucci, G. A. Synthesis of anthocyanidins-III: total synthesis of apigenidin and luteolinidin chlorides. *Tetrahedron,* 1981, *37,* 1481–1483.

Taleon, V. M.; Dykes, L.; Rooney, W. L.; and Rooney, L. W. Effect of genotype and environment on flavonoid concentration and profile of black sorghum grains. *J Cereal Sci,* **2012**, *56,* 470–475.

Taylor, J. R. N. Effect of malting on the protein and free amino nitrogen composition of sorghum. *J Sci Food Agric,* **1983***, 34,* 885–892.

Taylor, J. R. N.; Belton, P. S.; Beta, T.; and Duodu, K. G. Review: Increasing the utilization of sorghum, millets, and pseudocereals: Developments in the science of their phenolic phytochemicals, biofortification, and protein functionality. *J Cereal Sci,* **2013***, 59*(3), 257–275.

Taylor, J. R. N.; Belton, P. S.; Beta, T.; and Duodu, K. G. Increasing the utilisation of sorghum, millets and pseudocereals: developments in the science of their phenolic phytochemicals, biofortification and protein functionality. *J Cereal Sci,* **2014***, 59,* 257–275.

Towo, E.; Matuschek, E.; and Svanberg, U. Fermentation and enzyme treatment of tannin sorghum gruels: effects on phenolic compounds, phytate and *in vitro* accessible iron. *Food Chem,* **2006***, 94,* 369–376.

Trabelsi, N.; d'Estaintot, B. L.; Sigaud, G.; Gallois, B.; and Chaudière, J. Kinetic and binding equilibrium studies of dihydroflavonol 4-reductase from *Vitis vinifera* and its unusually strong substrate inhibition. *J Biophys Chem,* **2011***, 2*(3), 332–344.

Udachan, I. S.; Sahoo, A. K.; and Hend, G. M. Extraction and characterization of sorghum (*Sorghum bicolor L. Moench*) starch. *Int Food Res J,* **2012***, 19*(1), 315–319.

USDA (United States Department of Agriculture). *Basic Report: 20067, Sorghum grain. Nutrient Database for Standard Reference Release 28*, Agricultural Research Service, USDA. URL: http://ndb.nal.usda.gov/ndb/search/list. Accessed on August 18, 2017.

Vali, S. R.; Ju, Y.-H.; Kaimal, T. N. B. and Chern, Y.-T. A Process for the Preparation of Food-Grade Rice Bran Wax and the Determination of Its Composition. *J Am Oil Chem Soc,* **2005***, 82*(1), 57–64.

Van Hung, P. Phenolic Compounds of cereals and their antioxidant capacity. *Crit Rev Food Sci Nutr,* **2016***, 56*(1), 25–35.

Vauzour, D.; Rodriguez-Mateos, A.; Corona, G.; Oruna-Concha, M. J.; and Spencer, J. P. E. Polyphenols and human health: prevention of disease and mechanisms of action. *Nutrients,* **2010***, 2*(11), 1106–1131.

Visioli, F.; De La Lastra, C. A.; Andres-Lacueva, C.; Aviram, M.; Calhau, C.; Cassano, A.; D'Archivio, M.; Faria, A.; Favé, G.; Fogliano, V.; Llorach, R.; Vitagione, P.; Zoratti, M.; and Edeas, M. Polyphenols and human health: a prospectus. *Crit Rev Food Sci Nutr,* **2011***, 51,* 524–546.

Wang, M. -F.; Lian, H. Z.; Mao, L.; Zhou, J. P.; Gong, H. J.; Qian, B. Y.; Fang, Y.; and Li, J. Comparison of Various extraction methods for policosanol from rice bran wax and establishment of chromatographic fingerprint of policosanol. *J Agric Food Chem,* **2007,** *55,* 5552–5558.

Wang, Q.; Han, P.; Zhang, M.; Xia, M.; Zhu, H.; Ma, J.; Hou, M.; Tang, Z.; and Ling, W. Supplementation of black rice pigment fraction improves antioxidant and anti-inflammatory status in patients with coronary heart disease. *Asia Pac J Clin Nut,* **2007***, 16,* 295–301.

Wanga, T.; Hea, F.; and Chena, G. Improving bioaccessibility and bioavailability of phenolic compounds in cereal grains through processing technologies: a concise review. *J Funct Foods,* **2014***, 7,* 101–111.

Waniska, R. D.; Poe, J. H.; and Bandyopadhyay, R. Effects of growth conditions on grain molding and phenols in sorghum caryopsis. *J Cereal Sci,* **1989***, 10,* 217–225.

Waniska, R. D.; Rooney, L. W. Sorghum grain quality for increased utilization. In: Leslie, J. F. (Ed.), *Sorghum and Millets Diseases.* Iowa State Press, Ames, IA, USA, 2002, pages 327–335.

Watterson, J. J.; Butler, L. G. Occurrence of an unusual leucoanthocyanidin and absence of proanthocyanidins in sorghum leaves. *J Agric Food Chem*, **1983**, *31*, 41–45.

Wrolstad, R. E. Anthocyanin pigments—bioactivity and coloring properties. Symposium 12: Interaction of Natural Colors with Other Ingredients. *J Food Sci*, **2004**, *69*, C419-C421.

Wu, G.; Johnson, S.; Bornman, J.; Bennett, S.; Singh, V.; and Fang, Z. Effect of genotype and growth temperature on sorghum grain physical characteristics, polyphenol content and antioxidant activity. *Cereal Chem*, **2016**, *93*(4), 419–425.

Wu, X.; Prior, R. L. Identification and characterization of anthocyanins by high-performance liquid chromatography-electrospray ionization-tandem mass spectrometry in common foods in the United States: vegetables, nuts, and grains. *J Agric Food Chem*, **2005**, *53*, 3101–3113.

Xin, Z.; Edward, E. C.; Weiqun, W.; and Rajeshekar, C. B. Does organic production enhance phytochemical content of fruit and vegetables? Current knowledge and prospects for research. *HortTechnology*, **2006**, *16*(3), 449–456.

Yang, L.; Allred, K. F.; Geera, B.; Allred, C. D.; and Awika, J. M. Sorghum phenolics demonstrate estrogenic action and induce apoptosis in nonmalignant colonocytes. *Nutr Cancer*, **2012**, *64*, 419–427.

Yang, L.; Browning, J. D.; and Awika, J. M. Sorghum 3-deoxyanthocyanins possess strong phase II enzyme inducer activity and cancer cell growth inhibition properties. *J Agric Food Chem*, **2009**, *57*, 1797–1804.

Yousif, A.; Nheper, D.; and Johnson, S. Influence of sorghum flour addition on flat bread in vitro digestibility, antioxidant capacity and consumer acceptability. *Food Chem*, **2012**, *134*, 880–887.

Youssef, A. M. Extractability, fractionation and nutritional value of low and high tannin sorghum proteins. *Food Chem*, **1998**, *63*, 325–329.

CHAPTER 3

Effect of Processing on Bioactive Phytochemicals of Barley: A Cereal Grain with Potent Antioxidants and Potential Human Health Benefits

SUKHVINDER SINGH PUREWAL, MANINDER KAUR, ASHISH BALDI, PINDERPAL KAUR, and KAWALJIT SINGH SANDHU[*]

Department of Food Science & Technology, Maharaja Ranjit Singh Punjab Technical University, Bathinda 151001, Punjab, India

[*]*Corresponding author.*
E-mail: kawsandhu@rediffmail.com; kawsandhu5@gmail.com

ABSTRACT

Barley (*Hordeum vulgare*) is a rabi crop, its grains are small seeded and self-pollinating, mainly used as food and feed. It is grown over wide range of area due to its adaptability toward temperate climate conditions. Flour from barley grains is primarily used in the form of processed food products, bread preparation, breakfast snacks, and beverages (alcoholic and nonalcoholic). Being a rich source of bioactive phytochemicals and potent antioxidants, barley grains could be a preferred substrate for the production of nutraceuticals and functional foods of pharmaceutical importance. Barley grains are extensively studied for bioactive constituents and its flour is mainly used in food fortifications. Specific bioactive constituents present in barley grains are β-glucans, gallic acid, *o*-hydroxybenzoic acid (salicylic acid), vanillic acid, ferulic acid, *p*-coumaric acid, sinapinic acid, caffeic acid, tocopherols, catechin, quercetin, and alkylresorcinols. Knowledge of the proximate composition and bioactive profile could aid food and pharmacy industries in the design of barley based functional food products required to sustain healthy life style. Whole grains and fractions of barley are processed to improve nutritional efficiency using germination, roasting, solid state fermentation, thermal processing, and response surface methodology optimized conditions.

3.1 INTRODUCTION

Barley (*Hordeum vulgare* L.) have ranks 5th among the important cereal grains, they belong to the grass family Poaceae (Sharma and Gujral, 2010; Baba et al., 2016). This crop is grown mainly in temperate climates and during earlier stage of growth; barley requires 12–16 °C temperature whereas during the maturation stage it requires 30–32 °C. For maximal growth of barley plant, the preferred soil type varies from sodic to saline. Barley is grown by farmers (Figure 3.1), sometimes as main crop or in conjunction with other crops like rice, maize, pearl millet, sorghum, sugarcane, sesame, and cotton.

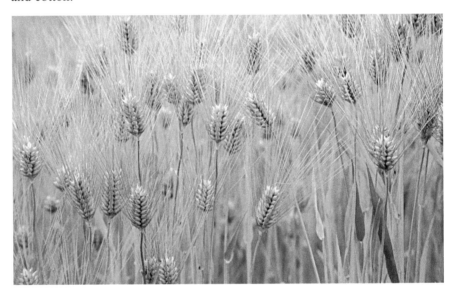

FIGURE 3.1   Standing barley (*Hordeum* vulgare) crop in field with the grains.

Grains are commonly used both as feed and food purposes; 80%–90% of the edible seeds are utilized as animal feed, chapatti's preparations, and other important food products. Apart from being important cereal grain, barley provides nutritional values including proximate composition (e.g., carbohydrates, proteins, fibers, etc.) vitamins, minerals, amino acids profile (Table

3.1) as well as bioactive phytochemicals like phenolic compounds, tannins, and flavonoids (Sharma and Gujral, 2010; Sandhu and Punia, 2017). Tables 3.2 and 3.3 compare the nutrient component of barley with other important cereal grains.

TABLE 3.1 Nutritional Value of Barley Grain [per 100 g (3.5 oz)]

Nutrients Components	Value	Nutrients Components	Value
Proximate		Vitamin B_5 (pantothenic acid)	0.282 mg
Energy	1473 kJ (352 kcal)	Vitamin B_6	0.260 mg
Carbohydrates	77.72 g	Vitamin B_9 (folate)	23 µg
Dietary fiber	15.6 g	Choline	37.8 mg
Fat	1.16 g	Vitamin E (α-tocopherol)	0.02 mg
Fatty acids		Vitamin K (phylloquinone)	2.2 µg
Saturated fatty acids	0.244 g	**Mineral Profile**	
MUFAs	0.149 g	Calcium (Ca)	29 mg
PUFAs	0.560 g	Iron (Fe)	2.50 mg
Protein	9.91 g	Magnesium (Mg)	79 mg
Vitamins Profile		Phosphorus (P)	221 mg
Vitamin A equiv.		Potassium (K)	280 mg
β-carotene	13 µg	Sodium (Na)	9 mg
Lutein and zeaxanthin	160 µg	Zinc (Zn)	2.13 mg
Vitamin B_1 (thiamine)	0.191 mg	Copper (Cu)	0.420 mg
Vitamin B_2 (riboflavin)	0.114 mg	Manganese (Mn)	1.322 mg
Vitamin B_3 (niacin)	4.604 mg	Selenium (Se)	37.7 6 µg
Amino Acids Profile			
Essential Amino Acids		Nonessential amino acids	
Arginine	0.496 g	Alanine	0.386 g
Histidine	0.223 g	Aspartic acid	0.619 g
Isoleucine	0.362 g	Cysteine	0.219 g
Leucine	0.673 g	Glutamic acid	2.588 g
Lysine	0.369 g	Glycine	0.359 g
Methionine	0.190 g	Proline	1.178 g
Phenylalanine	0.556 g	Serine	0.418 g
Threonine	0.337 g	Tyrosine	0.284 g
Tryptophan	0.165 g		
Valine	0.486 g		

MUFAs: monounsaturated fatty acids, PUFAs: polyunsaturated fatty acids.

Source: USDA (2018).

TABLE 3.2 Composition of Nutrient of Barley Grain with Comparison to Other Important Cereal Grains

Cereal Grains	Protein (g)	Fat (g)	Fiber (g)	Minerals (g)	Iron (mg)	Calcium (mg)	Calories (kcal)
Barley	9.91	1.16	15.6	–	2.50	29	352
Rice	6.8	2.7	0.2	0.6	0.7	10	362
Wheat	11.8	2	1.2	1.5	5.3	41	348
Sorghum	10.4	3.1	2	1.6	5.4	25	329
Corn	9.4	4.7	–	–	2.71	7	365

Sources: Modified from Kapri et al. (2017) and USDA (2018).

TABLE 3.3 Composition of Amino Acids of Barley Grain with Comparison to Other Important Cereal Grains

Amino Acids Composition	Barley and Other Cereal Grains (% of DM)			
	Barley	Wheat	Sorghum	Corn
Essential Amino Acids				
Arginine	4.1	5.7	5.7	5.8
Histidine	2.3	2.4	2.4	2.9
Isoleucine	5.0	3.4	3.4	3.2
Leucine	12.8	7.1	6.6	11.9
Lysine	2.4	2.8	4.0	3.1
Methionine	1.6	1.2	1.7	1.3
Phenylalanine	6.1	4.7	5.1	4.7
Valine	6.0	4.8	5.0	4.8
Nonessential Amino Acids				
Alanine	9.3	3.8	4.0	6.9
Aspartic	7.6	5.7	5.6	6.2
Glutamic	21.3	33.2	29.1	18.0
Glycine	3.6	4.4	3.8	3.7
Proline	8.4	11.2	9.6	8.8
Serine	4.9	5.0	4.2	4.6

Sources: Wu et al. (1984); Wu (1986, 1989); Wu and Sexson (1984).

Barley is required in daily food menu to sustain healthy life style and to maintain the level of antioxidants that combat oxidative stress. Numerous classes of bioactive phytochemicals are present in barley grains are in bound as well as free form (Gallegos-Infante et al., 2010). Barley is rich of different important bioactive compounds such as β-glucans (Izydorczyk et al., 2000;

Storsley et al., 2003; Andersson et al., 2004; Izydorczyk and Dextor, 2008; Lin et al., 2018; Martinez et al., 2018), gallic acid (Jende-Strid, 1985; Zhao et al., 2006; Carvalho et al., 2015; Suriano et al., 2018), o-hydroxybenzoic acid (salicylic acid) (Suriano et al., 2018), vanillic acid (Zielinski et al., 2001; Zhao et al., 2006; Irakli et al., 2011; Arigo et al., 2018; Martinez et al., 2018), ferulic acid (Jende-Strid, 1985; Yu et al., 2001; Klausen et al., 2010; Carvalho et al., 2015), p-coumaric acid (Bartolome and Gomez-Cordoves, 1999; Hernanz et al., 2001; Carvalho et al., 2015; Shen et al., 2015; Zhu et al., 2015; Arigo et al., 2018; Hajji et al., 2018; Rao et al., 2018; Suriano et al., 2018), sinapinic acid (Carvalho et al., 2015; Arigo et al., 2018; Martinez et al., 2018), caffeic acid (Jende-Strid, 1985; Yu et al., 2001; Carvalho et al., 2015), tocopherols (Goupy et al., 1999; Panfili et al., 2003; Falk et al., 2004; Moreau et al., 2007; Tsochatzis et al., 2012; Lachman et al., 2018; Martinez et al., 2018), catechin (Jende-Strid, 1985; Klausen et al., 2010; Carvalho et al., 2015), quercetin (Holtekjolen et al., 2006; Gangopadhyay et al., 2016; Arigo et al., 2018), and alkylresorcinols (Zarnowski et al., 2002; Zarnowski and Suzuki, 2004; Bordiga et al., 2016). Epidemiological studies support the additions of whole barley grain and processed products based on barley flour in breakfast menu for the reducing the possibility of cardiovascular diseases (CVD) (Sharma and Gujral, 2011; Gani et al., 2012; Zhao et al., 2014; Salar et al., 2017a). Increased interest in natural antioxidants attributes to radical scavenging capacity of phytochemicals especially phenolic compounds, flavonoids, and tannins in barley (Shahidi and Nackz, 1995; Kaur et al., 2018). Recently published scientific reports suggest that mixture of phytochemicals from cereal grains are required to slow down the damaging effects of disease causing free radicals in living organisms (Dvorakova et al., 2008; Gani et al., 2012; Carvalho et al., 2015; Baba et al., 2016; Hajji et al., 2018). Suggested food applications of barley flour (processed and unprocessed) could result in replacement of wheat flour in certain functional foods and bakery products along with other household recipes. Processing of barley grains could be achieved using germination (Sharma and Gujral, 2010), solid state fermentation (Sandhu and Punia, 2017), and thermal processing (Sharma and Gujral, 2011; Baba et al., 2016).

The aim of this chapter is to focus on different processing methods of barley, namely, fermentation, malting, steeping, germination, kilning, thermal processing, and effect of thermal processing on bioactive compounds and antioxidant property results of many researchers what they were confirmed in their experiments and what they were suggested for barley flour with improved nutritional properties. This chapter may serve as an easy approach for the designing of fortified food supplements and other important bakery products of barley flour.

3.2   PRODUCTION OF BARLEY IN INDIA AND WORLDWIDE

The data about the production of barley, area under cultivation, yield, and production in India and worldwide since last 10 years (2006–2016) were collected from the Crops: FAOSTAT database of Food and Agriculture Organization of United Nation (FAOUN) and depicted in Table 3.4 (FAOUN, 2016). At world level, India stands 22nd in terms of barley production (million tons). Major producer of barley in terms of production (million tons) was Russia followed by Germany, France, Canada, and Spain. At world level, the maximal production of barley was observed during the year 2008 (1537.95 million tons) and minimal production was observed during 2010 (123.30million tons) (Figure 3.2). As per data collected for India, the production of barley grains during the year 2016 was 1.51 million tons (Figure 3.2). The production was observed maximal during the year 2014 (1.83 million tons) whereas the minimal production was in year 2008 (1.20 million tons) (FAOUN, 2016). Within India major barley producing areas are Rajasthan, Uttar Pradesh, Madhya Pradesh, Haryana, Punjab, West Bengal, and Jammu and Kashmir.

TABLE 3.4   Area, Yield, and Production of Barley in India and the World Since 2006–2016

Years	Barley in National and International Scenario					
	In India			In World		
	Area	Yield	Production	Area	Yield	Production
2006	0.63	0.019	1.22	56.56	0.255	144.49
2007	0.65	0.021	1.33	54.90	0.024	131.13
2008	0.60	0.020	1.20	55.10	0.028	1537.95
2009	0.71	0.024	1.69	54.43	0.028	150.77
2010	0.62	0.022	1.36	47.41	0.026	123.30
2011	0.71	0.024	1.66	48.44	0.027	132.73
2012	0.64	0.025	1.62	49.84	0.027	132.21
2013	0.70	0.025	1.75	49.77	0.029	143.42
2014	0.67	0.027	1.83	49.62	0.029	144.49
2015	0.71	0.023	1.61	48.94	0.030	148.46
2016	0.59	0.023	1.51	46.92	0.030	141.28

Source: FAOUN (2016).

Note: Area (in million ha); Yield (in million hg/ha); Production (in million tons).

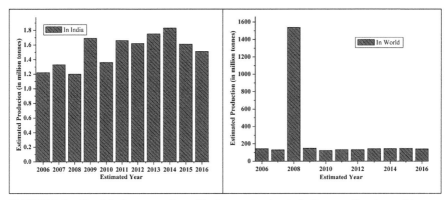

FIGURE 3.2   Graphical presentation of barley production in India as well as in world.

3.3   BIOACTIVE PHYTOCHEMICALS IN BARLEY

The term bioactive phytochemicals are used for mixture of bioactive compo-nents present in natural resources and these components possess solvent specific solubility (Dhull et al., 2016; Kaur et al., 2018; Singh et al., 2018). The chemical structure of some specific bioactive constituents present in barley grains are depicted in Figure 3.3. The type and amount of these specific bioactive components present in barley are presented in Table 3.5.

Whole barley grains and other counterparts (bran, husk, and milling fractions) possess a number of bioactive phytochemicals that include total phenolic compounds (TPC), condensed tannin content (CTC) (Sharma and Gujral, 2011; Salar et al., 2017a) followed by flavonoids (Tamagawa et al., 1999), tocopherols (Panfili et al., 2003), alkylresorcinols (Ross et al., 2003). TPC in the barley cultivars has been reported to range from 1.95 to 2.20 mg GAE/g dwb (Lahouar et al., 2014), 2.09 to 2.94 mg GAE/dwb (Salar et al., 2017a), and 3.07 to 4.43 mg FAE/g (Sharma and Gujral, 2010). Madhujith and Shahidi (2009) evaluated barley and found TPC value in the range from 2.63 to 4.51 mg FAE/g. The composition of TPC in natural resources may vary depending on the growing conditions (Temperature, pH, soil type, moisture content in soil, and fertilizer consumption followed by harvesting stage and time) (Salar et al., 2015; Salar and Purewal, 2017). The amount of TPC may also vary as per the quantification methods followed by various workers.

Grains contain various flavanols which include myricetin (0.28 mg/g), catechin (0.017 mg/g), and procyanidin B3 (0.105 mg/g) (Holtekjolen et al., 2006). Sharma and Gujral (2011) found total flavonoids content (TFC) in

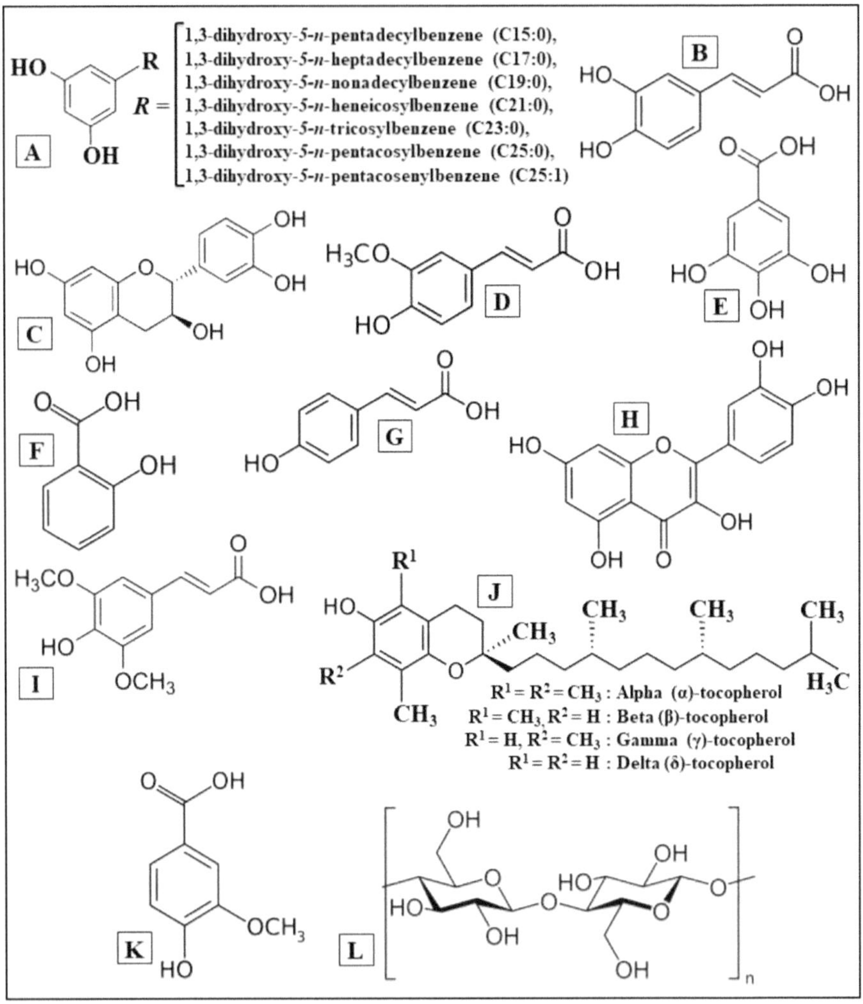

FIGURE 3.3 Chemical structure of some important bioactive components of barley grains. (A) Alkylresorcinols, (B) Caffeic acid, (C) Catechin, (D) Ferulic acid, (E) Gallic acid, (F) o-Hydroxybenzoic acid (salicylic acid), (G) p-Coumaric acid, (H) Quercetin, (I) Sinapinic acid, (J) Tocopherols, (K) Vanillic acid, and (L) β-Glucans.

barley in the range from 1.38 to 2.24 mg CE/g dwb. CTC in barley cultivars was observed to range from 0.40 to 0.99 mg CE/g dwb (Salar et al., 2017a) whereas Collins (1989) reported 0.74 mg/g tannins in barley. Presence of specific bioactive phytochemicals in barley was observed using HPLC and other specific techniques like HPTLC by various workers and their results

TABLE 3.5   Specific Bioactive Constituents Present in Barley

Bioactive Compounds	Reported Amounts	References
Total phenolic content	2.63–4.51 mg FAE/g	Madhujith and Shahidi (2009), Sharma and Gujral (2010)
Hydroxybenzoic		
o-Hydroxybenzoic acid	0.77 µg/g	Irakli et al. (2011)
Gallic acid	1.03–2.16 µg/g	Zhao et al. (2006), Irakli et al. (2011)
Protocatechuic acid	0.50 µg/g	Irakli et al. (2011)
Syringic acid	0.21–12.01 µg/g	Zielinski et al. (2001), Zhao et al. (2006), Irakli
Vanillic acid	0.63–3.57 µg/g	et al. (2011)
Hydroxycinnamic		
Caffeic acid	1.01–36 µg/g	Hernanz et al. (2001), Zhao et al. (2006), Quinde-Axtell and Baik (2006), Irakli et al. (2011)
Cinnamic acid	0.53 µg/g	Irakli et al. (2011)
Ferulic acid	6.24–567 µg/g	Zupfer et al. (1998), Hernanz et al. (2001), Zhao et al. (2006), Quinde-Axtell and Baik (2006), Dvorakova et al. (2008), Irakli et al. (2011)
p-Coumaric acid	0.97–29.7 µg/g	Zielinski et al. (2001), Quinde-Axtell and Baik (2006), Dvorakova et al. (2008), Irakli et al. (2011)
Sinapinic acid	1.60 µg/g	Irakli et al. (2011)
Tocols		
Alkylresorcinols	30–50 mg/kg	Garcia et al. (1997), Zarnowski et al. (2002), Mattila et al. (2005)
Carotenoid	15 µg/100 g	Choi et al. (2007)
Catechin	5.2–45.9 µg/g	Zhao et al. (2006), Holtekjolen et al. (2006), Dvorakova et al. (2008)
Kaempherol	12.7 µg/g	Holtekjolen et al. (2006)
Lignan	205 µg/g	Durazzo et al. (2009)
Myricetin	280 µg/g	Holtekjolen et al. (2006)
Procyanidin	105 µg/g	
Procyanidin	53.0 µg/g	
Prodelphindin	89.0 µg/g	
Prodelthinidin	102 µg/g	
Quercetin	17.4 µg/g	
Rutin	3.2 µg/g	
Tocopherol	25.1–75 mg/kg	Goupy et al. (1999), Panfili et al. (2003)
Tocotrienol	40 mg/kg	Panfili et al. (2003)

indicate the presence of gallic acid, ferulic acid, *o*-hydroxybenzoic acid, vanillic acid, syringic acid, *p*-coumaric acid followed by cinnamic and caffeic acid (Zupfer et al., 1998; Weidner et al., 1999; Hernanz et al., 2001; Quinde-Axtell and Baik, 2006; Zhao et al., 2006; Dvorakova et al., 2008; Lin et al., 2018).

3.4   EFFECT OF PROCESSING ON BIOACTIVE PHYTOCHEMICALS

Researchers/food scientists and food processing industries study bioactive phytochemicals and other important functional properties mainly due to health benefits associated with them. Despite the small size of grains, barley is a rich source of bioactive phytochemicals and potent antioxidants. Present scenario of research focused on conversion of bound bioactive phytochemicals of barley to free forms and changes in various functional properties after specific processing treatment. Effect of different processing methods on liberation of bioactive components from barley is presented in Table 3.6. Improvement/modulation in bioactive profile could be carried out using specific processing treatments like (1) fermentation, (2) malting, and (3) thermal processing.

3.4.1   FERMENTATION

In Asian and African regions, uses of cereal-grains-based food products are common. Barley could be a preferred source for food industries as the grains are rich in protein, fibers, and other important mineral nutrients. Grains contain a diversity of bioactive phytochemicals with radical scavenging potential. However, majority of these phytochemicals are present in bound form and for proper digestion in human intestinal region they should be present in free form. Conversion of bound bioactive phytochemicals into free form could be achieved by adopting solid state fermentation (SSF) process. SSF is widely used as a fruitful method for the production of functional fermented food for peoples and animal feed from a variety of natural substrates (Bhanja et al., 2009; Postemsky and Curvetto, 2015; Sandhu et al., 2016; Salar and Purewal, 2016; Salar et al., 2017b; Postemsky et al., 2017). As during SSF process the starter culture growing on steam cooked grains may produce specific enzymes like protease, α-amylase, pectinase, β-glucosidase, phytase, and xylanase. The activity of these enzymes during the SSF may results in breakdown of phytochemical complexes and releases

TABLE 3.6 Effect of Processing Methods on Liberation of Bioactive Phenolic Compounds from Barley

Substrate	Processing Type	Extraction Phase	Extraction Temperature	Extraction Time	Specific Bioactive Constituents	References
Barley cultivar Irina	Solvent extraction	Aqueous methanol (80.2%)	60.5 °C	38.3 min	Procyanidin dimer B, Procyanidin dimer C, Catechin, Prodelphinidin B, Catechin dihexoside, Caffeic acid, Coumaric acid, Quercetin, Ferulic acid	Gangopadhyay et al. (2016)
Barley husks (Ardhaoui Sfax, Ardhaoui Tataouine, Ardhaoui Medenine, Manel, Rihane, Konouz and Lemsi)	Acid hydrolysis Delignification Solvent extraction	H_2SO_4 (3%) NaOH (6.5%) Ethyl acetate	130 °C 25 °C	15 min 60 min 60 min	Gallic acid, Protocatechuic acid, Catechin, Syringic acid, p-coumaric acid, Naringin, Hyperoside (quercetin-3-ogalactoside), Rutin, 4,5-di-Ocaffeoyquinic acid, Naringenin, Cirsiliol, Apegenin, Sitosterol	Hajji et al. (2018)
Twenty-one hull-less and six hulled genotypes of barley	Solvent extraction Alkaline hydrolysis	(79.5% methanol, 19.5% Milli Q water and 1% formic acid) NaOH (2 mol/L)	Room temperature	12 h	β-Tocopherol, δ-Tocotrienol, 3,4-Dihydroxybenzoic acid, Vanillic acid, Syringic acid, Sinapinic acid, Syringaldehyde, Diferulic acid (decarboxylated form), Flavanols, p-Hydroxy-Benzoic acid, Syringic acid, Vanillic acid, Apigenin-6-C-arabinoside-8-Cglucoside	Martinez et al. (2018)
Whole kernel barley (Compass L1, Compass L2, Hindmarsh, LaTrobe, Westminster, Schooner and Gairdner)	Solvent extraction	Acetone, water and acetic acid solution (70:29.5:0.5 v/v/v)	25 °C	1 h	p-Coumaric acid isomer, Isoscoparin-2″-O-glucoside, Catechin dihexoside, Catechin-5-O-glucoside, Isoorientin-7-O-gentiobioside, Prodelpinidin B3, Prodelpinidin B, Procyanadin B2 and Apigenin 6-C-arabinoside 8-C-glucoside	Rao et al. (2018)

TABLE 3.6 *(Continued)*

Substrate	Processing Type	Extraction Phase	Extraction Temperature	Extraction Time	Specific Bioactive Constituents	References
Hulled barley cultivars (PL-172, PL-426, RD-2503, RD-2508, RD-2035, RD-2052, RD-2552, and DWR-28)	Sand roasting, microwave cooking and solvent extraction	Acidified methanol (HCl/ methanol/water, 1:80:10, v/v/v)	Room temperature	2 h	ND	Sharma and Gujral (2011)
Black highland barley	Solvent extraction	Chilled methanol (80%)	Room temperature	2 h	Ferulic acid, *p*-coumaric acid and catechin	Shen et al. (2015)
Colored barley	Solvent extraction	Methanol acidified with 1 N HCl (85:15; v/v)	Room temperature	18 min	Gallic acid, 3,4 Hydroxybenzoic acid, Chlorogenic acid, Caffeic acid, Syringic acid, *p*-coumaric acid, Ferulic acid, Cinnamic acid, Salicylic acid	Suriano et al. (2018)
Dehulled highland barley (*Zangqing 25* (ZQ25), *Zangqing 320* (ZQ320), *Changheiqingke* (CHQK) and *Dulihuang* (BQ))	Solvent extraction	Chilled acetone (80%) and distilled water	45 °C	–	Protocatechuic acid, Chlorogenic acid, Catechin, Caffeic acid, *p*-Coumaric acid, Ferulic acid	Zhu et al. (2015)
Barley malt rootlet	Steaming, Roasting, Enzyme Hydrolysis Solvent extraction	Acetone (80%)	220 °C 60 °C 50 °C 40 °C	120 s 3 min 120 min 1 h	ND	Budaraju et al. (2018)

TABLE 3.6 *(Continued)*

Substrate	Processing Type	Extraction Phase	Extraction Temperature	Extraction Time	Specific Bioactive Constituents	References
Barley grains	Solvent extraction Alkaline hydrolysis Acid hydrolysis	70% acetone/ water NaOH (4 M) Hydrochloric acid (1 M)	25 °C 45 °C	25 min 90 min	Gallic acid, Protocatechuic acid, Catechin, p-hydroxybenzoic acid, Gentisic acid, Vanillic acid, Caffeic acid, Epicatechin, Syringic acid, p-coumaric acid, Vanillin, Sinapinic acid, Ferulic acid, Taxifolin, Myricetin, Quercetin, Apigenin, Kaempferol	Arigo et al. (2018)

ND: Not detected. (Reprinted with permission from Singh et al., 2003. © John Wiley & Sons.)

them in their free form. Perhaps this may be the reason for the increment in bioactive phytochemicals after SSF. The steps during SSF include (Figure 3.4). Sandhu et al. (2016) reported that SSF positively affects the bioactive profile of barley grains. They observed the significant changes in bioactive compounds during the 5th day of fermentation with *Aspergillus awamori* (MTCC-548). In their study six different cultivars (cv.) of barley (PL-172, DWR-52, BH-393, BH-932, BH-902, and BH-885) were used for microbial transformation of bioactive constituents. SSF results in 1.37–1.78 fold increase in phenolic compounds. Percent increase in phenolic compounds after fermentation period was 37.51%–78.40% with maximum modulation in cv. PL-172 and minimal in BH-902. The results from their study support the use of SSF as an effective tool for the modulation of bioactive profile of barley grains. In addition to cereal grains, sometimes microorganisms themselves act as a source of potent antioxidants and during the fermentation of grains, the starter culture just adds the specific bioactive constituents to the fermented koji. Salar et al. (2017c) reported the presence of specific mycochemicals [coumarins, flavonoids, flavonon, reducing sugars, tannins, and phenolic compounds (*p*-coumaric acid, gallic acid, cinnamic acid, and ascorbic acid)] with potent antioxidant properties in *A. awamori* (MTCC-548) extracts.

3.4.2 MALTING OF BARLEY

Modulation of bioactive profile and physical characteristics of barley could be achieved in three different stages, they are: (1) steeping, (2) germination, and (3) kilning.

3.4.2.1 STEEPING

During the steeping process most of the soluble bioactive phytochemicals that are present in outer layer of whole grain barley come out through leaching.

3.4.2.2 GERMINATION

Germination of barley grains in the presence of specific moisture and dark conditions may results in activation of some specific kind of enzymes. The enzymatic activities (amylases and proteases) during the germination period

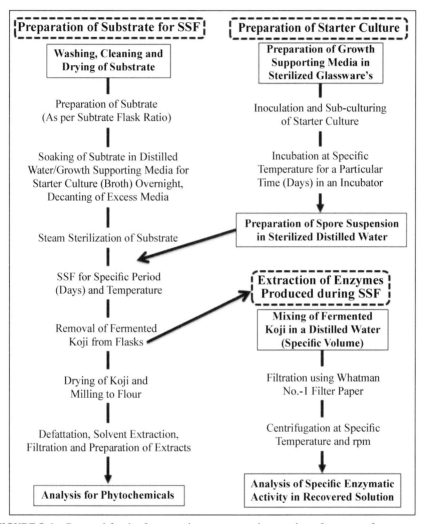

FIGURE 3.4 Protocol for the fermentation process and extraction of enzymes from fermented products.

result in hydrolysis of specific components present in endosperm. Conversion of insoluble complex of bioactive components into smaller simplest form is the major changes observed during germination which are actually required for the proper growth of seedlings. Germinated barley grains are useful in bakery and brewing and distillery industries as the kernels became soft and sweet in taste. Morphological and anatomical changes in barley grains up to specific period of time also occur during germination. Sharma and Gujral (2010) reported the effect of germination period on antioxidant and polyphenol oxidase activity (PPOA) of barley and its fractions. They observed that germination significantly improves the bioactive constituents of whole grain barley (12 h, 38.77%); bran (24 h, 23.89%) and refined flour (12 h, 36.16%) however, PPOA upon germination to 12 h results in initial decrease by 13%–59% for whole grain flour, 1.9%–59% for bran and 7%–46% for refined flour. Gallegos-Infante et al. (2010) studied the effect of germination period (24 h) on phenolic compounds among Mexican barley and observed a sharp decrease in phenolic content after germination.

3.4.2.3   KILNING

Kilning results in thermal modifications in germinated barley grains which impart specific flavor and induce specific coloration in finished malt and fractions.

3.4.3   EFFECT OF THERMAL PROCESSING

Baba et al. (2016) reported the effect of microwave roasting on antioxidant and anticancerous properties of extracts prepared from barley flour. They observed that microwave roasting significantly affects the bioactive phytochemicals of barley as confirmed by the improvement in DPPH [2,2-diphenyl-1-picrylhydrazyl] radical scavenging potential (DPPHRSP) and reducing power activity (RPA). A sharp decrease in TPC was observed among extracts prepared from roasted barley flour. TPC in extracts prepared in methanol, ethanol, and water from roasted barley flour decreased by 34%–121%. Percent (%) increase in DPPHRSP and RPA among extracts after microwave roasting was methanol (13%) > ethanol (8%) > water (6%) followed by 21.43% increase in ethanol followed by 21.37% in methanolic extracts and 15.23% in extracts prepared in water. Effect of sand roasting and microwave cooking on antioxidant properties of barley was observed by Sharma and Gujral (2011). Thermal processing results in decrease in TPC by 8.5%–49.6% and TFC by 24.5%–53.2% followed by increase in RPA and metal chelating activity by 77.5% and 79%, respectively.

3.4.4   EFFECT OF EXTRACTION CONDITIONS

Optimization and modeling of extraction conditions [extractions phase (phase type and concentration) temperature, duration of time] for the recovery of bioactive phytochemicals from various natural resources have been reported by many workers. Over the last few years, there has been a significant improvement in understanding the key factors that are responsible for leaching out of bioactive components from the experimental samples. Many reports are available on barley β-glucan which described different extraction conditions with significant results. Some of those studies are tabulated in Table 3.7, which will help to scientist, academia, and researchers in their further study and research.

For optimization of extraction parameters, an important statistical software response surface methodology (RSM) and Design Expert has been used by researchers (Liyana-Pathirana and Shahidi, 2005; Cheok et al., 2012; Nawaz et al., 2018). Statistical software provides specific tools that are quite helpful in emphasizing the relationship between various experimental variables. Central composite design is most commonly employed design to maximize the response (Silva et al., 2007; Banik and Pandey, 2008; Salar et al., 2016). RSM generated optimized conditions for the extraction of bioactive phytochemicals from experimental samples may vary depending on the type of natural resources and their specific parts selected the optimization. It also depends on the type of phytochemicals present in the experimental samples which finally determines the selection of appropriate extraction (Liyana-Pathirana and Shahidi, 2005; Salar and Purewal, 2017). RSM generated optimized conditions for various natural experimental samples were reported in many scientific reports; solid/liquid ratio (40%, 20.17 min) (Hayta and Iscimen, 2017); for purple corn (germination conditions 23 °C, 63 h) (Paucar-Menacho et al., 2017b); Kiwicha (*Amaranthus candatus*) (26 °C, 63 h) (Paucar-Menacho et al., 2017a); red rice (*Oryzae sativa*) (extraction time 10 min, 40 °C, phase concentration methanol 50%, solvent/solid ratio 2.5:1) (Setyaningsih et al., 2016); pearl millet (44.5 °C, ethanol 50%) (Salar et al., 2016), and microwave-assisted solvent extraction in rice (185 °C, 20 min, 100% MeOH, solvent/sample ratio 10:1) (Setyaningsih et al., 2015). RSM generated conditions are quite useful as it may help the workers in understanding various prospects of bioactive phytochemicals like antimicrobial potential, anticancerous, antioxidant, DNA damage protection, and *in vitro* cytotoxicity. RSM software is important from industrial point of view as it is helpful for reduction in use of noneffective organic solvents, provides exact extraction temperature ranges and timing as longer duration of extraction and heat generated in response to temperature results in hydrolytic degradation of bioactive phytochemical in natural resources (Odabas and Koca, 2016).

TABLE 3.7 Effect of Extraction Conditions on Barley β-Glucan

Study Report on Barley β-Glucan	Substrate	Extraction Methods	Extraction Conditions			
			Extraction Phase	Extraction Temperature (in °C)	Extraction Time	Extraction Yields (in %)
De Arcangelis et al. (2019)	Barley flour	Sequential extraction with water and sodium hydroxide (NaOH)	Water-extractable NaOH-extractable (NaE) Residual (Res)	Room temperature	17 h	51.7–82.2
Du et al. (2014)	Hull-less barley	Accelerated solvent extraction, ultrasound-assisted extraction, microwave-assisted extraction, and reflux extraction	Anhydrous ethanol	70	9 min	16.39
Limberger-Bayer et al. (2014)	Barley flour	Water extraction	Aqueous water with calcium carbonate (Ca_2CO_3) [(20%, p/v) at pH 7.56] suspended in ethanol	45.5	1.5 h	53.38
Sharma and Gujral (2013)	Hull-less barley	Pilot plant extraction	Sodium hydroxide (NaOH) and ethanol (80%) solvent	–	30 min	7.7–15.4
Zheng et al. (2011)	Hull-less barley	–	Aqueous sodium carbonate (20%) at pH 10	50	60 min	4.96–7.62
Ahmad et al. (2009)	Barley	Hot water extraction	–	–	90 min	5.4
Burkus and Temelli (2005)	Waxy barley	Alkali extraction	Aqueous ethanol at pH 9.4	53–55	–	71.1
Irakli et al. (2004)	Greek barley cultivars	Water extraction	Aqueous ethanol (95%, v/v)	85	2 h	5.93
Temelli (1997)	Barley	Water extraction	Aqueous water with sodium carbonate (Na_2CO_3) (20%, w/v) at pH of 7–10	40–55	30 min	5.54

TABLE 3.7 (Continued)

Study Report on Barley β-Glucan	Substrate	Extraction Methods	Extraction Conditions			
			Extraction Phase	Extraction Temperature (in °C)	Extraction Time	Extraction Yields (in %)
Saulnier et al. (1994)	Barley	Sequential treatment	Aqueous water	40	30 min	2.5
			Aqueous water with heat-resistant alpha-amylase	90	90 min	
			Aqueous water with 1 M sodium hydroxide (NaOH)	Room temperature	16 h	
Bhatty (1992)	Barley, barley bran, and flour	Dry-milled, water extract and freeze-dried	Aqueous ethanol (80%)	–	30 min	3.9–15.4
Fleming and Kawakami (1977)	Barley	Water extraction	Aqueous ethanol (80%)	40 and 100	1 h	0.71–7.24

(Reprinted with permission from Leguizamón et al., 2009. © John Wiley & Sons.)

3.5   VALUE-ADDED FOOD PRODUCTS OF BARLEY AND HUMAN HEALTH

Flour from barley grains are currently being used for the production of various gluten free fortified and other functional food products (Figure 3.5). As the products are rich source of potent antioxidants and they could be used as breakfast diet to sustain healthy life style. β-Glucan a specific type of soluble fiber present in barley grains makes them perfect source of health benefits (Table 3.8). Scientific reports suggest that β-glucan present in barley grains could lower low-density lipoproteins (LDL) cholesterol in living organisms. Consumption of even minor amount (3–5 g) of barley and products based on barley flour could lower down the LDL by 8%–10% (Maillard et al., 1996; Goupy et al., 1999). Sahu et al. (2015) prepared biscuits from normal barley flour and roasted barley and they observed that biscuits prepared from normal flour contains crude protein (4.52%), crude fiber (0.88%) followed by ash (1.52%), whereas biscuits prepared from roasted barley flour showed the presence of crude protein (3.12%), crude fiber (0.62%), and ash (1.31%). Beer is one of the alcoholic beverages that are most frequently used by people all around the world. Beer is a chemically complex product with combinations of mineral nutrients and potent antioxidants. Moura-Nunes et al. (2016) describe the phenolic profile of Brazilian beer for modeling antioxidant capacity. Food products designed from barley flour could be used in the management of type-2 diabetes and LDL. Being a rich source of niacin (a Vitamin B complex), products from barley could be used as natural edible vaccine to combat cardiovascular risk factors and minimize the level of bad lipoproteins.

3.6   FUTURE PROSPECTS

Increasing demand of functional food is a greater challenge to agricultural producers and food sector. Since the last 10 years (2008–2018), production of cereal grains has registered a rising trend which makes the pharmacological and food processing industries an important sector for human welfare. Worldwide priority is given to the research based on relationship of bioactive phytochemicals with the reduction of age related issues and other cardiovascular disorders. However, there is a need of more scientific and deep studies that can elaborate the use of important cereal grains like barley, pearl millet, and wheat for the production of edible vaccines from them. The identification of desirable features, role of extraction parameters, environmental

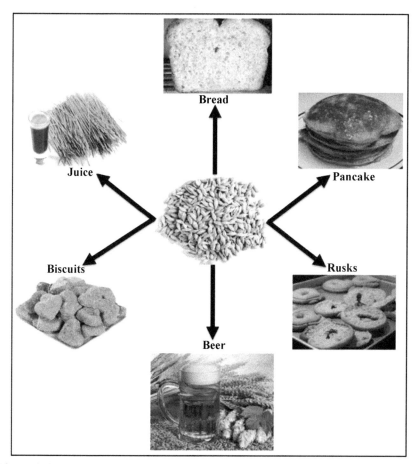

FIGURE 3.5 Functional and fortified food products prepared from barley flour.

conditions during the growth, processing parameters to evaluate various cultivars of barley; the assessment of cultivar and their interactions during oxidative stress could be a topic of greater concern for growing human race.

In addition, crops growing in specific conditions should be in adaptable with environmental conditions and agroclimatic approaches that lead a sharp increase in their production. More marketing schemes and training camps for farmers are required for the global transformation of knowledge and health benefits based on cereal grains. Lack of sufficient information about processing and handling of raw food material is a major factor responsible for the present gap between cereal grains and natural medicines production based on them. Taking into account the present scenario of cereal grains and

TABLE 3.8 Summary of Some Studies on Barley β-Glucan and Their Effect on Human Health and Disease

Years	Authors	Study Report	Does of β-Glucan	Value-Added Barley Products with β-Glucan	Findings/Remarks	Authors
1989	Newman and co-workers	Hypocholesterolemic effect on healthy men	9.6% per day	Whole-grain barley flour products like bars, bread, muffins, etc.	TC and LDLC reduction with 12% and 14%, respectively	Newman et al. (1989)
1991	McIntosh and co-workers	Plasma cholesterol concentrations in hypercholesterolemic men	8 g/day	Dietenriched with barley foods, namely, biscuits, flakes, muesli, spaghetti, and bran in bread	Reduction in TC and LDLC in moderately cholesterolemic men	McIntosh et al. (1991)
1994	Lupton and co-workers	Cholesterol-lowering effect on men and women	20 g/day	Barley bran flour in supplement meals	With 6.5% LDLC reduction.	Lupton et al. (1994)
1995	Lia and co-workers	Cholesterol excretion in ileostomy (men and women) subjects	12.4 g/day	Buns	Cholesterol excretion noted with significant increase	Lia et al. (1995)
1996	Ikegami and co-workers	Hypercholesterolemic and normolipemic in men and women	6.1 g/day	Mixture of cooked barley and rice	Significant decrease in cholesterol was noted for hypercholesterolemic subjects while there was no effect on normolipemic subjects	Ikegami et al. (1996)
1999	Bourdon and co-workers	Postprandial lipid, glucose, insulin, and cholecystokinin responses in healthy normolipemic men	5 g/day	Barley-enriched pasta	In healthy men, induced a significant reduction in insulinemia. Decrease in TC, change in insulin but not glucose response	Bourdon et al. (1999)

TABLE 3.8 (*Continued*)

Years	Authors	Study Report	Dose of β-Glucan	Value-Added Barley Products with β-Glucan	Findings/Remarks	Authors
2002	Cavallero and co-workers	Human glycemic response	0.1%–6.3% per day	Breads	A linear dose-dependent decrease in glycemic responses	Cavallero et al. (2002)
2003	Keogh and co-workers	CVD risk factors in mildly hypercholesterolemic men population	9.9 g/day	Snacks and food products like bread, cakes, muffins, or savory dishes	TC or LDLC was noted with no significant reduction and in fasting or postprandial glucose was noted with no significant change in mildly hypercholesterolemic men	Keogh et al. (2003)
	Li and co-workers	Glucose tolerance, lipid metabolism, and bowel function in women	8.9 g/day	Mixture of barley whole-grain diet added with cooked rice (7:3 ratio)	Significant reductions in TC and LDLC (with 14.5% and 21%, respectively) and was not seen in glucose tolerance	Li et al. (2003)
2004	Behall and co-workers	Lipids level in moderately hypercholesterolemic people	0.3, 3, or 6 g/day	Barley diets like pancakes, bars, hot cereal, etc.	Significant reduction in both TC (14%, 17%, and 17%) and LDL (17%, 17%, and 24%) cholesterol concentrations, respectively. This barley bioactive component can reduce CVD risk factors	Behall et al. (2004a)
		Lipids in mildly hypercholesterolemic men and women	3 or 6 g/day	Barley diets like pancakes, bars, hot cereal, etc.	Decrease in TC and LDLC, the higher intake in particular, more so in postmenopausal women and men	Behall et al. (2004b)
2005	Biorklund and co-workers	Serum lipoproteins and postprandial glucose and insulin concentrations	5 or 10 g/day	Beverages	Decrease in TC and LDLC, but not significant, possibly because of low molecular weight	Biorklund et al. (2005)

TABLE 3.8 *(Continued)*

Years	Authors	Study Report	Does of β-Glucan	Value-Added Barley Products with β-Glucan	Findings/Remarks	Authors
2006	Aman P.	Mildly hypercholesterolemic men and women	3 g/day	Activated barley in packages	LDLC decreased with 5%	Aman (2006)
	Dongowski and co-workers	Physiological effects on mildly hypercholesterolemic humans	7.2 g/day	Extruded whole-grain barley meal	Decreased LDLC with 6%	Dongowski et al. (2006)
2007	Hinata and co-workers	Diabetic (type 2) male prisoners in Fukushima Prison of Japan	18.7 g/day	Mixture of cooked rice and barley with 7:3 ratio	Reduction in TC (9.7%) and dramatically reduction in levels of fasting plasma glucose	Hinata et al. (2007)
	Keenan and co-workers	Blood lipids and other CVD risk factors in hypercholesterolemic men and women population	3 or 5 g/day	Concentrate with β-glucan in juice beverage and cereal	Reduction by 9%15% in LDLC	Keenan et al. (2007)
2008	Shimizu and co-workers	Serum cholesterol concentrations and visceral fat in Japanese men	7 g/day	Pearl barley and rice with 1:1 ratio	Significantly reduction in serum concentrations of TC and LDLC	Shimizu et al. (2008)
2009	Talati and co-workers	Serum lipids	3–10 g/day	Barley	Had significant reductions in TC, LDLC, and triglycerides	Talati et al. (2009)
	Vitaglione and co-workers	Energy intake and modifies plasma ghrelin and peptide YY concentrations	3% per day	β-Glucan-enriched bread	Significant reduction in energy intake and hunger; and increase in fullness and satiety	Vitaglione et al. (2009)
2010	Abumweis and co-workers	Meta-analyses of randomized clinical trials on lipid-lowering capacity	3–10 g/day	Barley	Had no effect on HDLC levels with different dietary backgrounds but significantly lowered TC and LDLC	Abumweis et al. (2010)
	Vitaglione and co-workers	Satiating effect	5.2% per day	Barley β-glucan enriched biscuits	Significantly suppressed appetite ratings in healthy adolescents	Vitaglione et al. (2010)

CVD: cardiovascular disease, HDLC: HDL (high-density lipoproteins) cholesterol, LDLC: LDL (low-density lipoproteins) cholesterol, TC: total cholesterol.

their processing suggest identification of key areas for future research and technology transfer from laboratory to common man.

3.7 CONCLUSIONS

Barley is a low cost, easily available staple food that is consumed for various health benefits in developing as well as developed countries. The main purpose of processing is the production of high quality functional food products for the welfare of human beings. In addition to improvement in texture and taste; shelf life processing is also required to maintain constant supply of products throughout the year. Processing results in season independent supply of food products and beverages that are based on raw barley grains. Among various processing adapted for cereal grains, SSF proved to be fruitful method as within a short span the technique results in tremendous improvements in texture, taste, and bioactive phytochemicals. SSF-based food products are thermally stable as after thermal processing the amount of specific phytochemicals remains higher as compared to untreated raw materials.

KEYWORDS

- **antioxidants**
- **barley**
- **extraction**
- **fermentation**
- **fortified food**
- **free radicals**
- **functional food**
- **germination**
- **kilning**
- **nutraceuticals**
- **oxidative stress**
- **phytochemicals**
- **roasting**
- **self-pollinating**

REFERENCES

Abumweis, S. S.; Jew, S. and Ames, N. P. β-Glucan from barley and its lipid-lowering capacity: a meta-analysis of randomized, controlled trials. *European J Clin Nutr*, **2010**, *64*(12), 1472–1480.

Ahmad, A.; Anjum, F. M.; Zahoor, T.; Nawaz, H. and Din, A. Physicochemical and functional properties of barley β-glucan as affected by different extraction procedures. *Int J Food Sci Techol*, **2009**, *44*, 181–187.

Aman, P. Cholesterol-lowering effects of barley dietary fiber in humans: scientific support for a generic health claim. *Scand J Food Nutr*, **2006**, *50*, 173–176.

Andersson, A. A. M.; Armö, E.; Grangeon, E.; Fredriksson, H.; Andersson, R. and Åman, P. Molecular weight and structure units of β-glucan in dough and bread made of hull-less barley milling fractions. *J Cereal Sci*, **2004**, *40*, 195–204.

Arigo, A.; Cesla, P.; Silarova, P.; Calabro, M. L. and Ceslova, L. Development of extraction method for characterization of free and bonded polyphenols in barley (*Hordeum vulgare* L.) grown in Czech Republic using liquid chromatography-tandem mass spectrometry. *Food Chem*, **2018**, *245*, 829–837.

Baba, W. N.; Rashid, I.; Shah, A.; Ahmad, M.; Gani, A.; Masoodi, F. A.; Wani, I. A. and Wani, S. M. Effect of microwave roasting on antioxidant and anticancerous activities of barley flour. *J Saudi Soc Agric Sci*, **2016**, *15*, 12–19.

Banik, R. M.; Pandey, D. K. Optimizing conditions for oleanolic acid extraction from *Lantana camara* roots using response surface methodology. *Indus Crop Prod*, **2008**, *27*, 241–248.

Bartolome, B.; Gomez-Cordoves, C. Barley spent grain: release of hydroxycinnamic acids (ferulic and *p*-coumaric acids) by commercial enzyme preparations. *J Sci Food Agric*, **1999**, *79*, 435–439.

Behall, K. M.; Scholfield, D. J. and Hallfrisch, J. Diets containing barley significantly reduce lipids in mildly hypercholesterolemic men and women. *Am J Clin Nutr*, **2004a**, *80*(5), 1185–1193.

Behall, K. M.; Scholfield, D. J. and Hallfrisch, J. Lipids significantly reduced by diets containing barley in moderately hypercholesterolemic men. *J Am Coll Nutr*, **2004b**, *23*(1), 55–62.

Bhanja, T.; Kumari, A. and Banerjee, R. Enrichment of phenolics and free radical scavenging property of wheat koji prepared with two filamentous fungi. *Bioresour Technol*, **2009**, *100*, 2861–2866.

Bhatty, R. S. Beta-glucan content and viscosities of barleys and their roller-milled flour and bran products. *Cereal Chem*, **1992**, *69*, 469–471.

Biorklund, M.; van Rees, A.; Mensink, R. P. and Onning, G. Changes in serum lipids and postprandial glucose and insulin concentrations after consumption of beverages with β-glucans from oats or barley: a randomised dose-controlled trial. *Eur J Clin Nutr*, **2005**, *59*(11), 1272–1281.

Bordiga, M.; Locatelli, M.; Travaglia, F.; Arlorio, M.; Reyneri, A.; Blandino, M. and Coisson, J. D. Alkylresorcinol content in whole grains and pearled fractions of wheat and barley. *J Cereal Sci*, **2016**, *70*, 38–46

Bourdon, I.; Yokoyama, W.; Davis P.; Hudson, C.; Backus, R.; Richter, D.; Knuckles, B. and Schneeman, B. O. Postprandial lipid, glucose, insulin, and cholecystokinin responses in men fed barley pasta enriched with β-glucan. *Am J Clin Nutr*, **1999**, *69*(1), 55–63.

Budaraju, S.; Mallikarjunan, K.; Annor, G.; Schoenfuss, T. and Raun, R. Effect of pre-treatments on the antioxidant potential of phenolic extracts from barley malt rootlets. *Food Chem*, **2018**, *266*, 31–37.

Burkus, Z.; Temelli, F. Rheological properties of barley β-glucan. *Carbohydr Polym*, **2005**, *59*, 459–465.

Carvalho, D. O.; Curto, A. F. and Guido, L. F. Determination of phenolic content in different barley varieties and corresponding malts by liquid chromatography-diode array detection-electrospray ionization tandem mass spectrometry. *Antioxidants*, **2015**, *4*, 563–576.

Cavallero, A.; Empilli, S.; Brighenti, F. and Stanca, A. M. High (1→3, 1→4)-β-glucan barley fractions in bread making and their effects on human glycemic response. *J Cereal Sci*, **2002**, *36*(1), 59–66.

Cheok, C. Y.; Chin, N. L.; Yusof, A. Y.; Talib, R. A. and Law, C. L. Optimization of total phenolic content extracted from *Garcinia mangostana* Linn. Hull using response surface methodology versus artificial neural network. *Indus Crop Prod*, **2012**, *40*, 247–253.

Choi, S.; Lee, S.; Kim, E.; Oh, J.; Yoon, K.; Parris, N.; Hicks, K. and Moreau, R. Antioxidant and antimelanogenic activities of polyamine conjugates from corn bran and related hydroxycinnamic acids. *J Agric Food Chem*, **2007**, 55, 3920–3925.

Collins, F. Oat phenolics: Avenanthramides, novel substituted N-cinnamoylanthranilate alkaloids from oat groats and hulls. *J Agric Food Chem*, **1989**, *37*, 60–66.

De Arcangelis, E.; Djurle, S.; Andersson, A. A. M.; Marconi, E.; Messia, M. C. and Andersson, R. Structure analysis of β-glucan in barley and effects of wheat β-glucanase. *J Cereal Sci*, **2019**, *85*, 175–181.

Dhull, S. B.; Kaur, P. and Purewal, S. S. Phytochemical analysis, phenolic compounds, condensed tannin content and antioxidant potential in Marwa (*Origanum majorana*) seed extracts. *Resour Effic Technol*, **2016**, *2*, 168–174.

Dongowski, G.; Huth, M. and Gebhardt, E. Physiological effects of a barley extrudate on humans. *Dtsch Lebensmitt Rundsch*, **2006**, *102*, 141–149.

Du, B.; Zhu, F. M. and Xu, B. J. β-Glucan extraction from bran of hull-less barley by accelerated solvent extraction combined with response surface methodology. *J Cereal Sci*, **2014**, *59*, 95–100.

Durazzo, A.; Azzini, E.; Raguzzini, A.; Maiani, G.; Finocchiaro, F.; Ferrari, B.; Gianinetti, A. and Carcea, M. Influence of processing on the lignans content of cereal based foods. *Tecnica Molitoria Int*, **2009**, *60*, 163–173.

Dvorakova, M.; Douanier, M.; Jurkova, M.; Kellner, V. and Dostalek, P. Comparison of antioxidant activity of barley (*Hordeum vulgare* L.) and malt extracts with the content of free phenolic compounds measured by high performance liquid chromatography coupled with Coul Array detector. *J Inst Brew*, **2008**, *114*, 150–159.

Falk, J.; Krahnstöver, A.; van der Kooij, T. A. W.; Schlensog, M.; Krupinska, K. Tocopherol and tocotrienol accumulation during development of caryopses from barley (*Hordeum vulgare* L.). *Phytochem*, **2004**, *65*, 2977–2985.

FAOUN (Food and Agriculture Organization of United Nation) (2016) Crops: FAOSTAT. Food and Agriculture Organization of United Nation, Rome, Italy. Accessed on 3 January 2018. URL: http://www.fao.org/faostat/en/#data/QC.

Fleming, M. and Kawakami, K. Studies of the fine structure of β-D glucans of barley extracted at different temperatures. *Carbohydr Res*, **1977**, *57*, 15–23.

Gallegos-Infante, J. A.; Rocha-Guzman, N. E.; Gonzalez-Laredo, R. F. and Pulido-Alonso, J. Effect of processing on the antioxidant properties of extracts from Mexican barley (*Hordeum vulgare*) cultivar. *Food Chem*, **2010**, *119*, 903–906.

Gangopadhyay, N.; Rai, D. K.; Brunton, N. P.; Gallagher, E. and Hossain, M. B. Antioxidant-guided isolation and mass spectrometric identification of the major polyphenols in barley (*Hordeum vulgare*) grain. *Food Chem*, **2016**, *210*, 212–220.

Gani, A.; Wani, S. M.; Masoodi, F. A. and Hameed, G. Whole-grain cereal bioactive compounds and their health benefits: a review. *J Food Process Tech*, **2012**, *3*(3), 1–10.

Garcia, S.; Garcia, C.; Heinzen, H. and Moyna, P. Chemical basis of the resistance of barley seeds to pathogenic fungi. *Phytochem*, **1997**, *44*, 415–418.

Goupy, P.; Hugues, M.; Boivin, P. and Amiot, M. J. Antioxidant composition and activity of barley (*Hordeum vulgare*) and malt extracts and of isolated phenolic compounds. *J Sci Food Agric*, **1999**, *79*, 1625–1634.

Hajji, T.; Mansouri, S.; Vecino-Bello, X.; Cruz-Freire, J. M.; Rezgui, S. and Ferchichi, A. Identification and characterization of phenolic compounds extracted from barley husks by LC-MS and antioxidant activity in vitro. *J Cereal Sci*, **2018**, *81*, 83–90.

Hayta, M.; Iscimen, E. M. Optimization of ultrasound-assisted antioxidant compounds extraction from germinated chickpea using response surface methodology. *LWT Food Sci Technol*, **2017**, *77*, 208–216.

Hernanz, D.; Nunez, V.; Sancho, A. I.; Faulds, C. B.; Williamson, G.; Bartolome, B. and Gomez-Cordove, C. Hydrocinnamic acids and ferulic acid dehydrodimers in barley and processed barley. *J Agric Food Chem*, **2001**, *49*, 4884–4888.

Hinata, M.; Ono, M.; Midorikawa, S. and Nakanishi, K. Metabolic improvement of male prisoners with type 2 diabetes in Fukushima Prison, Japan. *Diabetes Res Clin Pract*, **2007**, *77*, 327–332.

Holtekjolen, A. K.; Kinitz, C. and Knutsen, S. H. Flavanol and bound phenolic acid contents in different barley varieties. *J Agric Food Chem*, **2006**, *54*, 2253–2260.

Ikegami, S.; Tomita, M.; Honda, S.; Yamaguchi, M.; Mizukawa, R.; Suzuki, Y.; Ishii, K.; Ohsawa, S.; Kiyooka, N.; Higuchi, M. and Kobayashi, S. Effect of boiled barley-rice-feeding in hypercholesterolemic and normolipemic subjects. *Plant Foods Hum Nutr*, **1996**, *49*, 317–328.

Irakli, M.; Biliaderis, C. G.; Izydorczyk, M. S. and Papadoyannis, I. N. Isolation, structural features and rheological properties of water-extractable β-glucans from different Greek barley cultivars. *J Sci Food Agric*, **2004**, *84*, 1170–1178.

Irakli, M. N.; Victoria, F.; Samanidou, V. F.; Biliaderis, C. G. and Papadoyannis, I. N. Development and validation of an HPLC-method for determination of free and bound phenolic acids in cereals after solid-phase extraction. *Food Chem*, **2011**, *134*, 1624–1632.

Izydorczyk, M. S.; Dextor, J. E. Barley β-glucans and arabinoxylans: molecular structure, physicochemical properties, and uses in food products a review. *Food Res Int*, **2008**, 41, 850–868.

Izydorczyk, M. S.; Storsley, J. M.; Labossiere, D.; Macgregor, A. W. and Rossnagel, B. Variation in total and soluble β-glucan content in hulless barley: Effects of thermal, physical and enzymatic treatments. *J Agric Food Chem*, **2000**, *48*, 982–989.

Jende-Strid, B. Phenolic acids in grains of wild-type barley and proanthocyanidin-free mutants. *Cadsberg Res Commun*, **1985**, *50*, 1–14.

Kapri, M.; Verma, D. K.; Ajesh Kumar, V.; Billoria, S.; Mahato, D. K.; Yadav, B. S. and Srivastav, P. P. Modified pearl millet starch: a review on chemical modification, characterization, and functional properties. In: *Goyal, M. R. and Verma, D. K. (Eds.), Engineering Interventions in Agricultural Processing.* Volume 8, as part of book series on Innovations in Agricultural and Biological Engineering, Apple Academic Press, USA, 2017, pages 191–226.

Kaur, P.; Dhull, S. B.; Sandhu, K. S.; Salar, R. K. and Purewal, S. S. Tulsi (*Ocimum tenuiflorum*) seeds: in vitro DNA damage protection, bioactive compounds and antioxidant potential. *Food Measure,* **2018**, *12,* 1530–1538.

Kaur, P.; Purewal, S. S.; Sandhu, K. S.; Kaur, M.; Salar, R. K. Millets: a cereal grain with potent antioxidants and health benefits. *Food Measure,* **2018**, *13,* 793–806.

Keenan, J. M.; Goulson, M.; Shamliyan, T.; Knutson, N.; Kolberg, L. and Curry, L. The effects of concentrated barley β-glucan on blood lipids and other CVD risk factors in a population of hypercholesterolemic men and women. *British J Nutr,* **2007**, *97,* 1162–1168.

Keogh, G. F.; Cooper, G. J. S.; Mulvey, T. B.; McArdle, B. H.; Coles, G. D.; Monro, J. A. and Poppitt, S. D. Randomized controlled crossover study of the effect of a highly β-glucan-enriched barley on cardiovascular disease risk factors in mildly hypercholesterolemic men. *Am J Clin Nutr,* **2003**, *78,* 711–718.

Klausen, K.; Mortensen, A. G.; Laursen, B.; Haselmann, K. F.; Jespersen, B. M. and Fomsgaard, I. S. Phenolic compounds in different barley varieties: identification by tandem mass spectrometry (QStar) and NMR; quantification by liquid chromatography triple quadrupole-linear ion trap mass spectrometry (Q-Trap). *Nat Prod Commun,* **2010**, *5*(3), 407–414.

Lachman, J.; Hejtmánková, A.; Orsák, M.; Popov, M. and Martinek, P. Tocotrienols and tocopherols in colored-grain wheat, tritordeum and barley. *Food Chem,* **2018**, *240*(1), 725–735.

Lahouar, L.; Arem, A. E.; Ghrairi, F.; Chahdoura, H.; Salem, H. B.; Felah, M. E. and Achour, L. Phytochemical content and antioxidant properties of diverse varieties of whole barley (*Hordeum vulgare* L.) grown in Tunisia. *Food Chem,* **2014**, *145,* 578–583.

Li, J.; Kaneko, T.; Qin, L. Q.; Wang, J. and Wang, Y. Effects of barley intake on glucose tolerance, lipid metabolism, and bowel function in women. *Nutrition,* **2003**, *19,* 926–929.

Lia, A.; Hallmans, G.; Sandberg, A. S.; Sundberg, B.; Aman, P. and Andersson, H. Oat β-glucan increases bile acid excretion and a fiber-rich barley fraction increases cholesterol excretion in ileostomy subjects. *Am J Clin Nutr,* **1995**, *62,* 1245–1251.

Limberger-Bayer, V. M.; de Francisco, D.; Chan, A.; Oro, T.; Ogliari, P. J. and Barreto, P. L. M. Barley β-glucans extraction and partial characterization. *Food Chem,* **2014**, *154,* 84–89.

Lin, S.; Guo, H.; Gong, J. D.; Lu, M.; Lu, M. Y.; Wang, L.; Zhang, Q.; Qin, W. and Wu, D. T. Phenolic profiles, β-glucan contents, and antioxidant capacities of colored Qingke (Tibetan hulless barley) cultivars. *J Cereal Sci,* **2018**, *81,* 69–75.

Liyana-Pathirana, C.; Shahidi, F. Optimization of extraction of phenolic compounds from wheat using response surface methodology. *Food Chem,* **2005**, *93,* 47–56.

Lupton, J.; Robinson, M. C. and Morin, J. Cholesterol-lowering effect of barley bran flour and oil. *J Am Diet Assoc,* **1994**, *94,* 65–70.

Madhujith, T.; Shahidi, F. Antioxidant potential of barley as affected by alkaline hydrolysis and release of insoluble-bound phenolics. *Food Chem,* **2009**, *117,* 615–620.

Maillard, M. N.; Soum, M. H.; Boivin, P. and Berset, C. Antioxidant activity of barley and malt: relationship with phenolic content. *LWT Food Sci Tech,* **1996**, *29,* 238–244.

Martinez, M.; Motilva, M. J.; Hazas, M. C.; Romero, M. P.; Vaculova, K.; Ludwig, I. A. Phytochemical composition and β-glucan content of barley genotypes from two different geographic origins for human health food production. *Food Chem,* **2018**, *245,* 61–70

Mattila, P.; Pihlava, J. M. and Hellstrom, J. Contents of phenolic acids, alkyl- and alkenylresorcinols, and avenanthramides in commercial grain products. *J Agric Food Chem*, **2005**, *53*, 8290–8295.

McIntosh, G. H.; Whyte, J.; McArthur, R. and Nestel, P. J. Barley and wheat foods: influence on plasma cholesterol concentrations in hypercholesterolemic men. *Am J Clin Nutr*, **1991**, *53*, 1205–1209.

Moreau, R. A.; Wayns, K. E.; Flores, R. A. and Hicks, K. B. Tocopherols and tocotrienols in barley oil prepared from germ and other fractions from scarification and sieving of hulless barley. *Cereal Chem*, **2007**, *84*(6), 587–592.

Moura-Nunes, N.; Brito, T. C.; Fonseca, N. D.; Aguiar, P. F.; Monteiro, M.; Perrone, D. and Torres, A. G. Phenolic compounds of Brazilian beers from different types and styles and application of chemometrics for modeling antioxidant capacity. *Food Chem*, **2016**, *199*, 105–113.

Nawaz, H.; Shad, M. A. and Rauf, A. Optimization of extraction yield and antioxidant properties of *Brassica oleracea* Convar Capitata Var L. leaf extracts. *Food Chem*, **2018**, *242*, 182–187.

Newman, R. K.; Lewis, S. E.; Newman, C. W.; Boik, R. J. and Ramage, R. T. Hypocholesterolemic effect of barley foods on healthy men. *Nutr Rep Int*, **1989**, *39*, 749–760.

Odabas, H. I.; Koca, I. Application of response surface methodology for optimizing the recovery of phenolic compounds from hazelnut skin using different extraction methods. *Indus Crop Prod*, **2016**, *91*, 114–124.

Panfili, G.; Fratianni, A. and Irano, M. Normal phase high-performance liquid chromatography method for the determination of tocopherols and tocotrienols in cereals. *J Agric Food Chem*, **2003**, *51*, 3940–3944.

Paucar-Menacho, L. M.; Penas, E.; Duenas, M.; Frias, J. and Villauenga-Martinez, C. Optimizing germination conditions to enhance the accumulation of bioactive compounds and the antioxidant activity of kiwicha (*Amaranthus caudatus*) using response surface methodology. *LWT Food Sci Technol*, **2017a**, *76*, 245–252.

Paucar-Menacho, L. M.; Villaluenga-Martinez, C.; Duenas, M.; Frias, J. and Penas, E. Optimization of germination time and temperature to maximize the content of bioactive compounds and the antioxidant activity of purple corn (*Zea mays* L.) by response surface methodology. *LWT Food Sci Technol*, **2017b**, *76*, 236–244.

Postemsky, P. D.; Bidegain, M. A.; Gonzalez-Matute, R.; Figlas, N. D.; Cubitto, M. A. Pilot-scale bioconversion of rice and sunflower agro-residues into medicinal mushrooms and laccase enzymes through solid-state fermentation with *Ganoderma lucidum*. *Bioresour Technol*, **2017**, *231*, 85–93.

Postemsky, P. D.; Curvetto, N. R. Solid-state fermentation of cereal grains and sunflower seed hulls by *Grifola gargal* and *Grifola sordulenta*. *Int Biodeter Biodegrad*, **2015**, *100*, 52–61.

Quinde-Axtell, Z.; Baik, B. K. Phenolic compounds of barley grain and their implication in food product discoloration, *J Agric Food Chem*, **2006**, *54*, 9978–9984.

Rao, S.; Santhakumar, A. B.; Chinkwo, K. A.; Blanchard, C. L. Q-TOF LC/MS identification and UHPLC-Online ABTS antioxidant activity guided mapping of barley polyphenols. *Food Chem*, **2018**, *266*, 323–328.

Ross, A.; Shepherd, M.; Schupphaus, M.; Sinclair, V.; Alfaro, B.; Kamal-Eldin, A. and Aman, P. Alkylresorcinols in cereals and cereal products. *J Agric Food Chem*, **2003**, *51*, 4111–4118.

Sahu, U.; Kamlesh, P.; Sahoo, P.; Sahu, B. B.; Sarkar, P. C. and Prasad, N. Biscuit making potentials of raw and roasted whole grain flours: cereals and millets. *Asian J Dairy Food Res*, **2015**, *34*, 235–238.

Salar, R. K.; Purewal, S. S. and Bhatti, M. S. Optimization of extraction condition and enhancement of phenolic content and antioxidant activity of pearl millet fermented with *Aspergillus awamori* MTCC-548. *Resour Effic Technol*, **2016**, *2*, 148–157.

Salar, R. K.; Purewal, S. S. Improvement of DNA damage protection and antioxidant activity of biotransformed pearl millet (*Pennisetum glaucum*) cultivar PUSA-415 using *Aspergillus oryzae* MTCC 3107. *Biocatal Agric Biotechol* **2016**, *8*, 221–227.

Salar, R. K.; Purewal, S. S. Phenolic content, antioxidant potential and DNA damage protection of pearl millet (*Pennisetum glaucum*) cultivars of North Indian region. *Food Measure*, **2017**, *11*, 126–133.

Salar, R. K.; Sharma, P. and Purewal, S. S. In vitro antioxidant and free radical scavenging activities of stem extract of Euphorbia trigona Miller. *Tang [Humanitas Medicine]*, **2015**, *5*, 1–6.

Salar, R. K.; Purewal, S. S. and Sandhu, K. S. Relationships between DNA damage protection activity, total phenolic content, condensed tannin content and antioxidant potential among Indian barley cultivars. *Biocatal Agric Biotech*, **2017a**, *11*, 201–206.

Salar, R. K.; Purewal, S. S. and Sandhu, K. S. Fermented pearl millet (*Pennisetum glaucum*) with *in vitro* DNA damage protection activity, bioactive compounds and antioxidant potential. *Food Res Int*, **2017b**, *100*, 204–210.

Salar, R. K.; Purewal, S. S. and Sandhu, K. S. Bioactive profile, free-radical scavenging potential, DNA damage protection activity, and mycochemicals in *Aspergillus awamori* (MTCC 548) extracts: a novel report on filamentous fungi. *3 Biotech*, **2017c**, *7*, 164. DOI: https://doi.org/10.1007/s13205–017-0834–2.

Sandhu, K. S.; Punia, S. and Kaur, M. Effect of duration of solid state fermentation by *Aspergillus awamori* Nakazawa on antioxidant properties of wheat cultivars. *LWT Food Sci Techol*, **2016**, *71*, 323–328.

Sandhu, K. S.; Punia, S. Enhancement of bioactive compounds in barley cultivars by solid state fermentation. *Food Measure*, **2017**, *11*, 1355–1361.

Saulnier, L.; Gevaudan, S. and Thibault, J. F. Extraction and partial characterization of β-glucan from the endosperms of two barley cultivars. *J Cereal Sci*, **1994**, *19*, 171–178.

Setyaningsih, W.; Saputro, I. E.; Palma, M. and Barroso, C. G. Optimisation and validation of the microwave-assisted extraction of phenolic compounds from rice grains. *Food Chem*, **2015**, *169*, 141–149.

Setyaningsih, W.; Duros, E.; Palma, M. and Barroso, C. G. Optimization of the ultrasound-assisted extraction of melatonin from red rice (*Oryza sativa*) grains through a response surface methodology. *Appl Acoust*, **2016**, *103*, 129–135.

Shahidi, F.; Nackz, M. *Food Phenolics: Sources, Chemistry, Effects and Applications*, Technomic Publishing Company Inc., Lancaster, PA, 1995, pages 281–319.

Sharma, P.; Gujral, H. S. Antioxidant and polyphenol oxidase activity of germinated barley and its milling fractions. *Food Chem*, **2010**, *120*, 673–678.

Sharma, P.; Gujral, H. S. Effect of sand roasting and microwave cooking on antioxidant activity of barley, *Food Res Int*, **2011**, *44*, 235–240.

Sharma, P.; Gujral, H. S. Extrusion of hulled barley affecting β-glucan and properties of extrudates. *Food Bioproc Tech*, **2013**, *6*, 1374e1389.

Shen, Y.; Zhang, H.; Cheng, L.; Wang, L.; Qian, H.; Qi, X. In vitro and in vivo antioxidant activity of polyphenols extracted from black highland barley. *Food Chem,* **2015**, *194,* 1003–1012.

Shimizu, C.; Kihara, M.; Aoe, S.; Araki, S.; Ito, K.; Hayashi, K.; Watari, J.; Sakata, Y. and Ikegami S. Effect of high β-glucan barley on serum cholesterol concentrations and visceral fat area in Japanese men-a randomized, double-blinded, placebo-controlled trial. *Plant Foods Hum Nutr,* **2008**, *63*(1), 21–25.

Silva, E. M.; Rogez, H. and Larondelle, Y. Optimization of extraction of phenolics from *Inga edulis* leaves using response surface methodology. *Sep Purif Tech,* **2007**, *55,* 381–387.

Singh, S.; Kaur, M.; Sogi, D. S. and Purewal, S. S. A comparative study of phytochemicals, antioxidant potential and in-vitro DNA damage protection activity of different oat (*Avena sativa*) cultivars from India. *J Food Measur Character,* **2018**, *13,* 347–356.

Storsley, J. M.; Izydorczyk, M. S.; You, S.; Biliaderis, C. G. and Rossnagel, B. Structure and physicochemical properties of β-glucans and arabinoxylans isolated from hull-less barley. *Food Hydrocol,* **2003**, *17,* 831–834.

Suriano, S.; Iannucci, A.; Codianni, P.; Fares, C.; Russo, M.; Pecchioni, N.; Marciello, U. and Savino, M. Phenolic acids profile, nutritional and phytochemical compounds, antioxidant properties in colored barley grown in southern Italy. *Food Res Int,* **2018**, *113,* 221–233.

Talati, R.; Baker, W. L.; Pabilonia, M. S.; White, C. M. and Coleman, C. I. The effects of barley-derived soluble fiber on serum lipids. *Ann Family Med,* **2009**, *7*(2), 157–163.

Tamagawa, K.; Iizuka, A.; Ikeda, A.; Koike, H.; Naganuma, K. and Komiyama, Y. Antioxidative activity of proanthocyanidins isolated from barley bran. *Jpn Soc Food Sci Tech,* **1999**, *46,* 106–110.

Temelli, F. Extraction and functional properties of barley β-glucan as affected by temperature and pH. *J Food Sci,* **1997**, *62,* 1192–1201.

Tsochatzis, E. D.; Bladenopoulos, K. and Papageorgiou, M. Determination of tocopherol and tocotrienol content of Greek barley varieties under conventional and organic cultivation techniques using validated reverse phase high-performance liquid chromatography method. *J Sci Food Agric,* **2012**, *92,* 1732–1739.

USDA (United States Department of Agriculture). (2018). Full Report (All Nutrients) 2005, Barley, pearled, raw. Nutrient Database for Standard Reference Release 1, Agricultural Research Service, USDA. Accessed on 04 February 2019. URL: http://ndb.nal.usda.gov/ndb/search/list.

Vitaglione, P.; Lumaga, R. B.; Montagnese, C.; Messia, M. C.; Marconi, E. and Scalfi, L. Satiating effect of a barley beta-glucan-enriched snack. *J American Coll Nutr,* **2010**, *29*(2), 113–121.

Vitaglione, P.; Lumaga, R. B.; Stanzione, A.; Scalfi, L. and Fogliano, V. β-Glucan-enriched bread reduces energy intake and modifies plasma ghrelin and peptide YY concentrations in the short term. *Appetite,* **2009**, *53*(3), 338–344.

Weidner, S.; Amarowicz, R.; Karamac, M. and Dabrowski, G. Phenolic acids in caryopses of two cultivars of wheat, rye and triticale that display different resistance to pre-harvest sprouting. *Eur Food Res Tech,* **1999**, *210,* 109–113.

Wu, Y. V. Fractionation and characterization of protein-rich material from barley after alcohol distillation. *Cereal Chem,* **1986**, *63,* 142–145.

Wu, Y. V. Protein-rich residues from ethanolic fermentation of high lysine, dent, waxy and white corn varieties. *Cereal Chem,* **1989**, *66,* 506–509.

Wu, Y. V.; Sexson, K. R. and Lagoda, A. A. Protein-rich residue from wheat alcohol distillation: fractionation and characterization. *Cereal Chem,* **1984**, *61,* 423–427.

Wu, Y. V.; Sexson, K. R. Fractionation and characterization of protein-rich material from sorghum alcohol distillation. *Cereal Chem,* **1984**, *61,* 388–391.

Yu, J.; Vasanthan, T. and Temelli, F. Analysis of phenolic acids in barley by high-performance liquid chromatography. *J Agric Food Chem,* **2001**, *49*(9), 4352–4358.

Zarnowski, R.; Suzuki, Y. 5-n-Alkylresorcinols from grains of winter barley (*Hordeum vulgare* L.). *Z Naturforsch C,* **2004**, *59*(5–6), 315–317.

Zarnowski, R.; Suzuki, Y.; Yamaguchi, I. and Stanislaw, J. Alkylresorcinols in barley (*Hordeum vulgare*L. distichon) grains. *Z Naturforsch C,* **2002**, *57,* 57–62.

Zhao, H.; Dong, J.; Lu, J.; Chen, J.; Li, Y.; Shan, L.; Lin, Y.; Fan, W. and Gu, G. Effects of extraction solvent mixtures on antioxidant activity evaluation and their extraction capacity and selectivity for free phenolic compounds in barley (*Hordeum vulgare* L.). *J Agric Food Chem,* **2006**, *54,* 7277–7286.

Zhao, C.; Li, C.; Liu, S. and Yang, L. The galloyl catechins contributing to main antioxidant capacity of tea made from *Cammelia signensis* in China. *Sci World J,* **2014**, 1–11.

Zheng, X. L.; Li, L. M. and Wang, Q. Distribution and molecular characterization of β-glucans from hull-less barley bran, shorts and flour. *Int J Mol Sci,* **2011**, *12,* 1563–1574.

Zhu, Y.; Li, T.; Fu, X.; Abbasi, A. M.; Zheng, B.; Liu, R. H. Phenolics content, antioxidant and antiproliferative activities of dehulled highland barley (*Hordeum vulgare* L.). *J Funct Foods,* **2015**, *19,* 439–450.

Zielinski, H.; Kozowska, H. and Lewczuk, B. Bioactive compounds in the cereal grains before and after hydrothermal processing. *Innov Food Sci Emerg Technol,* **2001**, *2,* 159–169.

Zupfer, J. M.; Churchill, K. E.; Rasmusson, D. C. and Fulcher, R. G. Variation of ferulic acid concentration among diverse barley cultivars measured by HPLC and microspectrophotometry. *J Agric Food Chem,* **1998**, *46,* 1350–1354.

Part II
Phytochemistry of Medicinal Plants

CHAPTER 4

Phytochemicals in Giloy (*Tinospora cordifolia* L.): Structure, Chemistry, and Health Benefits

PRADYUMAN KUMAR[1], DEEPAK KUMAR VERMA[2], G. KIMMY, PREM PRAKASH SRIVASTAV, and KAWALJIT SINGH SANDHU

[1]Department of Food Engineering & Technology, Sant Longowal Institute of Engineering and Technology, Sangrur 148106, Punjab, India
E-mail: pradyuman2002@hotmail.com

[2]Agricultural and Food Engineering Department, Indian Institute of Technology Kharagpur, Kharagpur 721302, West Bengal, India
E-mails: deepak.verma@agfe.iitkgp.ernet.in, rajadkv@rediffmail.com

ABSTRACT

Giloy (*Tinospora cordifolia* L.) is a perennial shrubby creeper which belongs to Menispermaceae family and found in the many tropical regions of the world including India. *T. cordifolia* is one of the most important medicinal plants due to its properties which have been recommended as a potential solution for human health welfare and many diseases since thousands of years ago. The medicinal properties of *T. cordifolia* are because of the presence of several phytochemical compounds in its different parts such as root, stem, and leaves. Very few research works and reports are focused on therapeutic uses of *T. cordifolia* and its role in food health and pharmacological benefits. However, this plant needs more importance and attention. Therefore, authors have pointed out in this chapter on the knowledge of *T. cordifolia* and more emphasized on the development of its therapeutic use in food, health, and pharmacological industry.

4.1   INTRODUCTION

Plants are immense sources of human needs gifted by our Nature mother. The utilization of plants as medicine has been even proved with positive clinical treatments along with good patient acceptability. Year back, since thousand years ago till this 21st century, scientists and the general public have casted the importance of plants as new medicines and natural source of bioactive products (Kirtikar and Basu, 1933; Pendse et al., 1977, 1981; Lanfranco, 1992; Saleem et al., 2001; Tripathi and Tripathi, 2003; Bajpai et al., 2005; Singh, 2015). Still, up to 80% of people have believed mostly on plants and herbs to cure their diseases with traditional practices rather than the allopathic medication as reported by the World Health Organization (Tripathi and Tripathi, 2003). The United Nations Educational, Scientific and Cultural Organization report widely observed to the use of plants as traditional medicine for the maintenance of good health in most developing countries on the normative basis (UNESCO, 1996).

The newer and technological modern medicine has been blessed with the utilization of medicinal plants to provide numerous botanical therapeutic agents (Rani et al., 2014). Synthetic antibiotics develop resistance to the body; however, medicinal properties of plants are clinically effective and develop faster antimicrobial characteristics (Solanki, 2010). Different parts of such plants, viz., roots, branches/stems, barks, leaves, flower, and fruit are used for treatment; they are used in Ayurvedic medicine (Vani et al., 1997; Rege et al., 1999; Rani et al., 2014) due to the presence of huge amounts of various class of chemical compounds. Such chemical compounds include carvacrol, citral, flavonoids, geraniol, linalool, and phenolic acids, and these are well distributed in medicinal plants which may act independently or possess combined synergistic effect (Cai et al., 2004; Cartea et al., 2010; Nagavani and Rao, 2010; Subedi et al., 2014). Thus, it can be said that medicinal plants today have become the backbone of traditional medicine practices (Farnsworth, 1994).

Since centuries, an extensive number of medicinal plants have been selected, identified, and investigated for their biochemical and pharmaceutical properties throughout the globe including Asia, Europe, Africa, and so on for their prospective use against human disease. More than 1500 species of such plants are widely used in different countries, viz., Africa (Lemma, 1991; Mabona et al., 2013), Albania (Kathe et al., 2003, DSA, 2010), Bangladesh (Asadujjaman et al., 2013), Bulgaria (Kathe et al., 2003), China (Cai et al., 2004), Croatia (Kathe et al., 2003), Finland, France (Trouillas et al., 2003), Iraq (Molan et al., 2012), India (Devasagayam and Sainis, 2002; Auudy et al., 2003; Doss et al., 2008; Dixit and Ali, 2010; Rajurkar and Hande, 2011), Japan (Kinoshita et al., 2007; Changwei, 2009), Korea (Choi et al., 2002), Maxico (Calzada and Alanıs, 2007; Villa-Ruano et al., 2013), Nepal (Subedi et al., 2014), Pakistan (Saleem et al., 2001), Thailand (Chanwitheesuk et al., 2005), Turkey (Demiray et al., 2009), United Kingdom (Lanfranco, 1992), and so on. Scientific evidence reported that India is blessed with rich, diverse, and immense sources of plants estimated to be over 45,000 representing about 7% of the world's flora. Approximately 8000 species of them are medicinal plants (Table 4.1) which are used at household level by communities of the village, particularly those living in tribal areas, or in traditional medicine practicing systems, such as the Yearlong Ayurvedic treatments as a traditional medicine to cure the disease (Bodeker et al., 1997; Vaidya and Devasagayam, 2007; Singh, 2015). However, due to the lack of research only a few of them have been thoroughly explored for their therapeutic properties (Devasagayam and Sainis, 2002; Auudy et al., 2003; Doss et al., 2008; Dixit and Ali, 2010; Rajurkar and Hande, 2011; Chatterjee et al., 2013). Giloy (*Tinospora cordifolia* L.) is one of them known for a key player in medicine industries because of the therapeutic agents which are derived from this plant. The Giloy plant clinically is very much effective and safer alternative compared to synthetic chemicals due to the presence of a huge amount of different classes of phytochemicals. These phytochemicals are present in their different parts such as stems, leaves, and so on. They are well distributed and act either independently or with a combined synergistic effect on human health.

In this chapter, authors have discussed and focused on the chemistry, structure, and biological function of phytochemicals present in different plant parts of Giloy, which reveals to have the potent medicinal properties that can have potential side effect free alternative to synthetic chemicals for health beneficial use in the food and pharma industry.

TABLE 4.1 Some Important Indian Medicinal Plants Well Known for Rich Antioxidants and Its Potential

Scientific Name	Common Name	Family
Acacia catechu	Kair	Mimosaceae
Achyranthes aspera	Prickly Chaff-Flower	Amaranthaceae
Aegle marmelos	Bengal Quince, Bel	Rutaceae
Aglaia roxburghiana	Priyangu	Meliaceae
Allium cepa	Onion	Liliaceae
Allium sativum	Garlic	Amaryllidaceae
Aloe vera	Indian aloe, ghritkumari	Liliaceae
Amomum subulatum	Cardamom	Zingiberaceae

TABLE 4.1 *(Continued)*

Scientific Name	Common Name	Family
Andrographis paniculata	Creat, kariyat, Indian echinacea	Acanthaceae
Asparagus racemosus	Asparagus, wild asparagus, asparagus root, shatavari	Liliaceae
Azadirachta indica	Lilac, margosa tree, neem, neem chal	Meliaceae
Butea monosperma	Palas, dhak	Fabaceae
Brassica campestris	Field mustard	Cruciferae
Bauhinia purpurea	Butterfly tree	Caesalpiniaceae
Bacopa monnieri	Brahmi	Scrophulariaceae
Camellia sinensis	Tea	Theaceae
Capparis decidua	Karira	Capparaceae
Capsicum annuum	Chilli pepper	Solanaceae
Centella asiatica	Gotu kola	Mackinlayaceae
Cinnamomum verum	Cinnamon	Lauraceae
Commiphora mukul	Guggul	Burseraceae
Crataeva nurvala	Three-leaved caper, varuna	Capparidaceae
Curcuma longa	Turmeric	Zingiberaceae
Crocus sativus	Saffron	Iridaceae
Cymbopogon citratus	Lemongrass or oil grass	Poaceae
Emblica officinalis	Amla	Phyllanthaceae
Emilia sonchifolia	Cupid's shaving brush, lilac tasselflower	Asteraceae
Garcinia atroviridis	Asam gelugur	Clusiaceae
Garcinia kola	Bitter kola	Clusiaceae
Glycyrrhiza glabra	Yashti-madhu, yashti-madhuka, mulhathi, jethi-madh	Fabaceae
Hemidesmus indicus	Sariva	Apocynaceae
Hypericum perforatum	St John's wort	Hypericaceae
Indigofera tinctoria	Neelini	Fabaceae
Melissa officinalis	Lemon balm	Lamiaceae
Momordica charantia	Bitter gourd, bitter melon, bitter squash	Cucurbitaceae
Morus alba	White mulberry	Moraceae
Murraya koenigii	Curry leaf	Rutaceae
Nigella sativa	Kalonji, black cumin	Ranunculaceae
Ocimum sanctum	Holy basil, Tulsi	Lamiaceae
Picrorhiza kurroa	Kutki	Plantaginaceae
Piper betle	Paan	Piperaceae
Plumbago zeylanica	Chitrak (Chitraka)	Plumbaginaceae
Premna tomentosa	Woolly-leaved fire-brand teak	Lamiaceae
Punica granatum	Pomegranate	Lythraceae
Rubia cordifolia	Manjistha, Indian madder	Rubiaceae
Sesamum indicum	Sesame	Pedaliaceae
Sida cordifolia	Bala	Malvaceae
Swertia decussata	Kadu	Gentianaceae
Syzygium cumini	Jamun	Myrtaceae

TABLE 4.1   *(Continued)*

Scientific Name	Common Name	Family
Terminalia arjuna	Arjuna	Combretaceae
Terminalia bellirica	Baheda	Combretaceae
Tinospora cordifolia	Guduchi, Giloy	Menispermaceae
Trigonella foenum-graecum	Fenugreek	Fabaceae
Withania somnifera	Ashwagandha, Indian ginseng	Solanaceae
Zingiber officinalis	Ginger	Zingiberaceae

Sources: Modified from Devasagayam et al. (2001) and Tilak et al. (2005, 2006).

4.2   BOTANICAL DESCRIPTION AND DISTRIBUTION

Giloy (*Tinospora cordifolia* L.) is a perennial shrubby creeper, which belongs to the family Menispermaceae indigenous to tropical Asia, especially to the tropical areas of India ascending to an altitude of 300 to 1200 m above the mean sea level. Around 40 species of *Tinospora* are found in the arena of Southern Eastern Asia, Myanmar, Sri Lanka, Africa, and Australia; among them, four species are widely found in Indian tropical areas, viz., *T. cordifolia, T. crispa, T. glabra*, and *T. sinensis. T. cordifolia* is also called as Amrita, Chinna, Guduchi, and so forth in Hindi, and heart-leaved moonseed and Gilo in English (Nandkarni, 1954; Chopra et al., 1958; Devasagayam and Sainis, 2002; Sinha et al., 2004; Bhattacharyya and Bhattacharyya, 2013).

Scientific Classification	
Kingdom:	Plantae
(unranked):	Angiosperms
(unranked):	Eudicots
Order:	Ranunculales
Family:	Menispermaceae
Genus:	*Tinospora*
Species:	*T. cordifolia*

The plant of *T. cordifolia* is a succulent, deciduous, climbing, and glabrous shrub which is extensively found growing in dry forests throughout India (Nandkarni, 1954; Chopra et al., 1958). This plant thrives easily in plain regions and even found growing on some trees such as neem or mango (Figure 4.1A). It consists of succulent and fleshy stems recognized with its fleshy aerial roots with long filiform from the branches and corky dotted bark with grey-brown or creamy-white color (Figure 4.1B and C); heart-shaped leaves which are simple, alternate broadly ovate, membranous, juicy, shortly acuminate, and deeply cordate (Figure 4.1D). The flowers of Giloy are unisexual, small on separate plants, yellow or greenish-yellow in color on axillary, and terminal racemes in appearance and when the plant is leafless, they are found as solitary in the female and in the male plant are present in clustered form (Figure 4.1F); fruits are generally red in color as they ripen and possess drupes characteristics (Figure 4.1G). The drupes are ovoid, red, glossy, and succulent and the seeds are found in a curved form. In general, fruits have only one seed (Nandkarni, 1954; Chopra et al., 1958; Devasagayam and Sainis, 2002; Sinha et al., 2004; Bhattacharyya and Bhattacharyya, 2013). Guduchi plant can be easily grown in a wide range of soil such as sandy loam/loamy sand or loam to clay loam. The complete growth takes place when the soil has fair moisture content and it should be well drained. Generally, March to June month of the year is best suitable for flowering in Giloy while July month is for the setting of the fruit which matures during the cold season.

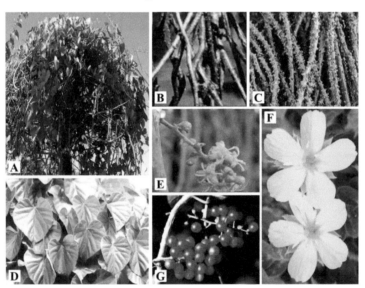

FIGURE 4.1   Giloy (*T. cordifolia* L.). (A) *T. cordifolia* thrived on a tree, (B) areal roots, (C) soft stem emerge out by roots, (D) thinly skinned wide leaves, (E) inflorescence, (F) yellow or green flowers, and (G) pea-sized red-colored fruits.

4.3   GILOY PHYTOCHEMICALS: STRUCTURE AND CHEMISTRY

The woody shrub of *T. cordifolia* is of pronounced concern to the scientists throughout the biosphere. The reason behind this is its different parts, viz., root, stem, and leaves have medicinal properties and reported for medicinal use. Among the different parts of *T. cordifolia,* the stem is comparatively more medicinally important (Anuman et al., 1988; Ghosal and Vishwakarma, 1997). The medicinal properties of the whole extract of *T. cordifolia* are because of the presence of various phytochemicals (Table 4.2), viz., arabinogalactan, berberine, bitter gilonin, β-sitosterol, chasmanthin, choline, clerodane furano diterpene, columibin, cordifol, cordifolide, diterpenes, diterpenoid furanolactone tinosporidine, furan lactones, glycoside, heptacosanol, magniflorine, nonglycoside gilonin gilosterol, palmarin, palmatine, phenolic lignans, phenyl propane glycosides, protoberberine, sesquiterpenoid, steroids, tembertarine, tinosporaside, tinosporic acid, tinosporide, tinosporin, tinosporine, tinosporol, and so on (Pendse et al., 1981; Anuman et al., 1988; Swaminathan et al., 1989; Gangan et al., 1994; Sipahimalani et al., 1994; Ghosal and Vishwakarma, 1997; Kapil and Sharma, 1997; Chintalwar et al., 1999; Singh et al., 2003). The chemicals b-sitosterol, clerodane furano diterpene, columbin, cordifol, cordifolide, diterpenoid furanolactone tinosporidine, heptacosanol, tinosporaside, tinosporide, and tinosporine are the major Giloy phytoconstituent (Anuman et al., 1988; Ghosal and Vishwakarma, 1997; Singh et al., 2003). Choline, berberine, tinosporin, magniflorine, tembertarine and palmatine reported in stem (Anuman et al., 1988; Ghosal and Vishwakarma, 1997) whereas protoberberine, tinosporic acid, tinosporide, and tinosporol in leaves (Swaminathan et al., 1989). The chemical structure of some important phytochemicals present in Giloy stem and leaves is shown in Figure 4.2.

TABLE 4.2 Phytochemicals Present in Different Parts of Giloy

Plant Part	Class of Phytochemicals	Active Compounds
Stem	Glycosides	18-Norclerodane glucoside, Cordifolioside (A, B, C, D, and E), Furanoid diterpene glucoside, Palmatosides (C and F), Syringin, Syringin-apiosylglycoside, Tinocordifolioside, Tinocordiside,
	Sesquiterpenoid	Tinocordifolin
Stem, root	Alkaloids	Berberine, Choline, Isocolumbin, Magnoflorine, Magnoflorine, Palmatine, Palmatine, Tembetarine, Tetrahydropalmatine, Tinosporin
Whole plant	Diterpenoid Lactones	Clerodane derivatives, Columbin, Furanolactone, Jateorine, Tinosporides, Tinosporon
	Aliphatic compound	Octacosanol, Heptacosanol Nonacosan-15-one dichloromethane
Root, whole plant	Others	3-(α,4-dihydroxy-3-methoxy-benzyl)-4-(4-compounds hydroxy-3-methoxy-benzyl)-tetrahydrofuran, Cordifelone, Cordifol, Giloin, Giloinin, Jatrorrhizine, *N*-transferuloyltyramine as diacetate, Tinosporic acid, and Tinosporidine

Source: Modified from Singh et al. (2003).

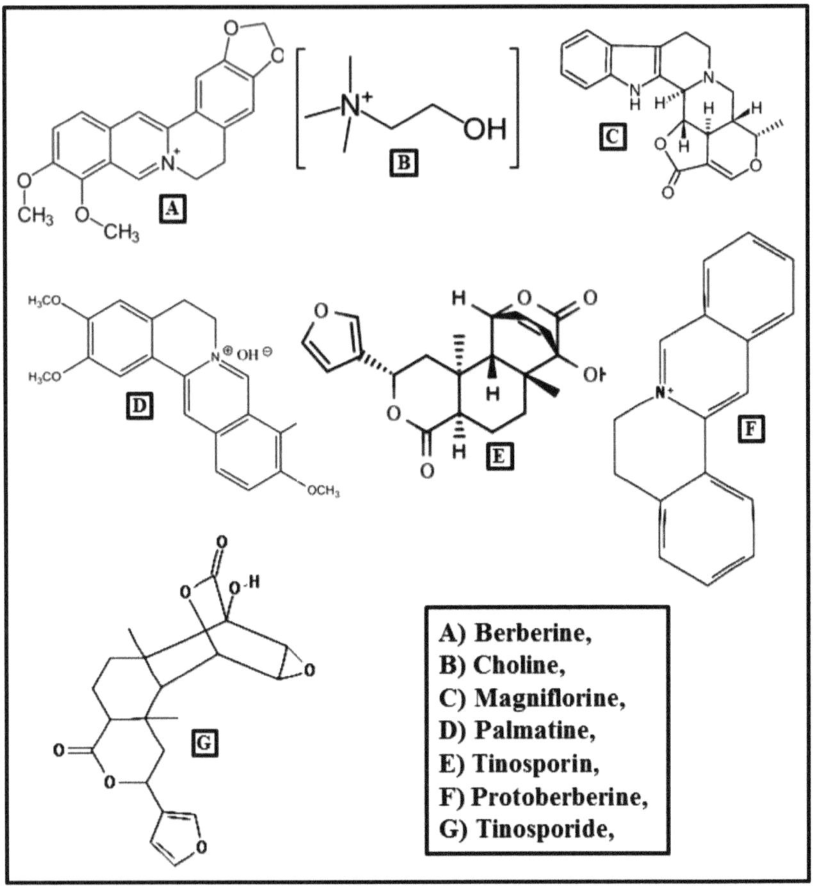

FIGURE 4.2   Structure of some important phytochemicals present in stem and leaves of Giloy.

4.4   CASE STUDY ON GILOY PHYTOCHEMICALS

4.4.1   IDENTIFICATION AND CHARACTERIZATION OF PHYTOCHEMICALS

Jhorar et al. (2016) studied the stem extract of *T. cordifolia* in methanol through gas chromatography-mass spectrometry (GC-MS) analysis and reported eight major peaks which showed the presence of 3-benzodioxolo[5,6-a]quinolizinium; 5,6-dihydro-9,10-dimethoxybezo[g]-1; cordifolioside A; difluorozene; palmitic acid (hexadecanoic acid); metholene; methyl10-trans,12-cis-octadecadienoate; nootkaton-11,12-epoxide; and vanillin lactoside (glycoside). Papitha et al. (2016) conducted the phytochemical screening of stem of *T.*

cordifolia extracts using solvents, viz., methanol, petroleum ether, chloroform, and ethyl acetate and reported the presence of phenols, alkaloids, saponins, terpenoids, flavonoids, carbohydrates, and tannins in it. Identification of four functional groups viz. alkyl halides (C–H), aromatics (C–H), secondary amines and amides (N–H), and α,β-unsaturated aldehydes and ketones (C=O) wryer carried out through Fourier-transform infrared spectroscopy analysis. The methanolic extract of *T. cordifolia* stem*,* when analyzed through GC-MS, reported 11 compounds (majorly phenol, 2,4-bis(1,1-dimethyl-ethyl; 3,7,11,15-tetramethyl-2-hexadecen-1-ol; 9-eicosene, (e)- and hexamethyl-cyclotrisiloxane) which are responsible for antibacterial, anticancer, anti-inflammatory, and antioxidant properties, respectively.

Albinjose et al. (2015) studied the GC-MS analysis of methanol extract, chloroform extract, and petroleum ether extract of stem of *T. cordifolia* and reported 40 compounds in total in all the three extracts, viz., 15 compounds detected in chloroform extract, 14 compounds detected in methanol extract, and 11 compounds detected in petroleum ether extract. The common compound found among all the three extracts was propanic acid, 2-(3-acetoxy-4,4,14-trimethylandrost-8-en-17-yl)- with varying retention times, viz., 23.57 for purified chloroform extract, 25.53 for purified methanol extract, and 16.05 for purified petroleum ether extract. Khan et al. (2015) characterized the stems of *T. cordifolia* using spectroscopical methods, viz., IR, ^{13}C, and ^{1}H-NMR (nuclear magnetic resonance) identified two compounds namely stigmasta-5,22,25-triene-2,3-diol and 1-octacosnol. They had reported the presence of –OH stretch (3300 cm[−1]), C–H stretching (2990 cm[−1]), aliphatic C–H stretching, C–O stretching vibration (1050 cm[−1]), alkyl long chain (720 cm[−1]), and alcohol (1720 cm[−1]) in 1-octacosnol, whereas the presence of –OH group (3450 cm[−1]), C–H stretching (2980 cm[−1]), >C=C< stretching (1640 cm[−1]), –CH$_2$– bending in aliphatic compound (1450 cm[−1]), –CH$_3$ group (1370 cm[−1]) and C–O stretching (1050 cm[−1]) in stigmasta-5,22,25-triene-2,3-diol. Yadav et al. (2015) reported the presence of bicyclo[3.1.1]heptane, 2,6,6-trimethyl; Hexadecanoic acid, methyl ester; *n*-hexadecanoic acid, and 9,12-octadecadienoic acid (Z, Z) in *T. cordifolia* extract when the analysis was performed using GC-MS.

Naik et al. (2014) conducted a study on chemical composition of essential oil isolated from *T. cordifolia* leaf by gas chromatography–flame ionization detector and GC-MS analysis and identified 27 volatile compounds with the help of National Institute for Standards and Technology library, Wiley GC-MS library, by comparing retention indices and by co-injection with the authentic compounds. The identified compounds in essential oil of *T. cordifolia* leaf include the highest amount of alcohols (32.1%) followed by phenols (16.6%), aldehydes (16.2%), fatty acids (15.7%), alkanes (8.3%), esters (3.2%), terpenes (1.2%), and other classes of compounds (4.8%). hydroquinone (16.6%), 2-hexenal (14.2%), palmitic acid (14.1%), 2-hexen-1-ol (11.5%), and phytol (11.4%) were found to be the major compounds.

4.4.2   TOTAL PHENOLIC CONTENT, FLAVONOID CONTENT, AND ANTIOXIDANT ACTIVITY

Bhagyasree et al. (2016) reported variation in total phenolic content (TPC) from 15.42 to 20.52 mg/g GAE. The highest antioxidant activity (AOA) (82.50%), DPPH (2,2-diphenyl-1-picrylhydrazyl): IC50 was found to be 46.80 µg/mL while total flavonoid content (TFC) was 30.40 µg RuE/mg. Jhorar et al. (2016) assessed the phytochemical screening and AOA of chloroform, ethanol, methanol, and water crude extracts of *T. cordifolia* and *Myristica fragrans* and reported that active compounds present in extracts of *M. fragrans* (Myristicin and eugenol) and *T. cordifolia* (palmatine and berberine) are responsible for their AOA. IC50 value for DPPH free radical scavenging activity for different extracts of *T. cordifolia* was found to be methanol extract (0.26 mg/mL), ethanol extract (3.83 mg/mL), chloroform extract (0.49 mg/mL), and aqueous extract (4.40 mg/mL) which showed that methanol extract of *T. cordifolia* had highest AOA.

Yadav et al. (2015) evaluated AOA, TPC, and TFC of *T. cordifolia* extract and reported that *T. cordifolia* extract had TPC of 3.12 µg GAE/mg sample, TFC of 36.80 µg CE/mL sample, and DPPH free radical scavenging activity was 45.80% and ferric reducing antioxidant power (FRAP) value of 394 µg butylated hydroxyl toluene (BE)/mg sample because of the presence of significant amount of phenolics, flavonoids, tannins, and saponins. Kumar and Sharma (2015) assessed the AOA of ethanolic extract of *T. cordifolia* plant's stem by Trolox equivalent antioxidant capacity (TEAC) assay and Ferric reducing ability of plasma assay and reported maximum ferrous sulphate equivalent (1785.66 µmol $Fe^{2+}E$/g of dried sample) and TEAC value (0.72 mmol Trolox E/g of dried sample) in ethanolic extract of stem of *T. cordifolia.*

Chauhan et al. (2014) evaluated the nutritional and phytochemical composition of the fresh stem of *T. cordifolia* along with other plants, viz., *Andrographis paniculata* leaves and roots, and *Boerhaavia diffusa* leaves which showed vitamin C in higher amount and minerals in leaves and that of fiber content in stems and roots. They had reported 0.033% berberine content in *T. cordifolia* and 1.8% andrographolide in *A. paniculata.* Radical scavenging activity was also possessed by these plant parts viz. leaves of *B. diffusa* (24.32%), leaves of *A. paniculata* (23.56%), and stem of *T. cordifolia* (21.72%). Naik et al. (2014) also studied the antioxidative ability of essential oil of *T. cordifolia* leaf extract and found strong AOA (IC$_{50}$ = 25±0.3 µg/mL) and dose-dependent reducing power activity. The study of Naik et al. (2014) found TPC of obtained essential oil which was 28 ± 0.4 mg GAE/g fresh leaves. Sharma et al. (2014) assessed the AOA potential of stem extracts of *T. cordifolia,* extracted with various solvents *viz.* acetone, aqueous benzene, chloroform, ethyl acetate, ethyl alcohol, hexane, and reported FRAP values in the range of 4981–6568 µmol ferrous sulfate equivalent/mg for chloroform, ethyl acetate, acetone, and ethyl alcohol extracts of *T. cordifolia* in rat liver homogenate. Upadhyay et al. (2014) assessed the antioxidant properties and TPC of ethanol and methanol extract of *T. cordifolia* bark and found ethanol extract had shown the higher DPPH free-radical scavenging ability (71.49%) as compared to methanol extract and 84.62 ± 0.12 mg/g TPC was found in ethanolic extract of *T. cordifolia* bark.

Ghate et al. (2013) examined the reactive oxygen species scavenging ability and AOA of 70% methanolic extract of *T. cordifolia* stem and reported carbohydrate (9.21 mg/100 mg extract glucose equivalent), alkaloid (45.11 mg/100 mg extract reserpine equivalent), ascorbic acid (0.61 mg/100 mg extract L-ascorbic acid equivalent), tannin (2.35 mg/100 mg extract catechin equivalent), phenolic (51.33 mg/100 mg GAE extract), and flavonoid compound (178.67 mg/100 mg QuE extract) along with TEAC value (0.257), IC$_{50}$ value for hydroxyl radical (128.86 µg/mL), superoxide (103.17 µg/mL), nitric oxide (51.98 µg/mL), hypochlorous acid (327.38 µg/mL), and lipid peroxidation (75.86 µg/mL). Grover et al. (2013) performed the quantitative and qualitative analysis of stem of *T. codiofolia* and reported a yield of 7.27% for petroleum ether stem extract and 12.05% for aqueous stem extract. Both the stem extracts were observed with the presence of carbohydrates, proteins, amino acids, alkaloids, glycosides, and tannins. Mishra et al. (2013) evaluated antioxidant and phytochemical screening of stem extract of *T. cordifolia* using different solvents and reported the presence of plants secondary metabolites including phenolics (8.75–52.50 catechol equivalent per gram), anthraquinones, terpenoids, and saponins. At a concentration of 10–40 µg/mL, 67%–95% ion chelating activity was possessed by aqueous stem extracts along with other solvents.

Bhalerao et al. (2012) studied in vitro AOA of ethanol extract of *T. cordifolia* grown with four different supporting trees viz. *Acacia leucophloea*, *Azadirachta indica*, *Butea monosperma*, and *Prosopis juliflora* and reported that *T. cordifolia* grown with the support of *A. indica* showed highest DPPH free-radical scavenging (86.36%), total AOA (2144 µM Fe(II)/g dry mass), antilipid peroxidation potential (96.8%) and TPC (21.5 mg/g dry weight). Devprakash et al. (2012) evaluated the AOA, TPC, and TFC of aqueous and ethanolic extract of *T. cordifolia* and reported that aqueous extract and ethanol extract at concentration of 50 µg/mL had TPC 17.23% w/w of total tannin and 15.48% w/w of total tannin whereas TFC 1.31% w/w of total quercetin and 0.90% w/w of total quercetin respectively. FRAP value recorded for aqueous extract and ethanol extract at the concentration of 500 µg/mL was 61.87 mg GAE/g extract and 52.21 mg GAE/g extract, respectively. DPPH: IC50 was found to be 205.24 µg/mL and 240.11 µg/mL in aqueous and ethanolic extract of *T. cordifolia.* Onkar et al. (2012) studied the traditional Ayurvedic formulation *T. cordifolia* and hydroalcoholic extract of the plant *Curculigo orchioides* (Kali Musali) in vitro for its AOA by different assay methods. In comparison with a standard, potent scavenging activity was revealed. The AOAs of plant extracts were found due to the presence of active constituents (viz., alkaloids, flavonoids, saponins, glycosides, and a lesser amount of phytosterols) either alone or in combination. Praveen et al. (2012) studied the AOA of *T. cordifolia* leaves extract by using different solvents viz. butanol, ethyl acetate, methanol, and water extract, and compared with the standard antioxidant. They found that although methanol possessed the highest AOA among different antioxidant assays at a concentration of 250 mg/mL in comparison to other solvents, it was lesser than that of standard antioxidant (butylated hydroxytoluene) at the same concentration. The phenolic contents of the different extracts were noted to be higher in methanol (44.36 mg/g) followed by ethyl acetate (38.73 mg/g), butanol (36.42 mg/g), and water (23.60 mg/g) extract.

Ilaiyaraja and Khanum (2011) demonstrated the TPC and AOA of stem and leaf of *T. cordifolia* using different solvents, viz., acetone, chloroform, ethyl acetate, hexane, methanol, and water and found that the extract with ethyl acetate of *T. cordifolia* stem had the highest amount of polyphenols (60.93 mg GAE/g extract) whereas methanolic extract of leaf of *T. cordifolia* had the highest amount of polyphenols (52.17 mg GAE/g extract) compared to other solvents. IC_{50} value in DPPH free-radical scavenging was found 0.60 mg for ethyl acetate stem extract and 0.54 mg for methanol leaf extract. FRAP value obtained from ethyl acetate stem extract and methanol leaf extract was 16.87 µg ferrous sulfate equivalent and 8.97 µg ferrous sulfate equivalents at 0.1 mg/mL concentration of extract respectively. They reported that stem extract was found to be a more effective source of antioxidants as compared to the leaf extract because of the presence of a higher amount of polyphenols in the stem of *T. cordifolia.* Yadav and Agarwala (2011) investigated the presence of phytochemicals and determined the TPC and TFC of the stem of *T. cordifolia* and reported *T. cordifolia* stem had 12.8 mg GAE/g sample of polyphenols and 6 mg QE/g sample of flavonoids due to the presence of phenols, tannins, saponins, and flavonoids.

Extract of *T. cordifolia* studied by Bhawya and Anilakumar (2010) for their AOA using different solvents, viz., ethanol, methanol, and water with different methods. Significant results were found with these solvents as compared to other solvents. Bhawya and Anilakumar, (2010) showed that methanol extract of *T. cordifolia* stem possessed higher AOA of 98.13% in DPPH radical scavenging (DPPH-RS) activity method followed by its ethanol extract (90.34%) in superoxide radical scavenging (SRS) method whereas in hydroxyl radical scavenging method, both the extracts represented good results (97.08% for methanol and 95.21% for ethanol extract) along with other solvents. There was also a significant increase in the reduction of ferrous ions and metal chelation of 60.62% for methanol followed by 57.62% and 40.89% for ethanol and aqueous extract. Sivakumar et al. (2010) also suggested from their study that methanol extract of *T. cordifolia* stem had increased ability toward different antioxidant assays viz. DPPH free-radical screening activity, SRS activity and reducing power assay due to the presence of 7.2% w/w total phenolics and 8.7% w/w total tannins. Premanath and Lakshmi Devi (2010) conducted in vitro models for studies on AOA of *T. cordifolia* leaves with different solvents, viz., chloroform, ethanol, hexane, methanol, and water for extraction of antioxidants and different in vitro models such as DPPH-RS activity, lipid peroxidation inhibitory (LPI) activity, SRS activity, total AOA, and total reducing power for antioxidant assays along with TPC and flavonoid content. The ethanol extract was reported to have the highest flavonoid and phenolic content of 0.52 ± 0.02 mg/g and 5.1 ± 0.25 mg/g, respectively, as compared to other solvent extracts and also exhibited the highest total AOA (41.4 ± 0.45 µM Fe(II)/g) when compared to other solvent extracts. Ethanol extract had exhibited IC_{50} value for LPI activity as 0.1 mg/mL and $IC50$ value for DPPH-RS activity was 0.5 mg/mL.

4.5   MEDICINAL PROPERTIES AND HEALTH BENEFITS OF GILOY

T. cordifolia is extensively used in medicines since times immemorial and prescribed in fevers, dyspepsia, diabetes, urinary problems, chronic diarrhea, jaundice, dysentery, and skin diseases. The uses of this medicinal plant as folk and tribal medicine by the people of different Indian provinces are shown in Table 4.3. Besides, it also has much biological significance in different therapeutic benefits viz. antioxidant, anticancer, anti-inflammatory, anti-aids, antidiabetic, antiallergic, antiulcer, and so on (Sarangi and Soni, 2013). Though its extracted is bitter in taste, *T. cordifolia* stem contains starch that is extremely nutritive, easily digestible, and is used to cure many diseases (Sinha et al., 2004). Extracts of *T. cordifolia* is having high biological importance in treating various ailments (Sharma et al., 2012).

It acts as an anti-stressing and antidepressant agent by enhancing the levels of antidepressing monoamines (viz. serotonin, norepinephrine, gamma-aminobutyric acid, and dopamine) by interacting with receptors of α-1 adrenergic, serotonergic, dopaminergic (D2) and metabotropic trans-membrane and/or by inhibition of monoamine oxidase in brain (Dhingra and Goyal, 2008; Sangeetha et al., 2011; Sharma et al., 2012). Thus in Ayurveda, it is also named as "*Medhya Rasayana*" (memory enhancer) and "*Bhrama*" (vertigo) (Dhingra and Goyal, 2008).

Different extracts of *T. cordifolia* show a great potential of hypoglycemic effect in traditional medicinal practices (Sudha et al., 2011). The extract of the whole plant of *T. cordifolia* also reported possessing antidiabetic activity (Sangeetha et al., 2011; Kinkar and Patil, 2015). Sangeetha et al. (2011) reported that regulation of blood glucose level might be achieved by promoting the secretion of insulin, eradicating oxidative stress and also by inhibiting gluconeogenesis and glycogenolysis through intake of *T. cordi-folia* extracts. Patel and Mishra (2011) reported that isoquinoline including palmatine, jatrorrhizine, and magnoflorine obtained from steam extract helps in showing insulin-releasing and insulin-mimicking effects.

T. cordifolia shows immune-modulatory attribute by improving the immune system and provides resistance to the body against infection (Kapil and Sharma, 1997; Manjrekar et al., 2000; Chintalwar et al., 1999; Bishayi et al., 2002; Subramanian et al., 2002). Cytotoxic effects of this herb are also reported due to the presence of alkaloids, glycosides, phenolics, diterpenoids lactones, steroids, sesquiterpenoid, polysaccharides, or aliphatic compounds or (Jahfar, 2003; Jagetia and Rao, 2006). Scientist studied that extracts of *T. cordifolia* show the potential of antimicrobial activity against different microbial species (Jeyachandran et al., 2003; Tambekar et al., 2009; Naray-anan et al., 2011; Sharma et al., 2012).

Leaves extract and root extract of *T. cordifolia* show strong free-radical scavenging potential against superoxide anion (O_2^-), hydroxyl

TABLE 4.3 Usages of Giloy (*Tinospora cordifolia*) in Indian Folk and Tribal Medicine

Indian Province	Peoples and Their Location	Remarks	Purpose for Treatments	Reference
Gujarat	The tribals of Khedbrahma region of North	Plant was used as food or medicine in their life of daily routine.	For the treatment of cancer	Bhatt and Sabnis (1987)
		The stem bark and root powder of *T. cordifolia* were used with milk.		
		Decoction of root	Used for the cure of dysentery and diarrhea	
		A decoction of old stems	Periodic fever was prefer for treatment	
Haryana	The people of Dhurala	Powder of Amrita (*T. cordifolia*) with the powder of Haritaki (*Terminalia chebula*) and Ajwain (*Trachyspermum ammi*) in equal proportion with salt was administered orally, once in early morning of the day	Kasa (cough) was treated	Anonymous (1999)
		A decoction of these drugs is also to be given in a dose of 50 mL		
Jammu and Kashmir	People of Jammu	Decoction of stem	Administered orally for the treatment of fever	Anonymous (1999)
	The Muslim tribals of Rajouri, Jammu (Tawi) comprising Gujjar and Backwals	Used the plant	In bone fracture	Jee et al. (1984)
Madhya Pradesh	The people of Deharwara Kolaras, Shivpuri district	A decoction of the stem is administered orally	In the case of twak roga (skin disease)	Anonymous (1999)

TABLE 4.3 (Continued)

Indian Province	Peoples and Their Location	Remarks	Purpose for Treatments	Reference
Maharashtra	The tribals of Bombay and its neighboring areas and the fishermen along the seacoast	Use *T. cordifolia* as drug	In the treatment of fever, jaundice, chronic diarrhea, and dysentery	Shah (1984)
	In Dahanu forest division, tribal races (viz. Agaris, Bhils, Dhodias, Dublas, Khakaris, Rimoshis, Thakurs, Vardaris, Vagharis, and Varlis)	Use the stem decoction with cold or hot water (about 34 gm) in the morning on an empty stomach as a tonic	In general debility	Shah et al. (1983)
Orissa	Inhabitants of Bhuvneshwar	Use the warm juice of root of *T. cordifolia*	Orally for the treatment of fever	Anonymous (1999)
Punjab	Local people of Patiala	Juice or decoction of leaves with honey	Administered orally in fever	Anonymous (1999)
	The local people of Patiala	Two drops of leaf juice of allied species of Guduchi	Dropped in the ear for the treatment of Karna Shula (pain in-ear)	Anonymous (1999)
Rajasthan	People of Bigwada	Decoction of stem	Administered orally for the treatment of fever	Anonymous (1999)
	The local women of Arjunpura	A paste of Guduchi (*T. cordifolia*) and five seeds of Krishna Marich (*Piper nigrum*)	Administered orally once daily in the morning in rakta pradar (leucorrhoea)	Anonymous (1999)
Uttar Pradesh	The tribals Baiga, living in the interior areas of Naugarh and Chakia block of Varanasi district	Make the paste of stem of the Guduchi (*T. cordifolia*) and the roots of Bhatkatiaya (*Solanum surattense*)	The pills are prepared and used in the treatment of fever for three days.	Singh and Maheshwari (1983)
	The inhabitants of Badala	Take the juice of stem orally with honey	for the treatment of swasa (Asthma)	Anonymous (1999)

radicals (·OH), nitric oxide (·NO) radical, and peroxynitrite anion (ONOO⁻) (Goel et al., 2002; Subramanian et al., 2002; Rawal et al., 2004; Sengupta et al., 2009). It also shows the potential of scavenging free radicals produced during aflatoxicosis and nephrotoxicity (induced by aflatoxin) (Gupta and Sharma, 2011). Stem extracts of *T. cordifolia* diminish the risk of reduced male fertility in rats when orally taken (Rao et al., 2005). In vitro studies of Jagetia et al. (1998) stated that extracts of *T. cordifolia* effectively kills the HeLa cells and thus having a potential of anti-neo-plastic properties.

Watery extracts of *T. cordifolia* efficiently acts as an anti-inflammatory agent in both induced edema and human arthritis. Its stem extract produces a significant effect in both acute and subacute inflammatory models and is more effective as compared with acetylsalicylic acid (Jana et al., 1999). Hence, it acts as an efficient anti-inflammatory agent (Pendse et al., 1977). Extracts of *T. cordifolia* also acts as a good hepatoprotective agent (Nagarkatti et al., 1994; Bishayi et al., 2002).

4.6   SUMMARY, CONCLUSION, AND FUTURE PROSPECT

T. cordifolia medicinal plant is a rich source of phytochemicals which is found in its various parts (viz., root, stem, and leaves) which has been described by Indian medicine system Ayurveda as a preventer of human health from several diseases with no side effect. In the last few decades, researchers and scientists are giving more importance, attention, and exploration to the numerous medicinal plants in the area of food, health, and medicine research. In these days, *T. cordifolia* due to high potential health benefits has become as an emerging medicinal plant for pharmacological and therapeutic use while extensive progress and development of its uses had already been described in the historical period of Indian medicine system "Ayurveda." However, there is either a lack of research or very few documented reports on the significance of this medicinal plant which immediately need more attention. Therefore, authors have considered opening a new door in this chapter with more emphasis on the knowledge, development, and scientific research of various aspects of *T. cordifolia* for food, health, and pharmacological industry which will help to give a new direction to all those peoples who are associated with this field.

KEYWORDS

- **antioxidant activity**
- **DPPH**
- **flavonoid content**
- **free-radical scavenging**
- **Giloy**
- **human health**
- **medicinal plants**
- **medicinal products**
- **phenolic content**
- **phytochemicals**
- **secondary metabolites**
- **therapeutic agents**
- **Tinospora cordifolia**

REFERENCES

Albinjose, J.; Jasmine, E.; Selvankumar, T.; Srinivasakumar K. P. Bioactive compounds of *Tinospora cordifolia* by gas chromatography-mass spectrometry (GC-MS). *Int J Multidiscip Res Dev,* **2015**, *2*(1), 88–97.

Anonymous. *An Appraisal of Tribal-Folk Medicine.* Central Council for Research in Ayurveda & Siddha: New Delhi, India, 1999, p. 350.

Anuman, J. H.; Amak, R.; Bhat, R.; Balakrishnan, S. B. A Clerodane Furano-Diterpene from *Tinospora cordifolia. J Nat Prod.* **1988**, *51*(2), 197–201.

Asadujjaman, M.; Hossain, M. A.; Karmakar, U. P. Assessment of DPPH free radical scavenging activity of some medicinal plants. *Archives,* **2013**, *1*, 161–165.

Auudy, B.; Ferreira, F.; Blasina, L.; Lafon, F.; Arredondo, F.; Dajas, R.; Tripathi, P. C. Screening of antioxidant activity of three Indian medicinal plants, traditionally used for the management of neurodegenerative diseases. *J Ethnopharmacol,* **2003**, *84*, 131–138.

Bajpai, M.; Pande, A.; Tewari, S. K.; Prakash, D. Phenolic contents and antioxidant activity of some food and medicinal plants. *Int J Food Sci Nutr,* **2005**, *56*(4), 287–291.

Bhagyasree, J. M.; Muralidhar. S. T.; Hrishikeshavan, H. J. Antioxidant and membrane stability studies in *Tinospora cordifolia. Imperial J Interdiscip Res,* **2016**, *2* (7), 1254–1260.

Bhalerao, B. M.; Kasote, D. M.; Nagarkar, B. E.; Jagtap, S. D.; Vishwakarma, K. S.; Pawar, P. K.; Maheshwari, V. L. Comparative analysis of radical scavenging and immunomodulatory activities of *Tinospora cordifolia* growing with different supporting trees. *Acta Biol Szeged,* **2012**, *56*(1), 65–71.

Bhatt, R. P; and Sabnis, S. D. Contribution to the ethnobotany of Khedbrahma region of North Gujarat. *J Econ Tax Bot*, **1987**, *9*(1), 139–146.

Bhattacharyya, C.; Bhattacharyya, G. Therapeutic potential of Giloe, *Tinospora cordifolia* (Willd.) Hook. f. & Thomson (Menispermaceae): the magical herb of Ayurveda. *Int J Pharmac Biol Arch*, **2013**, *4*(4), 558–584.

Bhawya, D.; Anilakumar, K. R. *In vitro* antioxidant potency of *Tinospora cordifolia* (gulancha) in Sequential Extracts. *Int J Pharmac Biol Arch,***2010**, *1*(5), 448–456.

Bishayi, B.; Roychowdhury, S.; Ghosh, S.; Sengupta, M. Hepatoprotective and immunomodulatory properties of *Tinospora cordifolia* in CCl_4 intoxicated mature albino rats. *J Toxicol Sci,* **2002**, *27*, 139–146.

Bodeker, G.; Bhat, K.K.S.; Burley, J.; Vantomme, P. *Non-wood Forest Products 11, Medicinal Plants for Forest Conservation and Health Care. Global Initiative for Traditional Systems (GIFTS) of Health*, Food and Agriculture Organization of the United Nations Rome, Italy, 1997. URL: http://www.fao.org/3/a-w7261e.pdf. Accessed on June 19, 2016.

Cai, Y.; Luo, Q.; Sun, M.; Corke, H. Antioxidant activity and phenolic compounds of 112 traditional Chinese medicinal plants associated with anticancer. *Life Sci*, **2004**, *74*: 2175–2184.

Calzada, F.; Alanıs, A. D. Additional antiprotozoal flavonol glycosides of the aerial parts of *Helianthemum glomeratum*. *Phytother Res,***2007**, *21*(1), 78–80.

Cartea, M. E.; Francisco, M.; Lema, M.; Soengas, P.; Velasco, P. Resistance of cabbage (Brassica oleracea capitata Group) crops to *Mamestra brassicae*. *J Econ Entom*, **2010**, *103*(5): 1866–1874.

Changwei, A. *Studies on antioxidant, antibacterial and anti-inflammatory active compounds from medicinal plants*. Ph.D. Thesis. United Graduate School of Agricultural Sciences, Kagoshima University, Kagoshima, Japan, 2009.

Chanwitheesuk, A.; Teerawutgulrag, A.; Rakariyatham, N. Screening of antioxidant activity and antioxidant compounds of some edible plants of Thailand. *Food Chem,* **2005**, *92*, 491–497.

Chatterjee, S.; Chatterjee, S.; Dutta, S. *Cassia alata*—an useful antimicrobial agent. *Med Arom Plants*, **2013**, *2*, e143. Doi: 10.4172/2167–0412.1000e143.

Chauhan, D. K.; Puranik, V.; Mishra, V. Analysis of Stem of *Tinospora cordifolia*, leaves of *Andrographis paniculata* and root and leaves of *Boerhaavia diffusa* for nutritional and phytochemical composition. *Int J Food Nutr Sci*, **2014**, *3*(4), 104–111.

Chintalwar, G.; Jain, A.; Sipahimalini, A.; Banerji, A.; Sumariwalla, P.; Ramakrishnan, R.; Sainis, K. An immunologically active arabinogalactan from *Tinospora cordifolia*. *Phytochem,* **1999**, *52*, 1089–1093.

Choi, C. W.; Kim, S. C.; Hwang, S. S.; Choi, B. K.; Ahn, H. J.; Lee, M. Y.; Park, S. H.; Kim, S. K. Antioxidant activity and free radical scavenging capacity between Korean medicinal plants and flavonoids by assay-guided comparison. *Plant Sci,* **2002**, *163*(6), 1161–1168.

Chopra, R. N.; Chopra, I. C.; Handa, K. L.; Kapur, L. D. *Indigenous Drugs of India*. 2nd ed., UN Dhar: Calcutta, India, 1958.

Demiray, S.; Pintado, M. E.; Castro, P. M. L. Evaluation of phenolic profiles and antioxidant activities of Turkish medicinal plants: *Tilia argentea, Crataegi folium* leaves, and *Polygonum bistorta* roots. *World Acad Sci Eng Tech*, **2009**, *54*, 312–317.

Devasagayam, T. P. A.; Kamat, J. P.; and Sreejayan, N. Antioxidant action of curcumin. In: Nesaretnam, K. and Packer, L. (Eds.), *Micronutrients and Health: Molecular Biological Mechanisms*. AOCS Press; USA, 2001, pp. 42–59.

Devasagayam, T. P.; Sainis, K. B. Immune system and antioxidants, especially those derived from Indian medicinal plants. *Indian J Exp Bio,* **2002**, *40*, 639–655.

Devprakash, S. K. K.; Subburaju, T.; Parag, S. M. Comparative antioxidant studies of ethanol extract and fresh aqueous extracts of *Tinospora cordifolia. Indian J Novel Drug Del,***2012**, *4*(1), 78–84.

Dhingra, D.; Goyal, P. K. Evidences for the involvement of monoaminergic and GABAergic systems in antidepressant-like activity of *Tinospora cordifolia* in mice. *Indian J Pharm Sci,* **2008**, *70*(6), 761–767.

Dixit, S.; Ali, H. Antioxidant potential some medicinal plants of central India. *J Cancer Therapy,* **2010**, *1*, 87–90.

Doss, A.; Doss, A.; Pichai, A.; Dhanabalan, R. *In vitro* antioxidant properties of certain indigenous medicinal plants from Western Ghats of India. *Int J Nutr Wellness,* **2008**, *7*(1), 1–5.

DSA (Development Solutions Associates). *The Medicinal and Aromatic Plants Value Chain in Albania,* USAID—Albania Agriculture Competitiveness (AAC) Program, 2010. URL: http://pdf.usaid.gov/pdf_docs/PA00JN4F.pdf. Accessed on June 18, 2016.

Farnsworth, N. R. Ethnopharmacology and Drug Development. *Ethnobot Sea New Drugs,* **1994**, *185*, 42–51.

Gangan, V. D.; Pradhan, P.; Sipahimalani, A. T.; Banerji, A. Cordifolisides A, B, C: norditerpene furan glycosides from *Tinospora cordifolia. Phytochemistry,* **1994**, *37*(3), 781–786.

Ghate, N. B.; Chaudhuri, D.; Mandal, R. In vitro assessment of *Tinospora cordifolia* stem for its antioxidant, free radical scavenging and DNA protective potentials. *Int J Pharm Bio Sci,***2013**, *4*(1), 373–388.

Ghosal, S.; Vishwakarma, R. A. Tinocordiside, a new rearranged cadinane sesquiterpene glycoside from *Tinospora Cordifolia. J Nat Prod,* **1997**, *60*(8), 839–841.

Goel, H. C.; Prem K. I.; Rana, S. V. S. Free radical scavenging and metal chelation by *Tinospora Cordifolia,* a possible role in radioprotection. *Indian J Exp Bio,* **2002**, *40*(6), 727–734.

Grover, D.; Dutta, S.; Farswan, A. S. *Tinospora Cordifolia*: pharmacognostical and phytochemical Screening. *Guru Drone J Pharm Res,* **2013**, *1*(1), 13–17.

Gupta, R.; Sharma, V. Ameliorative effects of *Tinospora Cordifolia* root extract on histopathological and biochemical changes induced by Aflatoxin-B 1 in mice kidney. *Toxicol Int,* **2011**, *18*(2), 94–98.

Ilaiyaraja, N.; Khanum, F. Antioxidant potential of *Tinospora cordifolia* extracts and their protective effect on oxidation of biomolecules. *Pharmacogn J,* **2011**, *3*(20), 56–62.

Jagetia, G. C.; Nayak, V.; Vidyasagar, M. S. Evaluation of the antineoplastic activity of Guduchi (*Tinospora cordifolia*) in cultured HeLa cells. *Cancer Lett,* **1998**, *127*(1), 71–82.

Jagetia, G. C.; Rao, S. K. Evaluation of cytotoxic effects of dichloromethane extract of Guduchi (*Tinospora cordifolia* Miers ex Hook F & THOMS) on cultured HeLa cells. *Evid Complement Altern Med,* **2006**, *3*(2), 267–272.

Jahfar, M. Glycosyl composition of polysaccharide from *Tinospora Cordifolia. Acta Pharmac (Zagreb, Croatia),* **2003**, *53*(1), 65–69.

Jana, U.; Chattopadhyay, R. N.; Shw, B. P. Preliminary studies on anti-inflammatory activity of *Zingiber officinale* Rosc., *Vitex negundo* Linn. and *Tinospora cordifolia* (Willid) Miers in albino rats. *Indian J Pharmacol,* **1999**, *31*, 232–233.

Jee, V.; Dar, G. H. and Bhat, G. M. Taxoethnobotanical studies of the rural areas in district Rajouri (Jammu). *J Econ Taxon Bot,* **1984**, *5*, 831–834.

Jeyachandran, R.; Xavier, T. F.; Anand, S. P. Antibacterial activity of stem extracts of *Tinospora cordifolia* (Willd) Hook.f and Thomson. *Anc Sci Life*, **2003**, *23*(1), 40–43.

Jhorar, R.; Kaur, A.; Mukherjee, T. K.; Batra, P. Phytochemical analysis and biological studies of Indian medicinal plants *Myristica fragrans* and *Tinospora cordifolia*. *Int J Adv Res*, **2016**, *4*(5), 245–258.

Kapil, A.; Sharma, S. Immunopotentiating compounds from *Tinospora cordifolia*. *J Ethnopharmacology*, **1997**, *58*(2), 89–95.

Kathe, W.; Heym, A.; Honnef, S. *Medicinal and Aromatic Plants in Albania, Bosnia-Herzegovina, Bulgaria, Croatia and Romania*. Federal Agency for Nature Conservation: Bonn, Germany, 2003.

Khan, N. M. M. U.; Akter, N.; Hossain, S.; Rahman, H. New stigmasterol and long chain alcohol from *Tinospora cordifolia*. *Int J Multidiscip Res Dev*, **2015**, *2*(8), 143–145.

Kinkar, S. B.; Patil, K. G. Antidiabetic Activity of *Tinospora cordifolia* (Fam: Menispermaceae) in alloxan treated albino rats. *Appl Sci J*, **2015**, *1*(5), 316–319.

Kinoshita, S.; Inoue, Y.; Nakama, S.; Ichiba, T.; Aniya, Y. Antioxidant and hepatoprotective actions of medicinal herb, Terminalia catappa L. from Okinawa island and its tannin corilagin. *Phytomedicine*, **2007**, *14*(11), 755–762.

Kirtikar, K. R.; Basu, B. D. Indian Medicinal Plants. In: Blatterss Canis, J. R. (Eds.), *Tinospora cordifolia*. Vol. I, Lalit Mohan: India, 1933, pp. 77–78.

Kumar, S.; Sharma, S. Anti-oxidant and anti-butyrylcholinesterase activity of an ethanolic extract of *Tinospora cordifolia*. *European J Pharm Med Res,* **2015**, *2*(4), 1263–1272.

Lanfranco, G. Popular Use of medicinal plants in the Maltese islands. *Insula*, **1992**, *1*, 34–35.

Lemma, A. *The Potentials and Challenges of Endod, the Ethiopian Soapberry Plant for Control of Schistosomiasis. Science in Africa: Achievements and Prospects*. American Association for the Advancement of Sciences (AAAS), Washington, DC, USA, 1991.

Mabona, U.; Viljoen, A.; Shikanga, E.; Marston, A.; Van Vuuren, S. Antimicrobial activity of southern African medicinal plants with dermatological relevance: from an ethnopharmacological screening approach, to combination studies and the isolation of a bioactive compound. *J Ethnopharmacol*, **2013**, *148*(1), 45–55.

Manjrekar, P. N.; Jolly, C. I.; Narayanan, S. Comparative studies of the immunomodulatory activity of *Tinospora Cordifolia* and *Tinospora Sinensis*. *Fitoterapia*, **2000**, *71*(3), 254–257.

Mishra, A.; Kumar, S.; Pandey, A. K. Scientific validation of the medicinal efficacy of *Tinospora cordifolia*. *Sci World J*, **2013**, *2013*, 1–8.

Molan, A. L.; Faraj, A. M.; Mahdy, A. S. Antioxidant activity and phenolic content of some medicinal plants traditionally used in Northern Iraq. *Phytopharmacology*, **2012**, *2*(2), 224–233.

Nagarkatti, D. S.; Rege, N. N.; Desai, N. K.; Dahanukar, S. A. Modulation of Kupffer cell activity by *Tinospora cordifolia* in liver damage. *J Postgrad Med*, **1994**, *40*(2), 65–67.

Nagavani, V.; Rao, T. R. Evaluation of Antioxidant Potential and Qualitative Analysis of Major Polyphenols by RP-HPLC in *Nymphaea nouchali* Burm flowers. *Int J Pharm Pharm Sci*, **2010**, *2*(4), 98–104.

Naik, D.; Dandge, C.; Rupanar, S. Determination of chemical composition and evaluation of antioxidant activity of essential oil from *Tinospora cordifolia* (Willd.) leaf. *J Essent Oil Bear Plants*, **2014**, *17*(2), 228–236.

Nandkarni, A. K. *Tinospora cordifolia. Indian Materia Medica*, 3rd ed., Popular Prakashan: Bombay, India, 1954, p. 1221.

148 Phytochemicals in Food and Health

Narayanan, A.; Raja, S.; Ponmurugan, K.; Kandekar, S.; Natarajaseenivasan, K.; Maripandi, A.; Mandeel, Q. Antibacterial activity of selected medicinal plants against multiple antibiotic resistant uropathogens: a study from Kolli Hills, Tamil Nadu, India. *Benef Microb*, **2011**, *2*(3), 235–243.

Onkar, P.; Bangar, J.; Karodi, R. Evaluation of antioxidant activity of traditional formulation *Giloy satva* and hydroalcoholic extract of the *Curculigo orchioides* Gaertn. *J Appl Pharm Sci*, **2012**, *2*(7): 209–213.

Papitha, R.; Lokesh, R.; Kaviyarasi, R.; Selvaraj, C. Phytochemical screening, FT-IR and gas chromatography mass spectrometry analysis of *Tinospora cordifolia* (Thunb.)Miers. *Int J Pharmacogn Phytochem Res,* **2016**, *8*(12), 2020–2024.

Patel, M. B.; Mishra, S. Hypoglycemic activity of alkaloidal fraction of *Tinospora cordifolia*. *Phytomedicine*, **2011**, *18*(12), 1045–1052.

Pendse, V. K.; Dadhich, A. P.; Mathur, P. N.; Bal, M. S.; Madan, B. R. Anti-inflammatory, immunosuppressive and some related pharmacological actions of the water extract of neem Giloe (*Tinospora cordifolia*): a preliminary report. *Indian J Pharm*, **1977**, *9*(3), 221.

Pendse, V. K.; Mahawar, M. M.; Khanna, N. K.; Somani, K. C.; Gautam S. K. Anti-inflammatory and related activity of water extract of *Tinospora cordifolia*. *Indian Drugs,* 1981, *19* (1): 14–21.

Praveen, N.; Thiruvengadam, M.; Kim, H. J.; Kumar, J. P.; Chung, I. M. Antioxidant activity of *Tinospora Cordifolia* leaf extracts through non-enzymatic method. *J Med Plants Res*, **2012**, *6*(33), 4790–4795.

Premanath, R.; Lakshmi Devi, N. Studies on anti-oxidant activity of *Tinospora cordifolia* (Miers.) leaves using *in vitro* models. *J Am Sci*, **2010**, *6*(10), 736–743.

Rajurkar, N. S.; Hande, S. M. Estimation of phytochemical content and antioxidant activity of some selected traditional Indian medicinal plants. *Indian J Pharmac Sci*, **2011**, *73*(2), 146–151.

Rani, A. A.; Punitha, S. M. J.; Rema, M. Anti-inflammatory activity of flower extract of Cassia auriculata –an i*n-vitro* study. *Int Res J Pharm Appl Sci*, 2014, *4*(1), 57–60.

Rao, P. R.; Kumar, V. K.; Viswanath, R. K.; Subbaraju, G. V. Cardio-protective activity of alcoholic extract of *Tinospora cordifolia* in ischemia-reperfusion induced myocardial infarction in rats. *Biol Pharm Bull*, **2005**, *28*(12), 2319–2322.

Rawal, A.; Muddeshwar, M.; Biswas, S. Effect of *Rubia Cordifolia, Fagonia Cretica* Linn, and *Tinospora Cordifolia* on free radical generation and lipid peroxidation during oxygen-glucose deprivation in rat hippocampal slices. *Biochem Biophy Res Comm*, **2004**, *324*(2), 588–596.

Rege, N. N.; Thatte, U. M.; Dahanukar, S. A. Adaptogenic properties of six rasayana herbs used in Ayurvedic medicine. *Phytother Res*, **1999**, *13*(4), 275–291.

Saleem, A.; Ahotupa, M.; Pihlaja, K. Total phenolics concentration and antioxidant potential of extracts of medicinal plants of Pakistan. *J Nat Sci C*, **2001**, *56*(11–12), 973–978.

Sangeetha, M. K.; Raghavendran, H. R. B.; Gayathri, V.; Vasanthi, H. R. *Tinospora cordifolia* attenuates oxidative stress and distorted carbohydrate metabolism in experimentally induced Type 2 diabetes in rats. *J Nat Med*, **2011**, *65*(3–4), 544–550.

Sarangi, M. K.; Soni, S. A review on Giloy: the magic herb. *Inventi Rapid: Planta Activa*, **2013**, *2*: 1–5.

Sengupta, S.; Mukherjee, A.; Goswami, R.; Basu, S. Hypoglycemic activity of the antioxidant saponarin, characterized as α-glucosidase inhibitor present in *Tinospora cordifolia*. *J Enzym Inhib Med Chem*, **2009**, *24*(3), 684–690.

Shah, G. L. Some Economically important plants of Salsette island near Bombay. *J Econ Taxon Bot*, **1984**, *5*, 753–765.

Shah, G. L.; Yadav, S. S.; and Badri, N. Medicinal plants from Dahanu forest division in Maharashtra state. *J Econ Taxon Bot,* **1983**, *5*, 141–151.

Sharma, A. K.; Kumar, S.; Pandey, A. K. Ferric reducing, anti-radical and cytotoxic activities of *Tinospora cordifolia* stem extracts. *Biochem Anal Biochem*, **2014**, *3,* 153. doi:10.4172/2161-1009.1000153.

Sharma, U.; Bala, M.; Kumar, N.; Singh, B.; Munshi, R. K.; Bhalerao, S. Immunomodulatory active compounds from *Tinospora cordifolia. J Ethnopharmacol*, **2012**, *141*(3), 918–926.

Singh, K. K.; and Maheshwari, J. K. Traditional phytotherapy amongst the tribals of Varanasi district, Uttar Pradesh. *J Econ Taxon Bot*, **1983**, *4*(3), 829–838.

Singh, R. Medicinal plants: a review. *J Plant Sci. Spec Issue: Med Plants*, **2015**, *3*(1–1), 50–55.

Singh, S. S.; Pandey, S. C.; Srivastava, S.; Gupta, V. S.; Patro, B.; Ghosh, A. C. Chemistry and medicinal properties of *Tinospora cordifolia* (Guduchi). *Indian J Pharmacol*, **2003**, *35*, 83–91.

Sinha, K.; Mishra, N. P.; Singh, J.; Khanuja, S. P. S. *Tinospora cordifolia* (Guduchi), a reservoir plant for therapeutic applications: a review. *Indian J Tradit Knowl*, **2004**, *3*(3), 257–270.

Sipahimalani, A. T.; Norr, H.; Wagner, H. Phenyl-propanoid and tetrahydroflourofuran lignan glycosides from the adaptogenic plant drugs *Tinospora cordifolia* and *Dryoetes rouxburghii*. *Planta Medica*, **1994**, *60,* 596.

Sivakumar, V.; Rajan, M. S. D.; Riyazullah, M. S. Preliminary phytochemical screening and evaluation of free radical scavenging activity of *Tinospora cordifolia. Int J Pharm Pharm Sci*, **2010**, *2*(4), 186–188.

Solanki, R. Some medicinal plants with antibacterial activity. *Int J Compr Pharm*, **2010**, *4*(1), 10–15.

Subedi, L.; Timalsena, S.; Duwadi, P.; Thapa, R.; Paudel, A.; Parajuli, K. Antioxidant activity and phenol and flavonoid contents of eight medicinal plants from Western Nepal. *J Tradit Chin Med*, **2014**, *34*(5), 584–590.

Subramanian, M.; Chintalwar, G. J.; Chattopadhyay, S. Antioxidant properties of a *Tinospora cordifolia* polysaccharide against iron-mediated lipid damage and γ-ray induced protein damage. *Red Rep*, **2002**, *7*(3), 137–143.

Sudha, P.; Zinjarde, S. S.; Bhargava, S. Y.; Kumar, A. R. Potent α-amylase inhibitory activity of Indian Ayurvedic medicinal plants. *BMC Complement Altern Med*, **2011**, *11*(1), 1–10.

Swaminathan, K.; Sinha, U. C.; Bhatt, R. K.; Sabata, B. K.; Tavale, S. S. Structure of tinosporide, a diterpenoid furanolactone from *Tinospora cordifolia* Miers. *Acta Crystallogr Sec C*, **1989**, *45*(1), 134–136.

Tambekar, D. H.; Khante, B. S.; Chandak, B. R.; Titare, A. S.; Boralkar, S. S.; Aghadte, S. N. Screening of antibacterial potentials of some medicinal plants from Melghat Forest in India. *Afr J Tradit Complement Alter Med*, **2009**, *6*(3), 228–232.

Tilak, J. C.; Adhikari, S.; Janardhanan, K. K.; Devasagayam, T. P. A.; Lakshmi, B. Antioxidant properties of select Indian medicinal plants in relation to their therapeutic effects. In: Yoshikawa, T., Hiramatsu, M.; and Packer, L. (Eds.), *Molecular Interventions in Lifestyle-Related Diseases*. CRC Press: Boca Raton, FL, 2005, pp. 303–317.

Tilak, J. C.; Devasagayam, T. P. A. Indian medicinal plants: a potential reservoir in health and disease. In: Kohli, K.; Gupta, M.; and Tejwani, S. (Eds.), *Contemporary Perspectives on Clinical Pharmacotherapeutics*. Elsevier: New Delhi, India, 2006, pp. 29–43.

Tripathi, L.; Tripathi, N. J. Role of biotechnology in medicinal plants. *Trop J Pharm Res*, **2003**, *2*(2), 243–253.

Trouillas, P.; Calliste, C. A.; Allais, D. P.; Simon, A.; Marfak, A.; Delage, C.; Duroux, J. L. Antioxidant, anti-inflammatory and antiproliferative properties of sixteen water plant extracts used in the Limousin countryside as herbal teas. *Food Chem*, **2003**, *80*(3), 399–407.

UNESCO (United Nations Educational, Scientific and Cultural Organization). *Culture and Health, Orientation Texts—World Decade for Cultural Development 1988–1997*. Document CLT/DEC/PRO 1996, Paris, France, 1996, p. 129.

Upadhyay, N.; Ganie, S. A.; Agnihotri, R. K.; Sharma, R. Free radical scavenging activity of *Tinospora cordifolia* (Willd.) Miers. *J Pharmacogn Phytochem*, **2014**, *3*(2), 63–69.

Vaidya, A. D. B.; Devasagayam, T. P. A. Current status of herbal drugs in India: an overview. *J Clin Biochem Nutr*, **2007**, *41*(1), 1–11.

Vani, T.; Rajani, M.; Sarkar, S.; Shishoo, C. J. Antioxidant properties of the Ayurvedic formulation Triphala and its constituents. *Int J Pharmacogn*, **1997**, *35*(5), 313–317.

Villa-Ruano, N.; Zurita-Vásquez, G. G.; Pacheco-Hernández, Y.; Betancourt-Jiménez, M. G.; Cruz-Durán, R.; Duque-Bautista, H. Anti-lipase and antioxidant properties of 30 medicinal plants used in Oaxaca, México. *Biol Res*, **2013**, *46*(2).153–160.

Yadav, R. N. S.; Agarwala, M. Phytochemical analysis of some medicinal plants. *J Phytol,* **2011**, *3*(12), 10–14.

Yadav, S.; Nand, P.; Gupta, R. K. Formulation and phytochemicals characterization of polyherbal (*Tinospora cordifolia, Gymnema sylvestre, Pterocarpus marsupium* and *Acacia arabica*) antidiabetic compressed tablet lozenges. *J Pharmacogn Phytochem*, **2015**, *4*(2), 244–253.

CHAPTER 5

Phytomedicinal Study on Brazilian Medicinal Plants for Their Potential in Chronic Diseases Treatment

MARCELO JOSÉ DIAS SILVA[1,*], LARISSA LUCENA PÉRICO,
MARCELO APARECIDO DA SILVA, DANIEL RINALDO,
ALESSANDRA GAMBERO, LOURDES CAMPANER DOS SANTOS,
CLÉLIA AKIKO HIRUMA-LIMA, WAGNER VILEGAS[1,*],
DEEPAK KUMAR VERMA, and MAMTA THAKUR

*[1]UNESP—São Paulo State University, Biosciences Institute,
Coastal Campus of São Vicente, Praça Infante Dom Henrique, s/n,
CEP 11330–900 São Vicente, São Paulo, Brazil*

**Corresponding authors.
E-mails: marcelofarmadias@gmail.com, vilegasw@gmail.com*

ABSTRACT

With the increase in life expectancy, the prevalence of chronic diseases of the digestive tract, such as peptic ulcers and inflammatory bowel disease, and the metabolic syndrome associated with the current obesity epidemic have increased in the population. High cost and adverse reactions have led to the search for herbal medicines. However, the market is more demanding, and it is necessary to look for safer and more effective alternatives that can prevent and cure these diseases. The two projects carried out by the group of Professor Wagner Vilegas ("Sustainable Use of Brazilian Biodiversity: Pharmacological and Chemical Prospection on Higher Plants" and "Standardized Extracts for the Treatment of Chronic Diseases") led to an extensive chemical and pharmacological screening of Brazilian plants with ethnopharmacological indications for the treatment of cancer, ulcers, inflammation, and diarrhea too. The first project aimed to investigate plant extracts more thoroughly under the chemical and pharmacological basis, whereas the second project was designed in order to standardize the method of preparation of the extracts, to evaluate the qualitative and quantitative chemical composition of the extracts according to pharmacopoeial standards, as well as to deeply investigate the mechanistic basis of the biological activities observed. Several alkaloids, flavonoids, terpenoids, saponins, fatty acids, catechins, tannins, and phenolic compounds were isolated, identified, and/or detected. Pharmacological studies have indicated that some of these medicinal species, commonly used by the population, have proven efficacy for various disorders, with promising results. Therefore, next steps intend the production of pharmaceutical formulations that must have effectiveness and safety of use, which will also facilitate the access to the population to these phytopreparations.

5.1   INTRODUCTION

In the context of the national and global panorama, the chronic diseases represent a serious problem in the public health system (Raghupathi and Raghupathi, 2018). The majority of the population all over the world uses "green medicine," traditional homemade preparations, to treat a wide variety of diseases. Throughout the world, herbal medicine has grown markedly. This is due to the growing loss of credibility in ordinary medicine, access to synthetic drugs, and the low availability of drugs distributed through the network service (Rakotomala et al., 2013; Gutierrez et al., 2014; Hsieh et al., 2015). The plants were also used as treatment of acute and chronic problems. Although, Brazil is considered to be have the most biodiversity hots pots of the medicinal plants (Table 5.1). In 2016, Dutra and coworkers published a review paper on Brazilian medicinal plants in which they described status of these plants, which is depicted in Figure 5.1 (Dutra et al., 2016). In Brazilian market, very few products are available and sold that are made by Brazilian origin medicinal plants and are used to treat different illnesses (Calixto, 2000). It is still severely restricted due to the lack of research and development, additional investments in the area of quality control and products standardized. Among them, top 20 products of Brazilian origin medicinal plants with their manufacturing companies are listed in Table 5.2. It should be remembered that the term "herbal medicine" already presupposes as an inherent quality profile. It is inconceivable idea of administering a medicine without the necessary production controls and quality to ensure their safety and security (Calixto, 2000; Ng et al., 2013; Choi et al., 2018). It is in this context that we will make the following discussion.

TABLE 5.1 Some Important Brazilian Medicinal Plants Well Known for Their Potential Uses in Diseases Treatment

Scientific Name	Family	Scientific Name	Family
Acosmium dasycarpum	Fabaceae	*Aeschynomene paniculata*	Fabaceae
Andira humilis	Fabaceae	*Annona crassiflora*	Annonaceae
Austroplenckia populnea	Celastraceae	*Baccharis dracunculifolia*	Asteraceae
Bauhinia curvula	Fabaceae	*Bixa orellana*	Bixaceae
Bowdichia virgilioides	Fabaceae	*Brosimum gaudichaudii*	Moraceae
Byrsonima coccolobifolia	Malpighiaceae	*Byrsonima intermedia*	Malpighiaceae
Byrsonima verbascifolia	Malpighiaceae	*Cabralea polytricha*	Meliaceae
Caryocar brasiliense	Caryocaraceae	*Casearia sylvestris*	Salicaceae
Copaifera langsdorffii	Fabaceae	*Dalbergia nigra*	Fabaceae
Davilla rugosa	Dilleniaceae	*Didymopanax macrocarpum*	Araliaceae
Dilodendron bipinnatum	Sapindaceae	*Emmotum nitens*	Metteniusaceae
Erythrina mulungu	Fabaceae	*Eugenia dysenterica*	Myrtaceae
Eugenia pitanga	Myrtaceae	*Guazuma ulmifolia*	Malvaceae
Hymenaea courbaril	Fabaceae	*Hymenaea stigonocarpa*	Fabaceae
Kielmeyera coriacea	Calophyllaceae	*Lafoensia pacari*	Lythraceae
Lantana camara	Verbenaceae	*Leonotis nepetaefolia*	Lamiaceae
Leonurus sibiricus	Lamiaceae	*Machaerium opacum*	Fabaceae
Miconia albicans	Melastomataceae	*Mimosa caesalpiniifolia*	Fabaceae
Momordica charantia	Cucurbitaceae	*Ocimum gratissimum*	Lamiaceae
Ouratea castaneifolia	Ochnaceae	*Plathymenia foliolosa*	Fabaceae
Plantago major	Plantaginaceae	*Pothomorphe umbellatum*	Piperaceae
Pouteria torta	Sapotaceae	*Qualea grandiflora*	Vochysiaceae
Qualea parviflora	Vochysiaceae	*Roupala heterophylla*	Proteaceae
Roupala montana	Proteaceae	*Rudgea viburnoides*	Rubiaceae
Sabicea brasiliensis	Rubiaceae	*Sclerolobium aureum*	Leguminosae
Senna occidentalis	Fabaceae	*Serjania marginata*	Sapindaceae
Solanum lycocarpum	Solanaceae	*Strychnos pseudoquina*	Loganiaceae
Stryphnodendron adstringens	Fabaceae	*Styrax camporum*	Styracaceae
Tabebuia caraiba	Bignoniaceae	*Terminalia catappa*	Combretaceae
Tabebuia ochracea	Bignoniaceae	*Tamarindus indica*	Fabaceae
Vochysia thyrsoidea	Vochysiaceae	*Zanthoxylum rhoifolium*	Rutaceae
Xylopia aromatica	Annonaceae	*Zeyhera digitalis*	Bignoniaceae

Sources: Modified from Alves et al. (2000) and Di Stasi et al. (2002).

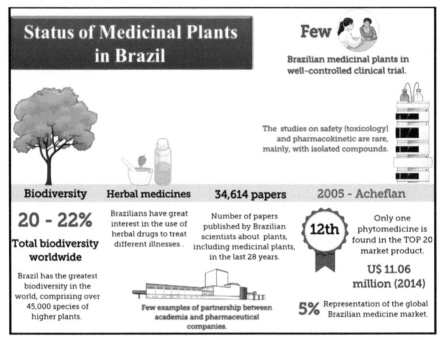

FIGURE 5.1 Status of Brazilian medicinal plants (Dutra et al., 2016). (Reprinted from Dutra, R. C.; Campos, M. M.; Santos, A. R. S.; and Calixto, J. B. Medicinal plants in Brazil: pharmacological studies, drug discovery, challenges and perspectives. *Pharm Res*, **2016**, *112*, 4–29 with permission. © 2016 Elsevier.)

TABLE 5.2 Brazilian Medicinal Plant's Products and Their Manufacturing Companies

Product Name	Manufacturing Company	Product Name	Manufacturing Company
Abrilar	Farmoquímica	Kaloba	Takeda
Acheflan	ACHÉ	Legalon	Takeda
Arlivry	Natulab	Naturetti	SANOFI-AVENTIS
Arpadol	APSEN FARMACÊUTICA	Pasalix	MARJAN FARMA
Calman	Ativus	Phitoss	Brasterápica
Eparema	Takeda	Plantaben	Takeda
Forfig	Eurofarma	Seakalm	Natulab
Ginkolab	Multilab	Tamarine	FARMASA
Ginkomed	CIMED	Tebonin	Takeda
Haar + Hair	INTEM Vitamed	Torante	Eurofarma

Source: Dutra et al. (2016) (adopted from Table 1 of Dutra, R. C.; Campos, M. M.; Santos, A. R. S.; and Calixto, J. B. Medicinal plants in Brazil: Pharmacological studies, drug discovery, challenges and perspectives. *Pharm Res, 2016, 112,* 4–29 with permission. © 2016 Elsevier.)

5.2 PHYTOMEDICINES AND DISEASE PREVENTION

The risk of chronic diseases may be higher when patients have other comorbidity factors such as obesity or chronic use of nonsteroidal anti-inflammatory drugs (NSAIDs) (Marcum and Hanlon, 2010). Table 5.3 indicates some chronic diseases with their variables (measure) and definitions (Raghupathi and Raghupathi, 2018). Studies have demonstrated that there is a relationship between obesity and the increased risk of peptic ulcers since obesity is associated with a chronic inflammatory process, which changes the intestinal microbiota and ruptures the epithelial barrier of the gastrointestinal mucosa (Boylan et al., 2014).

Peptic ulcers are acid injury of the digestive tract, which results from an imbalance between the protective (mucus, prostaglandins, sulfhydryl compounds, blood flow, nitric oxide, etc.) and aggressive (ethanol, stress, NSAIDs, smoking, infectious by the *Helicobacter pylori*, etc.) factors, resulting in mucosal break reaching the submucosa layer. Acid peptic disorders are very common in the United States, with 4 million individuals (new cases and recurrences) affected per year (Dell Vale., 2015).

Peptic ulcers occur more often in men than in women (Kurata et al., 1985). However, these differences are less pronounced after 45 years of age, probably because of the incidence of ulcers increases in women in the menopause period. Some papers report that differences in the incidence of the disease between the sexes are related to the sex hormones and that the female hormones exert a protective effect on ulcerations (El-Tablawy et al., 2012). Interestingly, pregnant women or women using contraceptive pills (estrogen/progesterone) present a reduction in the frequency of duodenal ulcers. In addition, duodenal ulcers follow a more severe course in postmenopausal women than in premenopausal women (Redchits and Petrov, 1995). Thus, similarly to other organs, estrogen may have a protective effect on the gastrointestinal tract (GI). In 2012, El-Tablawy and co-workers demonstrated that estrogen decreases gastric acid secretion and reduces formation of peptic ulcers, an effect that may provide a justification for therapy in the protection of the GI (El-Tablawy et al., 2012; Dong and Kaunitz, 2006), and suggested that the increase in incidence of peptic ulcers in women is related to their increasingly frequent participation in the labor market and in social activities. However, although there are beneficial arguments about the action of estrogen in peptic ulcer, studies are scarce and out of date, limiting to the understanding of the effect of estrogens on peptic ulcers and how they can directly affect processes that lead to its protection. Therefore, the entire study of herbal medicines to combat peptic ulcers should take into consideration the hormonal factors of its users in order to effectiveness of the action.

Recently, we demonstrated the antiulcer effect of hydroalcoholic extract from the leaves of *Eugenia punicifolia* against highly damaging agents such as NSAIDs and ethanol. The effect of this extract is modulated by female sex hormones and mediated by a reduction of neutrophil infiltration, decrease of lipid peroxidation, and increase in catalase activity and glutathione levels in the gastric mucosa (Périco et al., 2019). The importance and relevance of this study are that this is the first study to show that the effect of gastric healing of the medicinal plants is not the same in males and females.

Among the options available for antiulcer therapy are antacids, anticholinergics, H_2 receptor antagonists, proton pump inhibitors (PPIs), an eradication of *H. pylori* with triple drug therapy and cytoprotectors. Some drugs may cause adverse effects and also less effectiveness in the definitive treatment of ulcers (Jain et al., 2007). The antiulcer therapy changed dramatically with the discovery of the bacterium *H. pylori*, because disease was previously related to the secretion of acid and became investigated as an infectious disease. Acid suppressive therapy was substituted by antibiotic therapy (Malfertheiner et al., 2007). However, continued use of these drugs also produces side effects, resistance to antibiotics, osteoporosis, increased incidence of fractures, increased risk of pneumonia, diarrhea and iron deficiency, vitamin-B_{12} and thrombocytopenia. The literature reports that medicinal plants can be sources of substances capable of acting against *H. pylori* (Figure 5.2). Nevertheless, there are still very limited number of works that relate activities to the chemicals components present in the tested extracts depicted in Table 5.3.

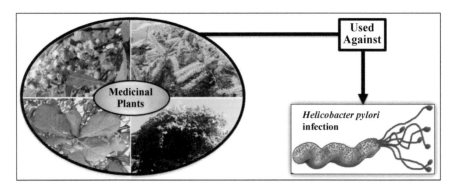

FIGURE 5.2   Medicinal plants used as an alternative approaches against *H. pylori* (Ayala et al., 2014).

TABLE 5.3 List of Some Chronic Diseases with Their Variables (Measure) and Definition

Subcategory of Chronic Disease	Variables (Measure)	Definition
Arthritis	Arthritis (%)	Prevalence of arthritis among adults aged ≥18 years; through 2013 to 2014
	Fair or poor health—arthritis (%)	Prevalence of fair or poor health among adults aged ≥18 years with arthritis— through 2013 to 2014
	Obesity—arthritis (%)	Prevalence of arthritis among adults aged ≥18 years who are obese— through 2013 to 2014
Asthma	Asthma (%)	Current asthma prevalence among adults aged ≥18 years, through 2012 to 2014
	Hospital—asthma (case per 100,000)	Hospitalizations for asthma
	Mortality—asthma (case per 100,000)	Asthma mortality rate through 2010 to 2014
Chronic Kidney Disease	Kidney (%)	Prevalence of chronic kidney disease among adults aged ≥18 years—through 2012 to 2014
	Mortality—kidney (case per 100,000)	Mortality with end stage renal disease, through 2010 to 2014
Chronic Obstructive Pulmonary Disease	Hospital—pulmonary (case per 100,000)	Hospitalization for chronic obstructive pulmonary disease as any diagnosis of 2010 and 2013
	Mortality—pulmonary (case per 100,000)	Mortality with chronic obstructive pulmonary disease as underlying cause among adults aged ≥45 years, through 2010 and 2014.
	Pulmonary (%)	Prevalence of chronic obstructive pulmonary disease among adults aged ≥18 years, through 2012 to 2014
Diabetes	Diabetes (%)	Prevalence of diagnosed diabetes among adults aged ≥18 years—through 2012–2014
	Hospital diabetes (number)	Hospitalization with diabetes as diagnosis; 2010 and 2013
	Mortality diabetes (case per 100,000)	Mortality rate due to diabetes listed as cause of death, through 2010–2014

Source: Raghupathi and Raghupathi (2018) (Partially adapted from Raghupathi, W. and Raghupathi, V. An empirical study of chronic diseases in the United States: a visual analytics approach to public health. *Int J Environ Res Public Health,* 2018, *15*(431), 1–24.)

In addition, although this disease has a chance of cure, its recurrence is almost 100% after two years of treatment discontinuation (Sone et al., 2008), which is related to poor quality of healing (Arakawa et al., 2012) (Table 5.4). The main projects of the group of Professor Wagner Vilegas seek medicinal plants with antiulcer effect that have a synergism of actions including antimicrobial, cytoprotective, anti-inflammatory, antisecretory, antioxidant, angiogenic, and healing.

Another disease that has a high incidence and prevalence is Inflammatory Bowel Disease (IBD) which basically encompasses Crohn's Disease (CD) and Ulcerative Colitis (Ulcerative Colitis, RCU). Although, CD and RCU have been historically studied together because they present same symptoms, damage to common structures, and therapeutic protocols, both are currently two different diseases. IBDs are associated with multiple pathogenic factors, such as genetic susceptibility, intestinal microbiota abnormalities, and deregulation immune responses (de Souza and Fiocchi, 2016).

In Brazil, according to the National Cancer Institute, colorectal cancer is the second main type of cancer in men and women in the Southeast region (INCA, 2014; Barbosa et al., 2015; Bray et al., 2018). The cost involved in treating IBDs is excessively high for the Brazilian reality, justifying the search for alternative therapies. Some medicinal plants have been studied and good results have been obtained in preclinical phases with characterization of anti-inflammatory and/or antioxidant activities or ability to alter the microbiota intestinal (Debnath et al., 2013; Ng et al., 2013).

A work carried out by the group of Professor Wagner Vilegas on species *Byrsonima intermedia* (Santos et al., 2012) and *Rhizophora mangle* (de Faria et al., 2012) presented antioxidant and anti-inflammatory activities on an experimental model of colitis induced by trinitrobenzenesulfonic acid (TNBS). Only one species of *Terminalia*, *Terminalia chebula*, has previously been studied in a model of colitis induced by acetic acid in rats which demonstrated antioxidant, anti-inflammatory, and immunomodulatory properties that was capable of promoting the healing of intestinal lesions (Gautam et al., 2013). We believe that at least chemotaxonomic principle and by the results obtained previously with *T. catappa*, anti-inflammatory and antiulcerogenic activities, the success rate of this plant in the fight against ulcerative colitis is promising.

Silva et al. (2017) evaluated mechanisms of action of phenolic compounds extracted from *Mimosa caesalpiniifolia* after TNBS-induced colitis with a focus on inflammatory markers. This model was accompanied by marked thickening of the colon wall, infiltration of polymorphonuclear leukocytes, and ulceration, resembling human Crohn's disease. The clinical findings of Silva and co-workers demonstrate that the administration of *M. caesalpiniifolia* at dose of 120 or 250 mg/kg were able to mitigate the noxious activities induced by experimental colitis. In the same way, histopathological findings revealed that rats treated with *Mimosa* at 120 or 250 mg/kg mitigate tissue damage

TABLE 5.4 List of Some Medicinal Plants with Their Plant Parts, Type of Materials, and Analysis Method Used Against *H. pylori* Infection

Medicinal Plants	Family	Used Plant Part	Material Types	Analysis Method	Reference
Achillea millefolium	Asteraceae	Areal part	MtE	In vitro	Mahady et al. (2005)
Agrimonia eupatoria	Rosaceae	Herb	EtE	In vitro	Cwikla et al. (2010)
Agrimonia pilosa	Rosaceae	Indefinite	AqE	MICM	Li et al. (2013)
Alchornea triplinervia	Euphorbiaceae	–	MtE and EaF	In vivo	Lima et al. (2008b)
Allium ascalonicum	Liliaceae	Leaf	MtE	In vitro	Adeniyi and Anyiam (2004)
Allium sativum	Liliaceae	Bulb	AqE	In vitro	Cellini et al. (1996)
Alpinia speciosa	Zingiberaceae	Root	EtE	CDM and MICM	Wang and Huang (2005)
Ambrosia confertiflora	Asteraceae	Dried plant	MtE	BMDM	Robles-Zepeda et al. (2011)
Amphipterygium adstringens	Anacardiaceae	Dried plant	MtE	BMDM	Robles-Zepeda et al. (2011)
		Bark	PeE	In vitro	Castillo-Juárez et al. (2007)
Anisomeles indica	Lamiaceae	Air-dried stems	EtE	In vitro	Lien et al. (2013)
		Leaves and stem	EtE	CDM and MICM	Wang and Huang 2005
Annona cherimola	Annonaceae	Leaves/stem	MtE	In vitro	Castillo-Juárez et al. (2009)
Apium graveolens	Apiaceae	Seeds	CAIE	In vitro	Zhou et al. (2009)
Artemisia ludoviciana	Asteraceae	Leaf	EtE	In vitro	Bork et al. (1997)
		Leaves/stem	AqE	In vitro	Castillo-Juárez et al. (2009)
Artocarpus obtusus	Moraceae	Stem bark	PA	In vitro	Sidahmed et al. (2013)
Bacopa monniera	Scrophulariaceae	Whole plant	BmE	In vitro using BMDM	Goel et al. (2003)
Bixa orellana	Bixaceae	Seed	EtE	In vitro	Cogo et al. (2010)
Bombax malabaricum	Malvaceae	Root	EtE	CDM and MICM	Wang and Huang (2005)
Byophyllum pinnatum	Crassulaceae	Dried plant	MtE	BMDM	Robles-Zepeda et al. (2011)
Byrsonima crassa	Malpighiaceae	Leaves	MtE and CfE	MICM	Bonacorsi et al. (2009)
Byrsonima fagifolia	Malpighiaceae	Leaves	MtE	In vitro using DDM and In vivo	Lima et al. (2008a)

TABLE 5.4 *(Continued)*

Medicinal Plants	Family	Used Plant Part	Material Types	Analysis Method	Reference
Byrsonima intermedia	Malpighiaceae	Leaves	MtE	In vitro and in vivo	Santos et al. (2012)
Calophyllum brasiliense	Clusiaceae	Stem bark	HEtE and DcmE	In vitro and in vivo using DDM and BMDM	Souza Mdo et al. (2009)
			HexE	In vitro and in vivo	Lemos et al. (2012)
Camellia sinensis	Theaceae	Shoot	MtE and WaE	In vitro	Hassani et al. (2009)
Carum carvi	Apiaceae	Fruit	MtE, DeE and PeBE	In vitro using DDM	Nariman et al. (2009)
Cassia obtusifolia	Leguminosae	Seed	EtE	UIA	Shi et al. (2011)
Castella tortuosa	Simaroubaceae	Dried plant	MtE	BMDM	Robles-Zepeda et al. (2011)
Chamomilla recutita	Asteraceae	Inflorescence	EtE	In vitro	Cogo et al. (2010)
Cistus laurifolius	Cistaceae	Leaves	CfE	In vitro	Ustün et al. (2006)
		Flowers	CfE	MICM	Yesilada et al. (1999)
Coptis chinensis	Ranunculaceae	Rhizome	AqE	MICM	Li et al. (2013)
Couterea latiflora	Rubiaceae	Dried plant	MtE	BMDM	Robles-Zepeda et al. (2011)
Cratoxylum arborescens	Hypericaceae	Stem bark	CfE, HexE and MtE	In vitro	Sidahmed et al. (2013)
Cuphe aaequipetala	Lythraceae	Aerial parts	AqE	In vitro	Castillo-Juárez et al. (2009)
Curcuma amada.	Zingiberaceae	Rhizome	EtE	In vitro	Zaidi et al. (2009)
Davilla elliptica and *D. nitida*	Dilleniaceae	Leaves	MtE	In vitro using DDM	Kushima et al. (2009)
Dysphania ambrosioides	Amaranthaceae	Dried plant	MtE	BMDM	Robles-Zepeda et al. (2011)
Eugenia caryophyllata	Myrtaceae	Flowers	AqE	MICM	Li et al. (2013)
Feijoa sellowiana	Myrtaceae	Fruit	AcE	In vitro	Basile et al. (2010)
Filipendula ulmaria	Rosaceae	Herb	EtE	In vitro	Cwikla et al. (2010)
Foeniculum vulgare	Apiaceae (Umbelliferae)	Seeds	MtE	In vitro	Mahady et al. (2005)

TABLE 5.4 *(Continued)*

Medicinal Plants	Family	Used Plant Part	Material Types	Analysis Method	Reference
Geranium wilfordii	Geraniaceae	Dried plant	EaF and EtE	In vitro	Zhang et al. (2010)
Glycyrrhiza glabra	Fabaceae	Root	DgE (GutGard)	In vitro	Puram et al. (2013)
			GgFs (GutGard)	In vitro using ADM and BMDM	Asha et al. (2013)
Guaiacum coulteri	Zygophyllaceae	Bark	MtE	In vitro	Castillo-Juárez et al. (2009)
Hancornia speciose	Apocynaceae	Bark	HAlE	In vitro and in vivo	Moraes Tde et al. (2008)
Hericium erinaceus	Hericiaceae	Mushrooms	EtE	In vitro	Shang et al. (2013)
Houttuynia cordata	Saururaceae	Indefinite	AqE	MICM	Li et al. (2013)
Hydrastis canadensis	Ranunculaceae	Root and rhizome	EtE	In vitro	Cwikla et al. (2010)
Ibervillea sonorae	Curcurbitaceae	Dried plant	MtE	BMDM	Robles-Zepeda et al. (2011)
Ilex paraguariensis	Aquifoliaceae	Green and roasted leaves	EtE	In vitro	Cogo et al. (2010)
Jatropha cuneate	Euphorbiaceae	Dried plant	MtE	BMDM	Robles-Zepeda et al. (2011)
Juglans regia	Juglandaceae	Woody fruit ridge	MtE	In vitro	Hajimahmoodi et al. (2011)
Kohleria deppeana	Gesneriaceae	Dried plant	MtE	BMDM	Robles-Zepeda et al. (2011)
Krameria erecta	Krameriaceae				
Larrea divaricata	Zygophyllaceae	Leaves and tender branches	AqE	In vitro	Stege et al. (2006)
Ludwigia repens	Onagraceae	Aerial parts	AqE	In vitro	Castillo-Juárez et al. (2009)
Magnolia officinalis	Magnoliaceae	Bark	EtE	UIA	Shi et al. (2011)
Mallotus philippensis	Euphorbiaceae	Powder covering fruits	EtE	In vitro	Zaidi et al. (2009)
Malva sylvestris	Malvaceae	Inflorescence and leaves	EtE	In vitro	Cogo et al. (2010)

TABLE 5.4 (Continued)

Medicinal Plants	Family	Used Plant Part	Material Types	Analysis Method	Reference
Marrubium vulgare	Lamiaceae	Dried plant	MtE	BMDM	Robles-Zepeda et al. (2011)
Mentha piperita	Lamiaceae	Leaves/stem	AqE	In vitro	Castillo-Juárez et al. (2009)
Mouriri elliptica	Melastomataceae	Leaves	MtE	In vivo	Moleiro et al. (2009)
Moussonia deppeana	Gesneriaceae	Leaves/stem	MtE	In vitro	Castillo-Juárez et al. (2009)
Myrisctica fragrans	Myristacaceae	Seeds/aerial parts Seeds	EtE	In vitro	Zaidi et al. (2009) Mahady et al. (2005)
Nigella sativa	Ranunculaceae	Seed	NsC	In vivo	Salem et al. (2010)
Origanum majorana	Lamiaceae	Aerial parts	MtE	In vitro	Mahady et al. (2005)
Paederia scandens	Rubiaceae	Whole plant	EtE	CDM and MICM	Wang and Huang (2005)
Passiflora incarnata	Passifloraceae	Aerial parts	MtE	In vitro	Mahady et al. (2005)
Pelargonium sidoides	Geraniaceae	Roots	PsE	In vitro	Beil and Kilian (2007); Wittschier et al. (2007)
Persea americana	Lauraceae	Leaves	MtE	In vitro	Castillo-Juárez et al. (2009)
Pteleopsis suberosa	Combretaceae	Bark	MtE	In vitro	Germanò et al. (1998)
Phyllanthus urinaria	Euphorbiaceae	Dried plant	CfE and MtE EtE	In vitro	Lai et al. (2008) Fang et al. (2008)
Pimpinella anisum	Apiaceae	Dried plant	MtE	BMDM	Robles-Zepeda et al. (2011)
Piper carpunya	Piperaceae	Leaves	PcFs EtE	In vitro	Shin et al. (2005) Quílez et al. (2010)
Pistacia lentiscus	Anacardiaceae	Mastic gum	Extract/acid and neutral fractions	In vitro and in vivo	Paraschos et al. (2007)
Plantago major	Plantaginaceae	Above-ground parts	EtE	In vitro	Cogo et al. (2010)
Plumbago zeylanica	Plumbaginaceae	Stem	EtE	CDM and MICM	Wang and Huang 2005
Pscalium decompositum	Asteraceae	Dried plant	MtE	BMDM	Robles-Zepeda et al. (2011)

TABLE 5.4 *(Continued)*

Medicinal Plants	Family	Used Plant Part	Material Types	Analysis Method	Reference
Psoralea corylifolia	Papilionaceae	Seeds	EtE	In vitro	Zaidi et al. (2009)
Punica granatum	Lythraceae	Fruit peel	MtE	In vitro	Hajimahmoodi et al. (2011); Moghaddam (2011)
Rosmarinus officinalis	Lamiaceae	Leaves	MtE	In vitro	Mahady et al. (2005)
Qualea parviflora	Vochysiaeceae	Bark	MtE	In vitro and in vivo	Mazzolin et al. (2010)
Rheum rhaponticum	Polygonaceae	Root	EtE	In vitro	Cogo et al. (2010)
Rhus chinensis	Anacardiaceae	Sumac	AqE	MICM	Li et al. (2013)
Salvia officinalis	Lamiaceae	Herb	EtE	In vitro	Cwikla et al. (2010)
Sclerocarya birrea	Anacardiaceae	Stem bark	CAcE	In vitro	Njume et al. (2011a, b)
Selaginella lepidophylla	Lycopodiaceae	Dried plant	MtE	BMDM	Robles-Zepeda et al. (2011)
Strychnos pseudoquina	Loganiaceae	Leaves	MtE/AIEF	In vitro and in vivo	Bonamin et al. (2011)
Taxodium mucronatum	Cupressaceae	Dried plant	MtE	BMDM	Robles-Zepeda et al. (2011)
Tecoma stans	Bignoniaceae				
Trachyspermum copticum	Apiaceae	Fruit	MtE, DeE and PeBE	In vitro using DDM	Nariman et al. (2009)
Xanthium brasilicum	Asteraceae	Aerial parts			
Zingiber officinale	Zingiberaceae	Rhizome	MtE	In vitro	Mahady et al. (2005)

Abbreviations: AcE: acetone extract, ADM: agar dilution method, AIEF: alkaloid-enriched fraction, AqE: aqueous extract, BMDM: broth microdilution method, BnE: *Bacopa monniera* extract, CAcE: crude acetone extract, CAIE: crude alcoholic extract, CDM: cup-plate diffusion method, CfE: chloroform extract, DCmE: dichloromethanic fraction, DDM: disk diffusion method, DeE: diethyl ether extract, DgE: deglycyrrhizinated extract, EaF: ethylacetate fraction, EtE: ethanol extract, GgFs: *Glycyrrhiza glabra* flavonoids, HAlE: hydroalcoholic extract, HEtE: hydroethanolic extract, HexE: hexane extract, MICM: minimum inhibitory concentration method, MtE: methanol extract, NsC: *Nigella sativa* capsules, PA: pyranocycloartobiloxanthone A, PcFs: *Piper carpunya* flavonoids, PeBE: petroleum benzene extract, PeE: petroleum ether extract, PsE: *Pelargonium sidoides* extract, UIA: urease inhibition assay, WaE: water extract.

induced by TNBS. Taken together, it seems that *M. caeasalpiniifolia* exerts either preventive or protective effects against experimental colitis in rats.

Rates of obesity are rising in patients with IBD, as in the general population; 15%–40% of adults with IBD are obese, and 20%–40% are overweight (Singh et al., 2017). IBD may be an independent risk factor for obesity that is driven by dysbiosis and aberrations in intestinal microbial metabolism (Winer et al., 2016; Karmiris et al., 2006). Treatments used for IBD, in particular corticosteroids and antitumor necrosis factor alpha therapies may also play a role in obesity (Singh et al., 2017). Inflammatory state can lead to impaired nutritional status of patients with IBD. Undernutrition is a major complication among these patients and it is strongly associated with worst prognostic and increased risk of clinical and surgical complications (Rocha et al., 2009). Factors associated with undernutrition in these patients are inadequate food intake, chronic inflammatory state with increased energy requirements, and losses from the GI (Elia et al., 2007; Rocha et al., 2009). On the other hand, the prevalence of overweight and obesity is increasing among these patients, especially in the last decades. Changes in dietary patterns are pointed out as one of the factors causing cardiovascular diseases and, therefore, this population needs careful nutritional follow-up in order to precociously detect patients that are under nutritional risk.

Excess weight has reached epidemic proportions in the world. In Brazil, cases of child malnutrition fall for each research, while the weight of Brazilian children exceeded the world average, demonstrating that childhood obesity is the new focus of health policies. Currently, 7% of the child population is malnourished, whereas 20% is obese (Silveira et al., 2010).

A report of Ministry of Health from Brazil on "surveillance of risk and protection factors for chronic diseases obtained by telephone investigation" revealed that 48.5% of the interviewed population was overweight or obese (NASHMH, 2011). In the beginning of few years back, a research done by the program my Healthy dish (Hospital das Clínicas, FM, USP, São Paulo) revealed that 66.3% of respondents in the city of São Paulo are overweight, 37.4% of them overweight and 28.9% patients with obesity, with 2.7% considered morbidly obese (Grade 3 obesity). Obesity is the critical factor for the establishment of the metabolic syndrome. Associated with obesity is the establishment of a low-grade chronic and systemic inflammation that evolves into a framework of insulin resistance and predispose this population to cardiovascular, metabolic, neurodegenerative diseases and to an increase in incidence of neoplasms (Christensen and Pike, 2015; Gallagher and LeRoith, 2015).

Restrictive diets that lead to weight loss are usually the therapy chosen by patients and clinicians, despite the limited long-term success. The synthetic medications available for the control of obesity are restricted to orlistat, which reduces the absorption of fat by the intestine and sibutramine, appetite suppressor drug, drugs with important adverse effects (Hassan and El-Gharib, 2015). Obese diabetic patients have oral hypoglycemic agents and drugs related to incretins, but these also have adverse effects, high cost, and little impact on the obesity control (Tabatabaei-Malazy et al., 2015). We have examples of natural products that have been employed in recent clinical studies such as *Camelia sinensis* and *Ilex paraguariensis*, suggesting that this is a promising field (Huang et al., 2014; Gambero and Ribeiro, 2015).

But still, the control of the expansion of adipose tissue and/or the establishment and control of inflammation in adipose tissue are therapeutic approaches that need to be explored more. Several species of *Terminalia* have been studied for their anti-obesogenics properties. Extracts obtained from the bark of the *Terminalia paniculatta* showed the ability to reduce body weight and improve glycemic control of rats fed with a hyperlipidic diet, suggesting an important antiadipogenic and antiobesogenic effect (Mopuri et al., 2015). *Terminalia chebula* and *Terminalia arjuna* are plants of Ayurveda medicine employed as safe antiobesogens (Gujarathi et al., 2014; Vasudeva et al., 2012).

Byrsonima crassifolia is traditionally used in the treatment of diabetes in Mexico, and its hexane extract showed great ability to control glycemia in experimental models of type 1 diabetes (Perez-Gutierrez et al., 2010; Gutierrez and Flores, 2014), being the same already demonstrated for *Rhizophora mucronata* (Pandey et al., 2014). Therefore, the species of the genus *Terminalia*, *Rhizophora*, and *Byrsonima* are important therapeutical indications for the combat of metabolic syndrome. In other words, these species may reveal a great potential for use in the control of the obesity epidemic and its comorbidities that have enacted the Brazilian public health system.

All these aspects emphasize, therefore, the need to search for new treatment alternatives and also the importance of conducting studies of new pharmacological targets with consequent expansion of the possibilities of establishing new therapeutic strategies.

5.3 PHYTOTHERAPY—AT A GLANCE

The study of phytotherapics is incomplete if the possibility of its constituents is not considered to present mutagenic and/or cytotoxic properties (Lapa,

2004). In fact, Brazilian legislation predicts that, prior to its registration, a phytotherapic potential should be evaluated for these activities. Plant preparations should be evaluated by in vivo and in vitro pharmacological assays, which demonstrate the alleged efficacy and safety of these plants. For its applicability, it is essential to consider the current norms approved by ANVISA (Agência Nacional de Vigilância Sanitária), a Brazilian Health Regulatory Agency. In this sense, the present study will perform the cytogenetic test for in vitro chromosomal damage (MN test) required in the "Guide for conducting nonclinical toxicology and pharmacologic safety studies necessary for the development of medications."

The definitions employed by ANVISA (NHSARRDC, 2014) for Phytotherapics consider two categories: the phytotherapic drug (MF) and the traditional phytotherapic product (PTP). The first (MF) is obtained with exclusive use of vegetable active raw materials whose safety and efficacy are based on clinical evidence and are characterized by the constancy of its quality. The second (PTP) is obtained with exclusive use of vegetable active materials whose safety and effectiveness are based on safe and effective usage data published in the scientific technical literature and which is designed to be used without the surveillance for diagnostic, prescription, or monitoring purposes. Additionally, PTP may not refer to diseases, disturbances, conditions, or actions considered severe, cannot contain raw materials in known toxic risk concentration and should not be administered by injectable and ophthalmic pathways.

The same resolution (NHSARRDC, 2014) maintained some definitions, such as the marker, which is "a substance or class of substances (e.g., alkaloids, flavonoids, fatty acids, etc.) used as a reference in the quality control of the plant raw material" and the phytotherapic, "preferably having a correlation with the therapeutic effect." However, it adds that "the marker may be of the active type, when related to the therapeutic activity of the phytocomplex, or analytical, when not demonstrated, to date, its relationship with the therapeutic activity of the phyto-complex."

Finally, NHSARRDC (2014) brings the concept of vegetable active pharmaceutical Insumo (IFAV): "plant active raw material, i.e., drug or vegetable derivative, used in the manufacturing process of a phytotherapic."

For MF and PTP, the need to ensure efficacy (pharmacologic evaluation) and safety (toxicological evaluation) is clear. Moreover, it is essential to know the chemical composition (chromatographic profile), the determination of the marker, the evaluation of seasonality, and the development of quantitative analytical methods validated for the quality control of the raw material (derivatives of plant or plant as extracts) and finished products (MF and PTP).

5.4 EXTRACTION AND ANALYSIS

5.4.1 EXTRACTION OF PHYTONUTRIENTS

The chemical composition of medicinal plants may vary because of many biotic and abiotic factors such as environmental stresses (such as salinity and alkalinity, temperatures, and diseases), geographic location (like growing areas, growing conditions, and time), water supply, handling, and availability of soil that tend to increase the phytochemical content. This implies possible alterations in their biological properties and pharmacological activity (Del Valle et al., 2015). Once known and characterized the vegetal raw material (dry and pulverized plant) both in the botanical and chemical aspects, and after developed qualitative and quantitative methods to monitor the chemical composition of the plant and its derivatives (extract, dyes, etc.), the phytopharmaceutical technology can collaborate to optimize the activity and/or application of the extracts. From the standardized material we can apply extraction techniques and especially drying to obtain phytopreparations (standardized dry extracts).

Obtaining the dry extract is an important technological step, because the product thus obtained can have greater chemical, physicochemical, and microbiological stability. In addition, the drying step can guarantee higher concentrations of the vegetable active pharmaceutical input, and greater ease of standardization. The standardized extracts in the dry form also have other advantages, because the longer the service life (chemical and microbiological stability), the greater the ease in transport and storage.

Spray drying (Figure 5.3) has been widely applied to obtain dry extracts with better technological characteristics and a higher concentration of constituents with biological activity (Oliveira and Petrovick, 2010). However, the drying conditions may influence the concentration of the marking substances, as observed for *Bidens pilosa* L., where the concentration of bioactive markers decreased with the increase of the inlet temperature of drying by spraying. In addition, the powders obtained at low inlet drying temperatures showed higher residual moisture and particle size, favoring fluidity properties (Cortés-Rojas et al., 2015).

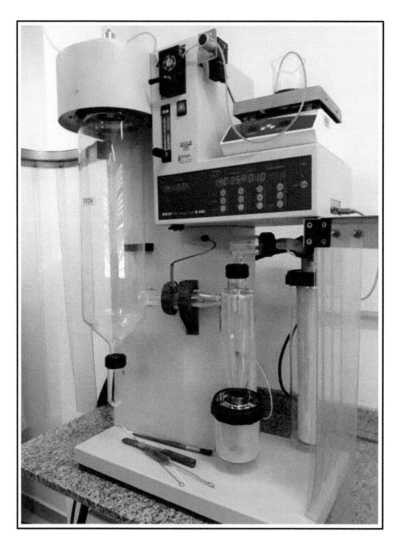

FIGURE 5.3   Laboratory setup of spray dryer instrument. (Picture credit: Laboratory of Medicinal and Phytotherapeutic Plants, Faculty of Pharmaceutical Sciences, UNIFAL—Univ Federal de Alfenas, Alfenas, Minas Gerais, Brazil).

The sprinkler drying technique has several advantages, such as higher physicochemical stability of the obtained product and ease of its derivation in other pharmaceutical forms. For the drying of plant extracts, the choice and proper use of adjuvants in the process are of fundamental importance, because this stage determines the stability and quality of the plants, and it may even affect the bioavailability characteristics (Oliveira and Petrovick, 2010). The process of drying by atomization (Spray Dryer) can, among other factors, increase the solubility and reduce the hygroscopicity of the samples (Daza et al., 2016).

Among various applications, atomization drying can provide greater solubility, bioavailability, and stability. For example, the guaraná extract *(Paullinia cupana Kunth, Sapindaceae)*, known for its potential antidepressants, presents low solubility, bioavailability, and stability, limiting its use. Studies conducted by Klein and collaborators in 2015 who used Spray-drying technique resulted in the obtaining of more stable dry (microencapsulated) extracts using maltodextrin and arabica gum as adjuvants. The microparticles obtained can protect the guaraná extract, maintaining its antioxidant capacity (Klein et al., 2015).

Finally, to better use these benefits and obtain extracts with appropriate technological characteristics, it is necessary to optimize the drying process for each formulation, because some properties of powders (dry extracts) obtained by atomization may be affected by the chemical nature of the plant extracts (Oliveira and Petrovick, 2010; Gallo et al., 2015).

5.4.2 ANALYSIS OF PHYTOPREPARATIONS

Among the several aspects to be considered, there is a need for chemical quality control, which is only possible after a thorough phytochemical study of the plant. A standardized phytopreparation is the one that presents a known content of the active principles and falls within pre-established criteria. This product presents characteristic marking substances and does not have foreign substances (Hostettman et al., 2003).

The biological activity of a plant species often does not depend on a substance but may be based on the synergistic interaction between the components present. For this reason, they are often more suitable for therapeutic use. Therefore, unlike a marker, the qualitative (identification of its components) and quantitative clinical profiles (content of each component of the mixture) of a plant may be more appropriate for the establishment of the chemical control of quality of phytopreparations.

In this context, ultraperformance liquid chromatography (UPLC) is a powerful tool for qualitative and quantitative analyzes of complex matrices, such as plant extracts. The photodiode array detector (PAD) provides spectra in the ultraviolet region of the separated substances, contributing some structural information that allows the identification of classes but is limited to those with chromophoric groups. The mass spectrometer (MS) is much more selective and may be more sensitive depending on the detection mode employed. It provides very important structural information and often allows one to evaluate the composition of a whole plant extract. Therefore, the use of coupled technique of UPLC–MS provides much greater agility, being an indispensable technique in the chemical characterization of a prepared phytopathogen. The UPLC–[PAD]–[MS]^n coupling favors the development of very reliable and selective qualitative and quantitative analyses, since it allows the confirmatory analysis of each detected peak (Harvey et al., 2015).

Quantitative analysis of a plant extract is valid and recommended if the method is validated, since it guarantees that the method used is accurate, specific, reproducible, and robust within an application range in which the analyte is analyzed. ANVISA (NHSARRE, 2003) describes the methods of validation of analytical and bioanalytical methods for the determination of drugs and their impurities. Most chemical studies use toxic solvents (acetonitrile and methanol). Depending on the routine of use, high-performance liquid chromatography (HPLC) or UPLC analyses can generate large amounts of toxic waste, as well as pose risks to the analyst's health and require costly treatments to avoid further contaminating nature (Behnoush et al., 2015).

5.5 GREEN CHEMISTRY IN THE CONTRIBUTION OF THE NATIONAL POLICY OF MEDICINAL AND PHYTOTHERAPEUTIC PLANTS

The studies on medicinal plants are aim to prioritize the scientific reports and the therapeutic results. In this case, there is a contradiction of terms: studies that aim to use toxic solvents/reagents that harm human beings and nature. This contradiction had at the same time the development of new strategies for the study of chemical studies (Lanardão et al., 2003) with a search for alternatives that produce a waste production, called green chemistry, clean chemistry, environmentally benign chemistry, yet, self-sustaining chemistry (Anastas and Warner, 1998). One of the actions was elaborated by ACS GCI—Guide of Selection of Green Solvents, much used in chromatographic investigations.

Today, the number of specific applications of chromatography in the studies of analysis of bioactive plant extracts is much lower than the total of published scientific reports on phytochemical studies and there is one of these models in nonexisting herbal industries. Recent studies have been carried out with hydroalcoholic extracts of *Bauhinia forficata, Casearina sylvestris,* and *Bidens pilosaed* and *Cynara scolymus* by green HPLC (use only water and ethanol in the mobile phase), newer than those using acetonitrile and methanol (Funari et al., 2014a, b; Souza et al., 2018).

In this context, the research group of Professor Wagner Vilegas intends to apply green chromatographic methods to analyze and standardize studied extracts, thus providing environmentally correct options for regulatory bodies for quality control of herbal medicines. For this, our group intends to evaluate the phytopreparations in the following steps:

1. Clean-up in cartridges;
2. Preliminary analyzes by chromatography (on plates and HPLC);
3. Evaluation of phytopreparates by UPLC–PAD– [MS]^n;
4. Development of methodologies for qualitative and quantitative analysis of phytopreparations.

All these studies are valid only if they are carried out with fully botanically identified plant species.

The content of this chapter converges to National Policy of Medicinal and Phytotherapeutic Plants (PNPMF) policies, which aims to "promote the formation of research groups working to address the main epidemiological needs identified in the country." The treatment of chronic diseases is one of the needs not only at the national level but also on a worldwide scale. In addition, the PNPMF guidelines include "fostering research, technological development and innovation based on Brazilian biodiversity, including adapted native and exotic plant species" and "fostering ethnopharmacological research (Lal and Junior, 2011) on medicinal plants traditionally used by the population."

This harmony is emphasized when considering the formation of human resources: PNPMF establishes that "The procedures adopted for Good Practices for Handling/Manufacture of Medicinal and Phytotherapeutic Plants imply technical and scientific training of the professionals involvements should elaborate guidelines of technical and scientific training in the areas of phytotherapeutic production." This is undoubtedly one of the central roles of the University and researchers involved in research projects, as we intend to foster the nucleation of "new research centers specialized in herbal and phytotherapeutic plants," as is the case of the research groups of the University Federal University of São Paulo (UNIFESP), Federal University of Alfenas, and São Paulo State University (UNESP). They all have highly qualified researchers in various fields of knowledge. However, only acting in a network will be able to nuclear new centers in the area of medicinal plants.

Still as a future result, also in line with PNPMF guidelines, it is hoped to generate a favorable environment for the future interaction between the potential of the academic sector and the demands of the productive sector, providing them with scientific and technical support to carry out research on advanced technologies, seeking complementarity between them regarding the stages of the production process, from the bench research phase to the production and commercialization of the product generated. "The guarantee of the quality, effectiveness, and safety of Brazilian herbal medicines will allow to increase the exports of phytotherapics and related inputs," adding value to the vegetal raw materials.

Under the social aspect, Professor Wagner Vilegas aims to expand the "therapeutic options offered to users of the "Health Unic System" (SUS), with a guarantee of access to herbal, herbal remedies, with safety, efficacy and quality (our emphasis) with a view to improving health care for the population and social inclusion."

The project standardized extracts for the treatment of chronic diseases had as objective to investigate medicinal plants that could be applicable in the treatment of chronic diseases: gastrointestinal diseases (ulcers, colitis, and IBD), inflammation, chronic pain, cancer, and diabetes. Extracts were evaluated under pharmacological and toxicological aspects. Under the supervision of Dr. Clélia Akiko Hiruma-Lima, five medicinal plants extract were evaluated, and they are as follows: (1) *Byrsonima intermedia* A. Juss., (2) *Terminalia catappa* L, (3) *Serjania marginata* Casar., (4) *Eugenia punicifolia* (Kunth) DC, and (5) *Arrabidaea brachypoda* (DC) Bureau.

5.6 CURRENT PROJECTS APPROVED BY THE SPONSORING BODY OF THE FOUNDATION FOR RESEARCH SUPPORT OF THE STATE OF SÃO PAULO (FAPESP), UNDER THE SUPERVISION OF PROFESSOR DR. WAGNER VILEGAS

Professor Wagner Vilegas, who received his bachelor's in Chemistry while master's and Ph.D. degree in Organic Chemistry, is currently serving as a professor at Coastal Campus of São Vicente, Biosciences Institute of UNESP—Universidade Estadual Paulista. The area of Professor Wagner Vilegas's research is Natural Products Chemistry that include sustainable use of Brazilian medicinal plants' biodiversity, pharmacological chemistry, and prospecting to superior plants and standardized their extracts for the treatment of chronic diseases. In this context, Professor Wagner Vilegas carried out many projects with his research teams in which they used some of the important Brazilian medicinal plants depicted in Figure 5.4. The species of these medicinal plants exhibited many biological activities (Table 5.5) due to presence of their chemical compounds (Figure 5.5). Table 5.6 indicated some sponsored research support by the state of São Paulo of Brazil and described in different sections.

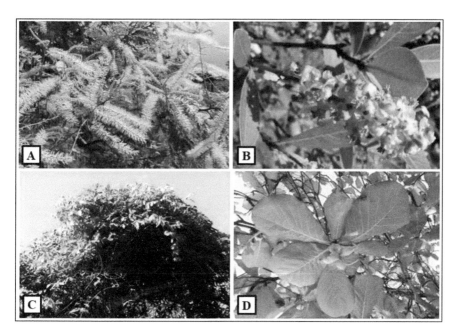

FIGURE 5.4   Important Brazilian medicinal plants used by Professor Wagner Vilegas and his teams in their research. (A) *Mimosa caesalpiniifolia*, (B) *Byrsonima intermedia*, (C) *Serjania marginata*, and (D) *Terminalia catappa*.

5.6.1   ALLELOPATHIC POTENTIAL OF MIMOSA SPP. FOR PHYTOMEDICINES DEVELOPMENT

The use of plants of the Brazilian flora as a source of active principles has been increasingly effective in the search for medicines. However, little has been done to transform this potential into new product development and patents. The present postdoctoral proposal will continue the studies of the thematic project "Standardized Herbal Medicine for the Treatment of Chronic Diseases" of FAPESP, with the species *Mimosa caesalpiniifolia* (Figure 5.4A) in the sense of developing a phytotherapeutic(s). Previous trials shown promising results for the development of phytomedications, with anti-inflammatory and antifungal activities. In addition to supporting activities and

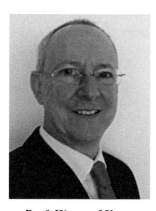

Prof. Wagner Vilegas

research conducted internally, a partnership with the University of Cadiz (UCA) of Spain will allow to evaluate the potential allelopathic extracts/ pure compounds of *Mimosa caesalpiniifolia* in the study of the phytotoxic activity the research group has different techniques and domain in "Studies in allelopathic plants and superior microorganisms" that in Brazil these studies are scarce. Allelopathy is a science that studies the interactions between plants and organisms in their environment mediated by chemical agents is a valuable source as medicinal potential. The group will enrich and complement the studies initially proposed by the thematic project and the present postdoctoral project.

5.6.2 STANDARDIZATION OF PHYTOMEDICINES FOR CHRONIC DISEASES TREATMENT

With increasing life expectancy, the prevalence of chronic diseases (peptic ulcers, inflammatory bowel disease, and metabolic syndrome) has risen among the population. High cost and adverse side effects have led to a search for herbal medicines. However, the market is more demanding, and a search of safer and effective alternatives to prevent and cure these diseases is needed. In this context, this project linked to the thematic project "Herbal Standardized for the Treatment of Chronic Diseases" of FAPESP aims to incorporate phytomedication plant extracts that have been studied by the group with potential antiulcer action and are viable for use as herbal medicines. For the project development, it will be necessary to assess the seasonal variability of plant species, to apply concepts of green chemistry, and further study of these new formulations in chronic diseases of the digestive tract and metabolic syndrome. For this, we need to develop and evaluate chemical, toxicological, and pharmacological, preparations of some of the plant species studied in previous projects that have shown therapeutic potential associated with safe use. The studies were conducted for species *Byrsonima intermedia* A. Juss. (Malpighiaceae), *Serjania marginata* Casar. (Sapindaceae), and *Terminalia catappa* L. (Combretaceae) and are depicted in **Figure 5.4**, which shows promising gastroprotective activity, anti-inflammatory, and no toxicity. The species *B. intermedia* and *S. marginata* still have significant results of antimutagenicity. Promising activities and ease of collection and/ or cultivation were two of the parameters that have guided us for the choice of these species.

TABLE 5.5 Biological Activities of Brazilian Medicinal Plants Used by Professor Wagner Vilegas and His Research Teams

Medicinal Plants Species	Biological Activity
Byrsonima spp.	Antidiabetic (Perez-Gutierrez et al., 2010; Pérez-Gutierrez and Ramirez, 2016), antidiarrhea (Figueiredo et al., 2005; Lima et al., 2008a; Santos et al., 2012), anti-inflammatory (Maldini et al., 2009; Moreira et al., 2011; Saldanha et al., 2016a, b), antimicrobial (Sannomiya et al., 2005a; Lima et al., 2008a; Bonacorsi et al., 2009; Bonacorsi et al., 2011; Santos et al., 2012), antioxidant (Mariutti et al., 2014), antiulcerogenic effect (Sannomiya et al., 2005b; Lima et al., 2008a; Santos et al., 2012; Bonacorsi et al., 2013; Santos et al., 2019), central nervous system depressant (Herrera-Ruiz et al., 2011), giardicidal (Amaral et al., 2006), mutagenic and antimutagenic (Cardoso et al., 2006; Sannomiya et al., 2007; Lira Wde et al., 2008; Lima et al., 2008a; Espanha et al., 2014), antitumoral (Carli et al., 2009), and antitubercular (Higuchi et al., 2011).
Mimosa spp.	Acetylcholinesterase (Trevisan and Macedo, 2003), antidiabetic (Ahmed et al., 2012), antifungal (Morais et al., 2012), anti-inflammatory (Rakotomala et al., 2013; Cruz et al., 2016), antimicrobial (Genest et al., 2008; Mohan et al., 2011), antinociceptive (Rejón-Orantes et al., 2013; Magalhães et al., 2018; Cruz et al., 2016), antioxidant (Nunes et al., 2008; Lin et al., 2011; Patro et al., 2016b), antiulcerogenic (Vinothapooshan and Sundar, 2010), cytotoxic and antitumor (Monção et al., 2015; Chowdhury et al., 2008), anticolitic (Silva et al., 2018), antigenotoxic (Silva et al., 2014); dermatoheliosis (Ijaz et al., 2019); wound healing (Choi et al., 2018); diuretic (Schlickmann et al., 2018); antianxiety, antidepressant, and memory-enhancing activities (Patro et al., 2016a) and pancreatitis (Kaur et al., 2016).
Serjania spp.	Antimicrobial (Lima et al., 2006; Cardoso et al., 2013; Périco et al., 2015), antifungal (Ekabo et al., 1996), anti-inflammatory (Napolitano et al., 2005; Gomig et al., 2008, Salinas-Sánchez et al., 2017), antioxidant (David et al., 2007), antiprotozoal (Mesquita et al., 2005), antispasmodic (Silva et al., 2012), antiulcer (Castelo et al., 2009; Castelo et al., 2009; Silva et al., 2012; Périco et al., 2015), larvicidal (Rodrigues et al., 2006), molluscicidal (Ekabo et al., 1996), trypanocidal (Polanco-Hernández et al., 2012), antimutagenic (Périco et al., 2015), antitoxicity (Silva Moreira et al., 2019), leishmanicidal (Alves Passos et al., 2017), and anti-alzheimer (Guimarães et al., 2015).
Terminalia spp.	Antiaging (Wen et al., 2011), antibacterial (Taganna et al., 2011; Dharmaratne et al., 2018; Allyn et al., 2018; Mandeville and Cock 2018; Bano et al., 2019), anticancer (Ko et al., 2002; Yang et al., 2010; Yeh et al., 2012; Pandya et al., 2013; Naitik et al., 2012; Sales et al., 2018; Lee et al., 2019), antidiabetic (Nagappa et al., 2003; Ahmed et al., 2005; Anand et al., 2015), antihepatotoxic (Lin et al., 1997), anti-inflammatory (Fan et al., 2004; Tanaka et al., 2018; Jayesh et al., 2018; Bag et al., 2019; Jitta et al., 2019), antimicrobial (Pawar and Pal, 2002; Kloucek et al., 2005; Nair and Chanda, 2008; Shinde et al., 2009), antimitochondrial (Tang et al., 2004), antimutagen (Chen et al., 2000), antinociceptive (Ratnasooriya et al., 2002), antioxidant (Lin et al., 2001; Chen and Li, 2006; Chyau et al., 2006; Kinoshita et al., 2007; Rajkumari et al., 2018; Huang et al., 2018; Kaneria et al., 2018; Sheng et al., 2018; Anokwuru et al., 2018), antiviral (Tan et al., 1991), hepato-protective (Gao et al., 2004; Tang et al., 2006; Kinoshita et al., 2007; Toppo et al., 2018; Bhattacharjee et al., 2019), modulatory (Aimola et al., 2014), radical scavenging (Lin et al., 2001; Tang et al., 2004), wound healing (Khan et al., 2014), antimicrobial (Pinheiro Silva et al., 2015), antiulcerogenic (Pinheiro Silva et al., 2015), gastric healing (Pinheiro Silva et al., 2015), antigenotoxicity (Beserra et al., 2018), antitoxicity (Beserra et al., 2018), neurotoxicity (Khalaf et al., 2019), cardiovascular (Liu et al., 2018; Shaik et al., 2018; Bhattacharjee et al., 2019; Mohanty et al., 2019), anticolitic (Cota et al., 2019), anxiolytic activity (Chandrasekhar et al., 2018), antifungal (Machado-Goncalves et al., 2018), anticholinergic (Kim et al., 2018), and antimycobacterial effects (Salih et al., 2018).

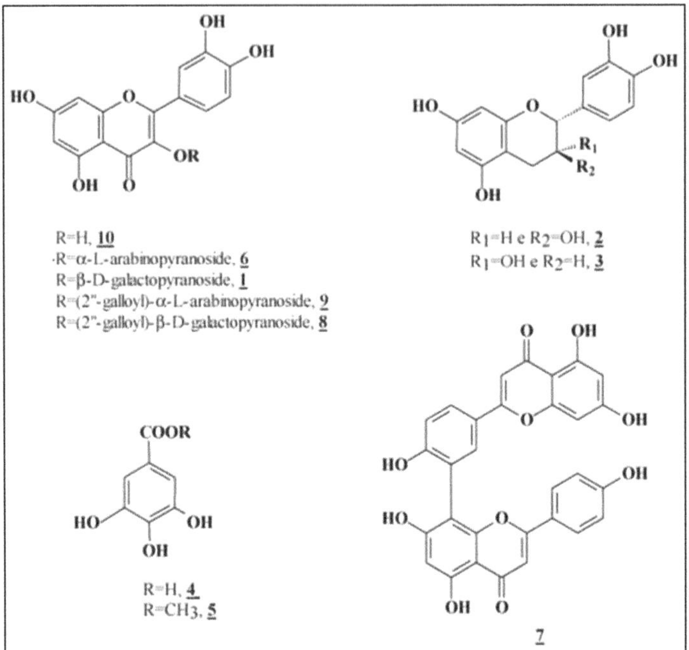

R=H, **10**
·R=α-L-arabinopyranoside, **6**
R=β-D-galactopyranoside, **1**
R=(2″-galloyl)-α-L-arabinopyranoside, **9**
R=(2″-galloyl)-β-D-galactopyranoside, **8**

R$_1$=H e R$_2$=OH, **2**
R$_1$=OH e R$_2$=H, **3**

R=H, **4**
R=CH$_3$, **5**

7

quercetin-3-*O*-β-D-galactopyranoside **1**, (+)-catechin **2**, (−)-epicatechin **3**, gallic acid **4**, methyl gallate **5**, quercetin-3-*O*-α-L-arabinopyranoside **6**, amentoflavone **7**, quercetin-3-*O*-(2″-*O*-galloyl)-β-galactopyranoside **8**, quercetin-3-*O*-(2″-*O*-galloyl)-α-arabinopyranoside **9** and quercetin **10**

FIGURE 5.5A Structures of chemical compounds reported in *Byrsonima intermedia* (Sannomiya et al., 2007). (Reprinted from Sannomiya, M.; Cardoso, C. R. P.; Figueiredo, M. E.; Rodrigues, C. M.; dos Santos, L. C.; dos Santos, F. V.; Serpeloni, J. M.; Cólus, I. M. S.; Vilegas, W.; and Varanda, E. A. Mutagenic evaluation and chemical investigation of *Byrsonima intermedia* A. Juss. leaf extracts. *J Ethnopharmacol*, **2007**, *112*(2), 319–326 with permission. © 2007 Elsevier.)

5.6.3 STANDARDIZATION OF PLANT EXTRACTS OF MIMOSA SPP. FOR PHYTOMEDICINES DEVELOPMENT

The uses of flora/plants as a source of active ingredients have been shown to be increasingly effective in the search for medicines. However, little has been done to turn this potential in developing new products and patents. This proposal for a postdoctoral project under the theme "Standardized Herbal for Treating Chronic Diseases" of FAPESP aims to give continuity to the studies with the species *Mimosa caesalpiniifolia* toward developing a phytotherapeutic in accordance with the requirements of current legislation.

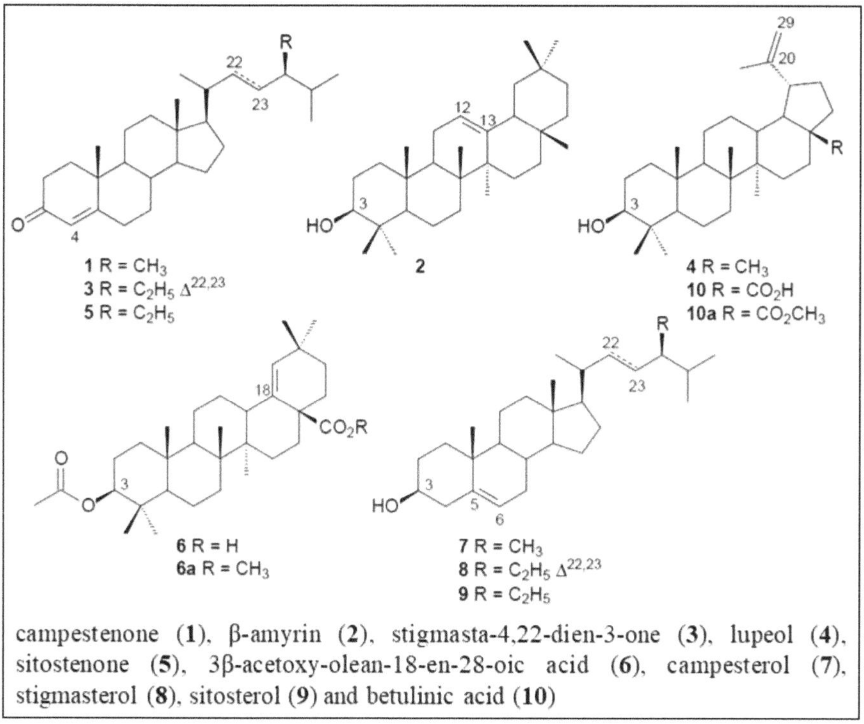
1 R = CH3
3 R = C2H5 Δ22,23
5 R = C2H5
2
4 R = CH3
10 R = CO2H
10a R = CO2CH3
6 R = H
6a R = CH3
7 R = CH3
8 R = C2H5 Δ22,23
9 R = C2H5
campestenone (1), β-amyrin (2), stigmasta-4,22-dien-3-one (3), lupeol (4), sitostenone (5), 3β-acetoxy-olean-18-en-28-oic acid (6), campesterol (7), stigmasterol (8), sitosterol (9) and betulinic acid (10)

FIGURE 5.5B Structures of chemical compounds reported in *Mimosa caesalpiniifolia* (Monção et al., 2015). (Reprinted from Monção, N. B. N.; Araújo, B. Q.; Silva, J. D. N.; Lima, D. J. B.; Ferreira, P. M. P.; Airoldi, F. P. S.; Pessoa, C.; and Citó, A. M. G. L. Assessing chemical constituents of *Mimosa caesalpiniifolia* stem bark: possible bioactive components accountable for the cytotoxic effect of *M. caesalpiniifolia* on human tumour cell lines. *Molecules* **2015**, *20*, 4204–4224 (http://creativecommons.org/licenses/by/4.0/).

Pharmacological tests shall be carried out with the compounds already isolated from *Mimosa caesalpiniifolia,* once in previous project these same compounds showed promising results for the development of plant health care, with anti-inflamatória and antifungal activities. The work will be transdisciplinary, with participants from various campus of UNESP and other universities (Institute of Bioscience of São Vicente, Institute of chemistry of Araraquara, and Institute of Bioscience of Botucatu), UEM (Department of Pharmacy—Palafito), UNIFESP (Institute of Bioscience of Baixada Santista) and UNIFAL/MG (Food and Drug Department). A partnership with the UCA of Spain will allow the exchange of methodologies and scientific information with Spanish group of chemists and pharmacologists in the field

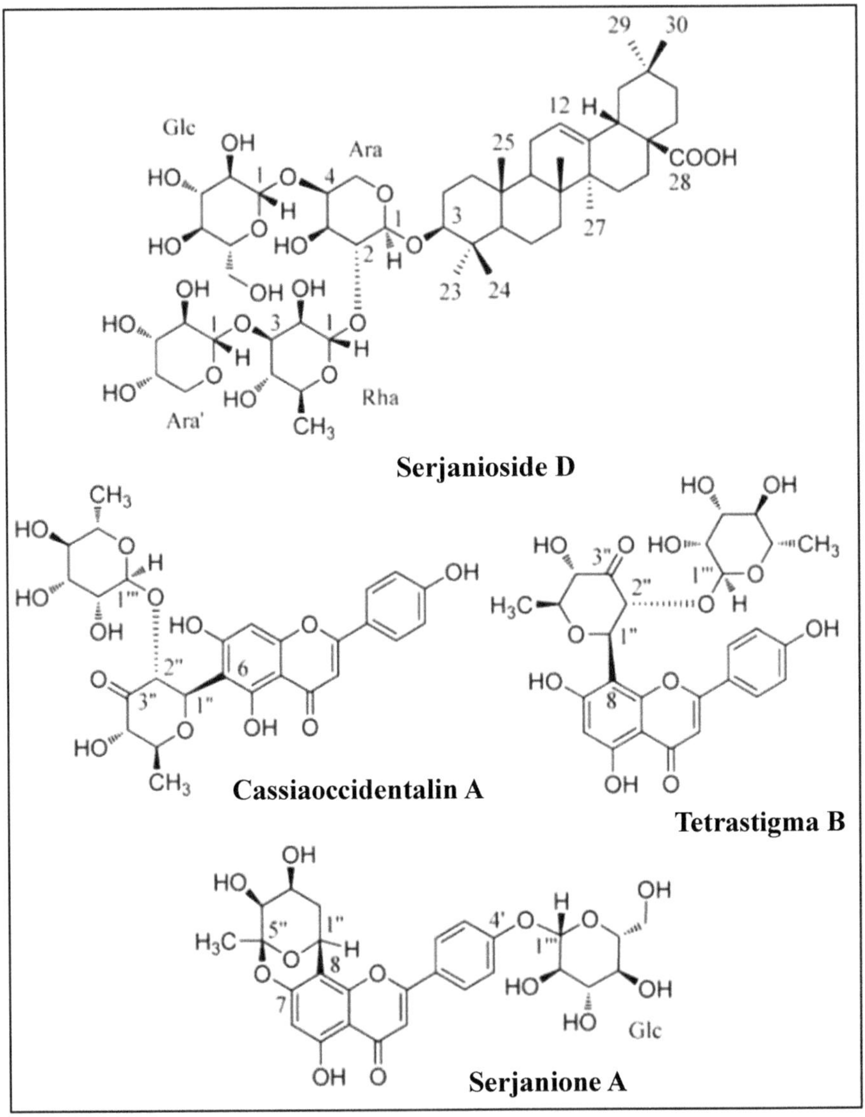

FIGURE 5.5C Structures of chemical compounds reported in *Serjania marginata* (Heredia-Vieira et al., 2015). (Reprinted from Heredia-Vieira, S. C.; Simonet, A. M.; Vilegas, W.; and Macías, F. A. Unusual C,O-fused glucosylapigenins from *Serjania marginata* leaves. *J Nat Prod*, **2015**, *78*, 77–84 with permission. 2015. © American Chemical Society.)

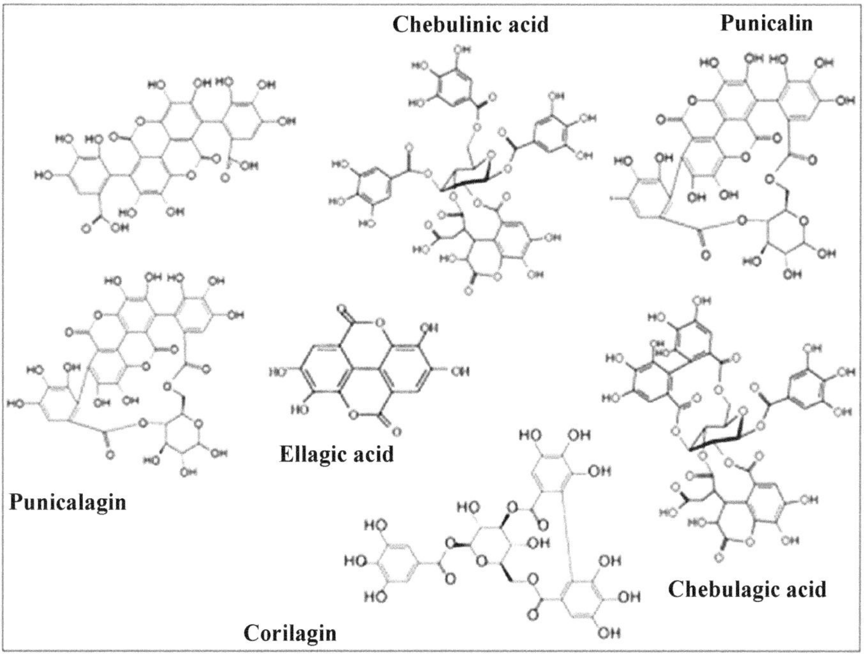

FIGURE 5.5D Structures of chemical compounds reported in *Terminalia catappa* (Dwevedi et al., 2016). (Reprinted from Dwevedi, A.; Dwivedi, R.; and Sharma, Y. K. Exploration of phytochemicals found in *Terminalia* sp. and their antiretroviral activities. *Pharmacogn Rev*, 2016, *10*(20), 73–83. Open access.)

TABLE 5.6 Current Approved Projects Under the Supervision of Professor Dr. Wagner Vilegas

Approved Projects	Period/Duration	Granted Finance	Researcher
Allelopathic potential of *Mimosa* spp. in the development of phytomedicines	15/09/2017 to 14/09/2018	US$ 42.734,11	Marcelo José Dias Silva
Standardization of phytomedicines for the treatment of chronic diseases	01/12/2017 to 31/07/2019	US$ 25.345,76	Ana Caroline Zanatta Silva
Standardization of plant extracts of *Mimosa* spp. development phytomedicines	01/05/2016 to 16/05/2019	US$ 50.598,89	Marcelo José Dias Silva

of product development, enriching and supplementing the objectives initially proposed by project and by this project linked to it.

5.7   CONCLUSION

The group of Professor Wagner Vilegas aims to produce phytopreparations from Brazilian plants to assist in the treatment of chronic diseases such as obesity, inflammation, and gastrointestinal diseases. The mastery of the processes of extraction and preparation of phytopreparations generates innovations that enable the destination of these materials for the phytotherapic production sector. The industrial manufacturing of a phytotherapic can only occur after the execution of the guarantee of the chemical and pharmacological integrity of its active principles. This type of innovation (science based) is what allows to increase the possibilities of the phytotherapic industries and the like to apply structured knowledge in universities. There are recurring discussions in scientific events about the absence of Brazilian products in the market, and one of the causes is the lack of continuity of studies of the plant extracts oriented by the pharmaceutical technology. The interruption of these studies is precisely one of the barriers that block the introduction of innovative products in the market.

KEYWORDS

- **biological activities**
- **chronic diseases**
- **disease prevention**
- **herbal medicines**
- **medicinal plants**
- **pharmacological studies**
- **phytomedicines**
- **phytopreparations**
- **plant's products**

REFERENCES

Abdel-Aziz, H.; Kelber, O.; Lorkowski, G.; and Storr, M. Evaluating the multitarget effects of combinations through multistep clustering of pharmacological data: the example of the commercial preparation Iberogast. *Planta Medica*, **2017**, *83*(14/15): 1130–1140.

Adeniyi, B. A.; and Anyiam, F. M. *In vitro* anti-*Helicobacter pylori* potential of methanol extract of *Allium ascalonicum* Linn. (Liliaceae) leaf: susceptibility and effect on urease activity. *Phytother. Res.* **2004**, *18*, 358–361.

Ahmed, S. M.; Vrushabendra Swamy, B. M.; Gopkumar, P.; Dhanapal, R.; and Chandrashekara, V. M. Anti-Diabetic Activity of *Terminalia catappa* Linn. leaf extracts in alloxan-induced diabetic rats. *Iran J Pharmacol Ther*, **2005**, 4, 36–39.

Ahmed, T.; Imam, K. M. S. U.; Rahman, S.; Mou, S. M.; Choudhury, M. S.; Mahal, M. J.; Jahan, S.; Hossain, M. S.; and Rahmatullah, M. Antihyperglycemic and antinociceptive activity of Fabaceae family plants—an evaluation of *Mimosa pigra* L. stems. *Adv Nat Sci*, **2012**, *6*, 1490–1495.

Aimola, I. A.; Inuwa, H. M.; Nok, A. J.; and Mamman, A. I. Induction of foetal haemoglobin synthesis in erythroid progenitor stem cells: mediated by water-soluble components of *Terminalia catappa*. *Cell Biochem Funct*. **2014**, 32, 361–367.

Allyn, O. Q.; Kusumawati, E.; and Nugroho, E. A. Antimicrobial Activity of *Terminalia catappa* brown leaf extracts against *Staphylococcus aureus* ATCC 25923 and *Pseudomonas aeruginosa* ATCC 27853. *F1000Res*, **2018**, *7*(1406), 1–9.

Alves, T. M. A.; Silva, A. F.; Brandão, M.; Grandi, T. S. M.; Smânia, E. F. A.; Júnior, A. S.; and Zani, C. L. Biological screening of Brazilian medicinal plants. *Mem Inst Oswaldo Cruz,* **2000**, *95*(3), 367–373.

Alves Passos, C. L.; Rodríguez, R.; Ferreira, C.; Costa Soares, D.; Vieira Somner, G.; Hamerski, L.; da Cunha Pinto, A.; Moraes Rezende, C.; and Saraiva, E. M. Anti-leishmania amazonensis activity of *Serjania lethalis* A. St.-Hil. *Parasitol Int*, **2017**, *66*(1), 940–947.

Amaral, F. M. M.; Ribeiro, M. N. S.; Barbosa-Filho, J. M.; Reis, A. S.; Nascimento, F. R. F.; and Macedo, R. O. Plants and chemical constituents with giardicidal activity. *Rev Bras Farmacogn*, **2006**, *16*(Suppl.), 696–720.

Anand, A. V.; Divya, N.; and Kotti, P. P. An updated review of *Terminalia catappa*. *Pharmacogn Rev*. **2015**, *9*, 93–98.

Anastas, P. T.; and Warner, J. C. Green chemistry: theory and practice. Oxford University Press, New York, 1998.

Anokwuru, C.; Sigidi, M.; Boukandou, M.; Tshisikhawe, P.; Traore, A.; and Potgieter, N. Antioxidant activity and spectroscopic characteristics of extractable and non-extractable phenolics from *Terminalia sericea* Burch. ex DC. *Molecules*, **2018**, *23*(6), 1–17.

Arakawa, T.; Watanabe, T.; Tanigawa, T.; Tominaga, K.; Fujiwara,Y.; Morimoto, K. Quality of ulcer healing in gastrointestinal tract: its pathophysiology and clinical relevance. *World J Gastroenterol*, **2012**, *18*, 4811–4822.

Asha, M. K.; Debraj, D.; Prashanth, D.; Edwin, J. R.; Srikanth, H. S.; Muruganantham, N.; Dethe, S. M.; Anirban, B.; Jaya, B.; Deepak, M.; and Agarwal, A. *In vitro* anti-*Helicobacter pylori* activity of a flavonoid rich extract of *Glycyrrhiza glabra* and its probable mechanisms of action. *J Ethnopharmacol,* **2013**, *145*, 581–586.

Bag, P. K.; Roy, N.; Acharyya, S.; Saha, D. R.; Koley, H.; Sarkar, P.; and Bhowmik, P. *In vivo* fluid accumulation-inhibitory, anticolonization and anti-inflammatory and *in vitro* biofilm-inhibitory activities of methyl gallate isolated from *Terminalia chebula* against fluoroquinolones resistant *Vibrio cholerae*. *Microb Pathogen*, **2019**, *128*, 41–46.

Bano, S.; Intisar, A.; Rauf, M.; Ghaffar, A.; Yasmeen, F.; Zaman, W. U.; Intisar, U.; Kausar, G.; Muhammad, N.; and Aamir, A. Comparative analysis of oil composition and antibacterial activity of aerial parts of *Terminalia arjuna* (Roxb.). *Nat Prod Res*, **2019**, *8*, 1–4.

Barbosa, I. R.; de Souza, D. L.; Bernal, M. M.; and do C Costa, Í. Cancer mortality in Brazil: temporal trends and predictions for the year 2030. *Medicine* **2015**, *94*(16), e746. DOI: 10.1097/MD.0000000000000746

Basile, A.; Conte, B.; Rigano, B.; Senatore, B.; and Sorbo, S. Antibacterial and antifungal properties of acetonic extract of *Feijoa sellowiana* fruits and its effect on *Helicobacter pylori* growth. *J Med Food*, **2010**, *13*, 189–195.

Behnoush, B.; Sheikhazadi, A.; Bazmi, E.; Fattahi, A.; Sheikhazadi, E.; and Saberi Anary, S. H. Comparison of UHPLC and HPLC in benzodiazepines analysis of postmortem samples: a case-control study. *Medicine*, **2015**, *94*(14), e640. DOI: 10.1097/MD.0000000000000640

Beil, W.; and Kilian, P. EPs 7630, an extract from *Pelargonium sidoides* roots inhibits adherence of *Helicobacter pylori* to gastric epithelial cells. *Phytomed*, **2007**, *14*(Suppl 6), 5–8.

Beserra, A. M. S. E. S.; Vilegas, W.; Tangerina, M. M. P.; Ascêncio, S. D.; Soares, I. M.; Pavan, E.; Damazo, A. S.; Ribeiro, R. V.; and Martins, D. T. O. Chemical characterisation and toxicity assessment *in vitro* and *in vivo* of the hydroethanolic extract of *Terminalia argentea* Mart. leaves. *J Ethnopharmacol*, **2018,** *227*: 56–68.

Bhattacharjee, B.; Pal, P. K.; Ghosh, A. K.; Mishra, S.; Chattopadhyay, A.; and Bandyopadhyay, D. Aqueous bark extract of *Terminalia arjuna* protects against cadmium-induced hepatic and cardiac injuries in male Wistar rats through antioxidative mechanisms. *Food Chem Toxicol*, **2019**, *124*, 249–64.

Bonacorsi, C.; da Fonseca, L. M.; Raddi, M. S.; Kitagawa, R. R.; and Vilegas, W. Comparison of Brazilian plants used to treat gastritis on the oxidative burst of *Helicobacter pylori*-stimulated neutrophil. *Evid Based Complement Altern Med*, **2013**, *2013*, 1–8.

Bonacorsi, C.; Raddi, M. S. G.; Carlos, I. Z.; Sannomiya, M.; and Vilegas, W. Anti-*Helicobacter pylori* activity and immunostimulatory effect of extracts from *Byrsonima crassa* Nied. (Malpighiaceae). *BMC Complement Altern Med*, **2009**, *9*(1), 1–7.

Bonacorsi, C.; Raddi, M. S. G.; da Fonseca, L. M.; Sannomiya, M.; and Vilegas, W. Effect of *Byrsonima crassa* and phenolic constituents on *Helicobacter pylori*-induced neutrophils oxidative burst. *Int J Mol Sci*, **2011**, *13*(1), 133–141.

Bonamin, F.; Moraes, T. M.; Kushima, H.; Silva, M. A.; Rozza, A. L.; Pellizzon, C. H.; Bauab, T. M.; Rocha, L. R. M.; Vilegas, W.; and Hiruma-Lima, C. A. Can a *Strychnos* species be used as antiulcer agent? ulcer healing action from alkaloid fraction of *Strychnos pseudoquina* St. Hil. (Loganiaceae). *J Ethnopharmacol*, **2011**, *138*, 47–52.

Bork, P. M.; Schmitz, M. L.; Kuhnt, M.; Escher, C. and Heinrich, M. Sesquiterpene lactone containing Mexican Indian medicinal plants and pure sesquiterpene lactones as potent inhibitors of transcription factor NF-kappaB. *FEBS Lett.*, **1997**, *402*, 85–90.

Boylan, M. R.; Khalili, H.; Huang, E. S.; and Chan, A. T. Measures of Adiposity Are Associated With Increased Risk of peptic ulcer. *Clin Gastroenterol Hepatol*, **2014**, *12*(10), 1688–1694.

Bray, F.; Ferlay, J.; Soerjomataram, I.; Siegel. L.; Torre, L. A.; and Jemal, A. Global cancer statistics 2018: GLOBOCAN estimates of incidence and mortality worldwide for 36 cancers in 185 countries. *CA: Cancer J Clin*, **2018**, *68*, 394–424.

Calixto, J. B. Efficacy, safety, quality control, marketing and regulatory guidelines for herbal medicines (phytotherapeutic agents). *Brazilian J Med Biol Res, 2000, 33,* 179–189.

Cardoso, C. A. L.; Coelho, R. G.; Honda, N. K.; Pott, A.; Pavan, F. R.; and Leite, C. Q. F. Phenolic compounds and antioxidant, antimicrobial and antimycobacterial activities of *Serjania erecta* Radlk. (Sapindaceae). *Brazilian J Pharm Sci,* **2013,** *49*(4), 775–782.

Cardoso, C. R.; de Syllos Cólus, I. M.; Bernardi, C. C.; Sannomiya, M.; Vilegas, W.; and Varanda, E. A. Mutagenic activity promoted by amentoflavone and methanolic extract of Byrsonima crassa Niedenzu. *Toxicology,* **2006,** *225*(1), 55–63.

Carli, C. B.; de Matos, D. C.; Lopes, F. C.; Maia, D. C.; Dias, M. B.; Sannomiya, M.; Rodrigues, C. M.; Andreo, M. A.; Vilegas, W.; Colombo, L. L.; and Carlos, I. Z. Isolated flavonoids against mammary tumour cells LM2. *Z Naturforsch C,* **2009,** *64*(1–2), 32–36.

Castelo, A. P.; Arruda, B. N.; Coelho, R. G.; Honda, N. K.; Ferrazoli, C.; Pott, A. and Hiruma-Loma, C. A. Gastroprotective effect of *Serjania erecta* Radlk (Sapindaceae): involvement of sensory neurons, endogenous nonprotein sulfhydryls, and nitric oxide. *J Med Food,* **2009,** 12(6), 1411–1415.

Castillo-Juárez, I.; Rivero-Cruz, F.; Celis, H., Romero, I.; Anti-*Helicobacter pylori* activity of anacardic acids from *Amphipterygium adstringens*. *J Ethnopharmacol,* **2007,** *114,* 72–77.

Castillo-Juárez, I.; Violeta González, V.; Jaime-Aguilar, H.; Martinez, G.; Linares, E.; Bye, R.; and Romero, I. Anti-*Helicobacter pylori* activity of plants used in Mexican traditional medicine for gastrointestinal disorders. *J Ethnopharmacol,* **2009,** 122(2), 402–405.

Cellini, L.; Di Campli, E.; Masulli, M.; Di Bartolomeo, S.; and Allocati, N. Inhibition of *Helicobacter pylori* by garlic extract (*Allium sativum*). *Immunol Med Mic,* **1996,** *13,* 273–277.

Chandrasekhar, Y.; Phani Kumar, G.; Navya, K.; Ramya, E. M.; and Anilakumar, K. R. Tannins from *Terminalia chebula* fruits attenuates GABA antagonist-induced anxiety-like behaviour via modulation of neurotransmitters. *J Pharm Pharmacol, 2018, 70*(12), 1662–1674.

Chen, P. S.; and Li, J. H. Chemopreventive effect of punicalagin, a novel tannin component isolated from *Terminalia catappa* on H-ras-transformed NIH3T3 cells. *Toxicol Lett,* **2006,** *163,* 44–53.

Chen, P. S.; Li, J. H.; Liu, T. Y.; and Lin, T. C. Folk medicine *Terminalia catappa* and its major tannin component, punicalagin, are effective against bleomycin-induced genotoxicity in Chinese hamster ovary cells. *Cancer Lett,* **2000,** *52,* 115–122.

Choi, J.; Park, Y. G.; Yun, M. S.; and Seol, J. W. Effect of herbal mixture composed of *Alchemilla vulgaris* and Mimosa on wound healing process. *Biomed Pharmacother, 2018, 106,* 326–332.

Chowdhury, S. A.; Islam, J.; Rahaman, M. M.; Rahman, M. M.; Rumzhum, N. N.; Sultana, R.; and Parvin, M. N. Cytotoxicity, antimicrobial and antioxidant studies of the different plant parts of *Mimosa pudica*. *Stamford J Pharm Sci,* **2008,** *1,* 80–84.

Christensen, A.; and Pike, C. J. Menopause, obesity and inflammation: interactive risk factors for Alzheimer's disease. *Front Aging Neurosci,* **2015,** *7*(130), 1–14.

Chyau, C. C.; Ko, P. T.; and Mau, J. L. Antioxidant properties of aqueous extracts from *Terminallia catappa* leaves. *LWT—Food Sci Technol,* **2006,** *39,* 1099–1108.

Cogo, L. L.; Monteiro, C. L. B.; Miguel, M. D.; Miguel, O. G.; Cunico, M. M.; Ribeiro, M. L.; Camargo, E. R.; Kussen, G. M. B.; Nogueira, K. S.; and Costa, L. M. D. Anti-*Helicobacter pylori* activity of plant extracts traditionally used for the treatment of gastrointestinal disorders. *Braz J Microbiol,* **2010,** *41,* 304–309.

Cortés-Rojas, D. F.; Souza, C. R. F.; and Oliveira, W. P. Optimization of spray drying conditions for production of *Bidens pilosa* L. dried extract. *Chem Eng Res Des*, **2015**, *93*, 366–376.

Cota, D.; Mishra, S.; and Shengule, S. Beneficial role of *Terminalia arjuna* hydro-alcoholic extract in colitis and its possible mechanism. *J Ethnopharmacol*, **2019**, *230*, 117–25.

Cruz, M. P.; Andrade, C. M.; Silva, K. O.; de Souza, E. P.; Yatsuda, R.; Marques, L. M.; David, J. P.; David, J. M.; Napimoga, M. H.; and Clemente-Napimoga, J. T. Antinoceptive and anti-inflammatory activities of the ethanolic extract, fractions and flavones isolated from *Mimosa tenuiflora* (Willd.) Poir (Leguminosae). *PLoS One*, **2016**, *11*(3): e0150839. https://doi.org/10.1371/journal.pone.0150839.

Cwikla, C.; Schmidt, K.; Matthias, A.; Bone, K. M.; Lehmann, R.; and Tiralongo, E. Investigations into the antibacterial activities of phytotherapeutics against *Helicobacter pylori* and *Campylobacter jejuni*. *Phytother Res*, **2010**, *24*, 649–656.

David, J. P.; Meira, M.; David, J. M.; Brandão, H. N.; Branco, A.; Agra, M. F.; Barbosa, M. R. V.;Queiroz, L. P.; and Giulietti, A. M. Radical scavenging, antioxidant and cytotoxic activity of Brazilian Caatinga plants. *Fitoterapia*, **2007**, 78(3), 215–218.

Daza, L. D.; Fujita, A.; Favaro-Trindade, C. S.; Rodrigues-Ract, J. N.; Granato, D.; and Genovese, M. I. Effect of spray drying conditions on the physical properties of *Cagaita* (*Eugenia dysenterica* DC.) fruit extracts. *Food Bioprod Process*, **2016**, 97, 20–29.

de Faria, F. M.; Luiz-Ferreira, A.; Socca, E. A.; de Almeida, A. C.; Dunder, R. J.; Manzo, L. P.; da Silva, M. A.; Vilegas, W.; Rozza, A. L.; Pellizzon, C. H.; Dos Santos, L. C.; and Souza Brito, A. R. Effects of *Rhizophora mangle* on experimental colitis induced by TNBS in rats. *Evid Based Complement Altern Med*, **2012**, *2012*(753971), 1–11. DOI:10.1155/2012/753971

de Souza, S.; and Fiocchi, C. Immunopathogenesis of IBD: current state of the art. *Nat Rev Gastroenterol Hepatol*, **2016**, *13*(1), 13–27.

Debnath, T.; Kim, da H. and Lim, B. O. Natural products as a source of anti-inflammatory agents associated with inflammatory bowel disease. *Molecules*, **2013**, *18*(6), 7253–7270.

Del Valle, J. C.; Buide, M. L.; Camimiro-Soriguer, I.; Whithall, J. B.; and Narbona, E. On flavonoid accumulation in different plant parts: variation patterns among individuals as population in the shore campion (*Silene littorea*). *Front Plant Sci*, **2015**, 6(9), 1–13. DOI: 10.3389/fpls.2015.00939

Dharmaratne, M. P. J.; Manoraj, A.; Thevanesam, V.; Ekanayake, A.; Kumar, N. S.; Liyanapathirana, V.; Abeyratne, E.; and Bandara, B. M. R, *Terminalia bellirica* fruit extracts: in-vitro antibacterial activity against selected multidrug-resistant bacteria, radical scavenging activity and cytotoxicity study on BHK-21 Cells. *BMC Complement Altern Med*, **2018**, *18*(325), 1–12.

Di Stasi, C. L.; Oliveira, G. P.; Carvalhaes, M. A.; Queiroz-Junior, M.; Tien, O. S.; Kakinami, S. H.; and Reis, M. S. Medicinal plants popularly used in the Brazilian Tropical Atlantic Forest. *Fitoterapia*, **2002**, *73*, 69–91.

Dong, M. H.; and Kaunitz, J. D. Gastroduodenal mucosal defense. *Curr Opinion Gastroenterol*, **2006**, *22*(6), 599–606.

Dutra, R. C.; Campos, M. M.; Santos, A. R. S.; and Calixto, J. B. Medicinal plants in Brazil: pharmacological studies, drug discovery, challenges and perspectives. *Pharmacol Res*, **2016**, *112*, 4–29.

Dwevedi, A.; Dwivedi, R.; and Sharma, Y. K. Exploration of phytochemicals found in *Terminalia* sp. and their antiretroviral activities. *Pharmacogn Rev*, 2016, *10*(20), 73–83.

Ekabo, O. A.; Farnsworth, N. R.; Henderson, T. O.; Mao, G.; and Mukherjee, R. J. Antifungal and Molluscicidal Saponins from *Serjania salzmanniana*. *Nat Prod*, **1996**, *59*, 431–435.

El-Tablawy, N. M. S.; Omran, M. M.; Khowailed, A. A.; and Tantawy, E. E. M. A. Effect of Estrogen on basal, charbacol stimulated acid secretion and Indomethacin induced ulcer in female albino rats. *Med J Cairo Univ*, **2012**, *80*(1), 533–544.

Espanha, L. G.; Resende, F. A.; de Sousa, L. N. J.; Boldrin, P. K.; Nogueira, C.H.; de Camargo, M. S.; De Grandis, R. A.; dos Santos, L. C.; Vilegas, W.; and Varanda, E. A. Mutagenicity and antimutagenicity of six Brazilian *Byrsonima* species assessed by the Ames test. *BMC Complement Altern Med*, **2014**, *14*(182), 1–10.

Fan, Y. M.; Xu, L. Z.; Gao, J.; Wang, Y.; Tang, X. H.; Zhao, X. N.; and Zhang, Z. X. Phytochemical and anti-inflammatory studies on *Terminalia catappa. Fitoterapia*, **2004**, 75, 253–260.

Fang, S. H.; Rao, Y. K.; and Tzeng, Y. M. Anti-oxidant and inflammatory mediator's growth inhibitory effects of compounds isolated from *Phyllanthus urinaria. J Ethnopharmacol*, **2008**, *116*, 333–340.

Figueiredo, M. E.; Michelin, D. C.; Sannomiya, M.; Silva, M. A.; Santos, L. C.; Almeida, L. F. R.; Souza-Brito, A. R. M.; Salgado, H. R. N.; and Vilegas, W. Avaliação química e anti-diarréica das folhas de *Byrsonima cinera* DC. (Malpighiaceae). *Rev Bras Cienc Farm*, **2005**, *41*, 79–83.

Funari, C. S.; Carneiro, R. L.; Andrade, A. M.; Cavalheiro, A. J.; and Hilder, E. F. Green chromatographic fingerprinting: an environmentally friendly approach for the development of separation methods for fingerprinting complex matrices. *J Sep Sci*, **2014a**, *37*, 37–44.

Funari, C. S.; Carneiro, R. L.; Cavalheiro, A. J.; and Hilder, E. F. A trade off between separation, detection and sustainability in liquid chromatographic fingerprinting. *J Chromatogr A*, **2014b**, *1354*, 34–42.

Gallagher, E. J.; and LeRoith D. Obesity and diabetes: the increased risk of cancer and cancer-related mortality. *Physiol Rev*, **2015**, *95*(3), 727–748.

Gallo, L.; Ramírez-Rigo, M. V.; Piña, J.; and Bucalá, V. A comparative study of spray-dried medicinal plant aqueous extracts. Drying performance and product quality. *Chem Eng Res Design*, **2015**, *104*, 681–694.

Gambero, A.; and Ribeiro, M. L. The positive effects of yerba maté (Ilex paraguariensis) in obesity. *Nutrients*, **2015**, *7*(2), 730–750.

Gao, J.; Tang, X.; Dou, H.; Fan, Y.; Zhao, X.; and Xu, Q. Hepatoprotective activity of *Terminalia catappa* L. leaves and its two triterpenoids. *J Pharm Pharmacol*, **2004**, 56, 1449–1455.

Gautam, M. K.; Goel, S.; Ghatule, R. R.; Singh, A.; Nath, G.; and Goel, R. K. Curative effect of *Terminalia chebula* extract on acetic acid-induced experimental colitis: role of antioxidants, free radicals and acute inflammatory marker. *Inflammopharmacology*, **2013**, 21(5), 377–383.

Genest, S.; Kerr, C.; Shah, A.; Rahman, M. M.; Saif-E-Naser, G. M. M.; Nigam, P.; Nahar, L.; and Sarker, S. D. Comparative bioactivity studies on two *Mimosa* species. *Bol Latinoa Caribe Plant Med Aromat*, **2008**, *7*, 38–43.

Germanò, M. P.; Sanogo, R.; Guglielmo, M.; Pasquale, R.; Crisafi, G.; and Bisignano G. Effects of *Pteleopsis suberosa* extracts on experimental gastric ulcers and *Helicobacter pylori* growth. *J Ethnopharmacol*, **1998**, *59*(3), 167–172.

Goel, R. K.; Sairam, K.; Babu, M. D.; Tavares, I. A.; and Raman, A. *In vitro* evaluation of *Bacopa monniera* on anti-*Helicobacter pylori* activity and accumulation of prostaglandins. *Phytomedicine*, **2003**, *10*, 523–527.

Gomig, F.; Pietrovski, E. F.; Guedes, A.; Dalmarco, E. M.; Calderari, M. T.; Guimarães, C. L.;Pinheiro, R. M.; Cabrini, D. A.; and Otuki, M. F. Topical anti-inflammatory activity of *Serjania erecta* Radlk (Sapindaceae) extracts. *J Ethnopharmacol*, **2008**, *118*(2), 220–224.

Guimarães. C. C.; Oliveira, D. D.; Valdevite, M.; Saltoratto, A. L.; Pereira, S. I.; França Sde, C.; Pereira, A. M.; and Pereira, P. S. The glycosylated flavonoids vitexin, isovitexin, and quercetrin isolated from *Serjania erecta* Radlk (Sapindaceae) leaves protect PC12 cells against amyloid-β25–35 peptide-induced toxicity. *Food Chem Toxicol*, **2015**, *86*, 88–94.

Gujarathi, R. A.; Dwivedi, R.; and Vyas, M. K. An observational pilot study on the effect of *Gomutra Haritaki*, diet control and exercise in the management of Sthaulya (obesity). *Ayu*, **2014**, *35*(2), 129–134.

Gutierrez, R. M.; Flores, J. M. Effect of chronic administration of hexane extract of *Byrsonima crassifolia* seed on B-cell and pancreatic oxidative parameters in streptozotocin-induced diabetic rat. *Afr J Tradit Complement Altern Med*, **2014**, *11*(2), 231–236.

Hajimahmoodi, M.; Shams-Ardakani, M.; Saniee, P.; Siavoshi, F.; Mehrabani, M.; Hosseinzadeh, H.; Foroumadi, P.; Safavi, M.; Khanavi, M.; Akbarzadeh, T.; Shafiee, A.; and Foroumadi, A. *In vitro* antibacterial activity of some Iranian medicinal plant extracts against *Helicobacter pylori*. *Nat Prod Res*, **2011**, *25*, 1059–1066.

Harvey, A. L.; Edrada-Ebel, R, A.; and Quinn, R. J. The re-emergence of natural products for drug discovery in the genomics era. *Nat Rev Drug Discov*, **2015**. *14*(2), 111–129.

Hassan, H. A.; and El-Gharib, N. E. Obesity and clinical riskiness relationship: therapeutic management by dietary antioxidant supplementation—a review. *Appl Biochem Biotechnol*, **2015**, *176*(3), 647–669.

Hassani, A. R.; Ordouzadeh, N.; Ghaemi, A.; Amirmozafari, N.; Hamdi, K.; and Nazari, R. *In vitro* inhibition of *Helicobacter pylori* urease with non and semi fermented *Camellia sinensis*. *Indian J Med Microbiol*, **2009**, *27*, 30–34.

Heredia-Vieira, S. C.; Simonet, A. M.; Vilegas, W.; and Macías, F. A. Unusual C,O-fused glucosylapigenins from *Serjania marginata* leaves. *J Nat Prod*, **2015**, *78*, 77–84.

Herrera-Ruiz, M.; Zamilpa, A.; González-Cortazar, M.; Reyes-Chilpa, R.; León, E.; Garcia, M. P.; Tortoriello, J.; and Huerta-Reyes, M. Antidepressant effect and pharmacological evaluation of standardized extracts of flavonoids from *Byrsonima crassifolia*. *Phytomedicine*, **2011**, *18*, 1255–1261.

Higuchi, C. T.; Sannomiya, M.; Pavan, F. R.; Leite, S. R. A.; Sato, D. N.; Franzblau, S. G.; Sacramento, L. V. S.; Vilegas, W.; and Leite, C. Q. F. *Byrsonima fagifolia* niedenzu apolar compounds with antitubercular activity. *Evid Based Complement Altern Med*, **2011**, *2011*, 1–5.

Hostettman, K.; Queiroz, E. F.; and Vieira, P. C. *Active Principles of Higher Plants*. Universidade Federal de São Carlos (UFSCar), São Carlos, Brazil, 2003.

Huang, J.; Wang, Y.; Xie, Z.; Zhou, Y.; Zhang, Y.; and Wan, X. The anti-obesity effects of green tea in human intervention and basic molecular studies. *Eur J Clin Nutr*, *68*(10), **2014**, 1075–1087.

Huang, Y.-H.; Wu, P.-Y.; Wen, K.-C.; Lin, C.-Y.; and Chiang, H.-M. Protective effects and mechanisms of *Terminalia catappa* L. methenolic extract on hydrogen-peroxide-induced oxidative stress in human skin fibroblasts. *BMC Complement Altern Med*, **2018**, *18*(266), 1–9.

Ijaz, S.; Shoaib Khan, H. M.; Anwar, Z.; Talbot, B.; and Walsh, J. J. HPLC profiling of *Mimosa pudica* polyphenols and their non-invasive biophysical investigations for anti-dermatoheliotic and skin reinstating potential. *Biomed Pharmacother*, **2019**, *109*, 865–875.

INCA (Instituto Nacional do Câncer). *Estimate 2014: Incidence of Cancer in Brazil. Instituto Nacional do Câncer*, Rio de Janeiro, Brazil, 2014, page 124. URL: https://www.inca.gov.br/

Jain, K. S.; Shah, A. K.; Bariwal, J.; Shelke, S. M.; Kale, A. P.; Jagtap, J. R.; and Bhosale, A. V. Recent advances in proton pump inhibitors and management of acid-peptic disorders. *Bioorg Med Chem*, **2007**, *15*, 1181–1205.

Jayesh, K.; Karishma, R.; Vysakh, A.; Gopika, P.; and Latha, M. S. *Terminalia bellirica* (Gaertn.) Roxb fruit exerts anti-inflammatory effect via regulating arachidonic acid pathway and pro-inflammatory cytokines in lipopolysaccharide-induced RAW 264.7 macrophages. *Inflammopharmacology*, **2018**, 1–10. DOI: 10.1007/s10787–018-0513-x.

Jitta, S. R.; Daram, P.; Gourishetti, K.; Misra, C. S.; Polu, P. R.; Shah, A.; Shreedhara, C. S.; Nampoothiri, M.; and Lobo, R. *Terminalia tomentosa* bark ameliorates inflammation and arthritis in Carrageenan induced inflammatory model and Freund's adjuvant-induced arthritis model in rats. *J Toxicol,* **2019**, 2019, 1–11.

Kaneria, M. J.; Rakholiya, K. D.; Marsonia, L. R.; Dave, R. A.; and Golakiya, B. A. Nontargeted metabolomics approach to determine metabolites profile and antioxidant study of Tropical Almond (*Terminalia catappa* L.) fruit peels using GC-QTOF-MS and LC-QTOF-MS. *J Pharm Biomed Anal*, **2018**, *160*, 415–427.

Kaur, J.; Sidhu, S.; Chopra, K.; and Khan, M. U. Protective effect of *Mimosa pudica* L. in an L-arginine model of acute necrotising pancreatitis in rats. *J Nat Med*, **2016**, *70*(3), 423–434.

Khalaf, A. A.; Galal, M. K.; Ibrahim, M. A.; Abd Allah, A. A.; Afify, M. M.; and Refaat, R. The *Terminalia laxiflora* modulates the neurotoxicity induced by fipronil in male albino rats. *Biosci Rep*, **2019**, *39*(3), 1–10.

Khan, A. A.; Kumar, V.; Singh, B. K.; and Singh, R. Evaluation of wound healing property of *Terminalia catappa* on excision wound models in Wistar rats. *Drug Res*, **2014**, *64*, 225–228.

Kim, M. S.; Lee, D. Y.; Lee, J.; Kim, H. W.; Sung, S. H.; Han, J. S.; and Jeon, W/K. *Terminalia chebula* extract prevents scopolamine-induced amnesia via cholinergic modulation and anti-oxidative effects in mice. *BMC Complement Altern Med*, **2018**, *18*(136), 1–11.

Kinoshita, S.; Inoue, Y.; Nakama, S.; Ichiba, T.; and Aniya, Y. Antioxidant and hepatoprotective actions of medicinal herb, *Terminalia catappa* L. from Okinawa Island and its tannin corilagin. *Phytomedicine*, **2007**, *14*, 755–762.

Klein, T.; Longhini, R.; Bruschi, M. L.; and Mello, J. C. P. Microparticles containing guaraná extract obtained by spray-drying technique: development and characterization. *Rev Bras Farmacogn*, **2015**, *25*(3), 292–300.

Kloucek. P.; Polesny. Z.; Svobodova. B.; Ikova. E.; and Kokoska. L. Antibacterial screening of some Peruvian medicinal plants used in Calleria District. *J Ethnopharmacol*, **2005,** *99*, 309–312.

Ko, T. F.; Weng, Y. M.; and Chiou, R. Y. Squalene content and antioxidant activity of Terminalia catappa leaves and seeds. *J Agric Food Chem*, **2002**, *50*, 5343–5348.

Kurata, J. H.; Haile, B. M.; and Elashoff, J. D. Sex differences in peptic ulcer disease. *Gastroenterology*, **1985**, *88*, 96–100.

Kushima, H.; Nishijima, C. M.; Rodrigues, C. M.; Rinaldo, D.; Sassá, M. F.; Bauab, T. M.; Stasi, L. C.; Carlos, I. Z.; Brito, A. R.; Vilegas, W.; and Hiruma-Lima, C. A. *Davilla elliptica* and *Davilla nitida*: gastroprotective, anti-inflammatory immunomodulatory and anti-*Helicobacter pylori* action. *J Ethnopharmacol*, **2009**, *123*, 430–438.

Lai, C. H.; Fang, S. H.; Rao, Y. K.; Geethangili, M.; Tang, C. H.; Lin, Y. J.; Hung, C. H.; Wang, W. C.; and Tzeng, Y. M. Inhibition of *Helicobacter pylori*-induced inflammation in human gastric epithelial AGS cells by *Phyllanthus urinaria* extracts. *J Ethnopharmacol,* **2008**, *118,* 522–526.

Lal, R.; and Junior, W. F. S. *Where Biodiversity, Traditional Knowledge, Health and Livelihoods Meet: Institutional Pillars for the Productive Inclusion of Local Communities (Brazil Case Study).* International Policy Centre for Inclusive Growth (IPC-IG) jointly supported by Poverty Practice, Bureau for Development Policy, UNDP and the Government of Brazil. Working Paper Number 81, 2011, pages 1–30. URL: http://www.ipc-undp.org/pub/IPCWorkingPaper81.pdf

Lanardão, E. J.; Freitag, R. A.; Dabdoub, M. J.; Batista, A. C. F.; and Silveira, C. C. Green chemistry—Os 12 principios da quimica verde e sua inserção nas atividades de ensino e pesquisa. *Quím Nova,* **2003**, *26,* 123–129.

Lapa A. J. Pharmacology and Toxicology of Natural Products. In: Simões, C. M. O. et al. (Eds.). *Pharmacognosy: From the Plant to the Medicine.* 5th Ed., Faculty of Education, Federal University of Rio Grande do Sul (UFRGS), Porto Alegre, Brazil, 2004, pages 247–262.

Lee, C. Y.; Yang, S. F.; Wang, P. H.; Su, C. W.; Hsu, H. F.; Tsai, H. T.; and Hsiao, Y. H. Antimetastatic effects of *Terminalia catappa* leaf extracts on cervical cancer through the inhibition of matrix metalloprotein-9 and MAPK pathway. *Environ Toxicol,* **2019**, *34*(1), 60–66.

Lemos, L. M.; Martins, T. B.; Tanajura, G. H.; Gazoni, V. F.; Bonaldo, J.; Strada, C. L.; Silva, M. G.; Dall'oglio, E. L.; de Sousa Júnior, P. T.; and Martins, D. T. Evaluation of antiulcer activity of chromanone fraction from *Calophyllum brasiliesnse* Camb. *J Ethnopharmacol,* **2012**, *141,* 432–439.

Li, M.; Wang, J.; and Xu, Z. Studied Chinese herbs on *Helicobacter pylori. Int J Microb Rev,* **2013**, *1,* 6–10.

Lien, H. M.; Wang, C. Y.; Chang, H. Y.; Huang, C. L.; Peng, M. T.; Sing, Y. T.; Chen, C. C.; and Lai, C. H. Bioevaluation of *Anisomeles indica* extracts and their inhibitory effects on *Helicobacter pylori*-mediated inflammation. *J Ethnopharmacol,* **2013**, *145,* 397–401.

Lima, M. R. F.; Luna, J. S.; Santos, A. F.; Andrade, M. C. C.; Sant'Ana, A. E. G.; Genet, J. P.; Marquez, B.; Neuville, L.; and Moreau, N. Anti-bacterial activity of some Brazilian medicinal plants. *J Ethnopharmacol,* **2006**, *105*(1–2), 137–147.

Lima, Z. P.; Calvo, T. R.; Silva, E. F.; Pellizzon, C. H.; Vilegas, W.; Brito, A. R.; Bauab, T. M.; and Hiruma-Lima, C. A. Brazilian medicinal plant acts on prostaglandin level and *Helicobacter pylori. J Med Food,* **2008b**, *11,* 701–708.

Lima, Z. P.; dos Santos Rde, C.; Torres, T. U.; Sannomiya, M., Rodrigues, C. M.; dos Santos, L. C.; Pellizzon, C. H.; Rocha, L. R.; Vilegas, W.; Souza Brito, A. R.; Cardoso, C. R.; Varanda, E. A.; de Moraes, H. P.; Bauab, T. M.; Carli, C.; Carlos, I. Z.; and Hiruma-Lima, C. A. *Byrsonima fagifolia*: an integrative study to validate the gastroprotective, healing, antidiarrheal, antimicrobial and mutagenic action. *J Ethnopharmacol,* **2008a**, *120,* 149–160.

Lima, Z. P.; dos Santos Rde, C.; Torres, T. U.; Sannomiya, M.; Rodrigues, C. M.; dos Santos, L. C.; Pellizzon, C. H.; Rocha, L. R.; Vilegas, W.; Souza Brito, A. R.; Cardoso, C. R.; Varanda, E. A.; de Moraes, H. P.; Bauab, T. M.; Carli, C.; Carlos, I. Z.; and Hiruma-Lima, C. A. *Byrsonima fagifolia*: an integrative study to validate the gastroprotective, healing, antidiarrheal, antimicrobial and mutagenic action. *J Ethnopharmacol,* **2008c**, *120*(2), 149–160.

Lin, C. C.; Chen, Y. L.; Lin, J. M.; and Ujiie, T. Evaluation of the antioxidant and hepatoprotective activity of *Terminalia catappa*. *Am J Chin Med*, **1997**, *25*, 153–161.

Lin, C. C.; Hsu, Y. F.; and Lin T. C. Antioxidant and free radical scavenging effects of the tannins of *Terminalia catappa* L. *Anticancer Res*, **2001**, *21*, 237–243.

Lin, L. C.; Chiou, C. T.; and Cheng, J. J. 5-Deoxyflavones with cytotoxic activity from Mimosa diplotricha. *J Nat Prod*, **2011**, *74*, 2001–2004.

Lira Wde, M.; dos Santos, F. V.; Sannomiya, M.; Rodrigues, C. M.; Vilegas, W.; and Varanda, E. A. Modulatory effect of *Byrsonima basiloba* extracts on the mutagenicity of certain direct and indirect-acting mutagens in *Salmonella typhimurium* assays. *J Med Food,* **2008**, *11*(1), 111–119.

Liu, T. Y.; Ho, L. K.; Tsai, Y. C.; Chiang, S. H.; Chao, T. W.; Li, J. H.; and Chi, C. W. Modification of mitomycin C-induced clastogenicity by *Terminalia catappa* L. *in vitro* and *in vivo*. *Cancer Lett*, **1996**, *105*(1), 113–118.

Liu, W.; Mu, F.; Liu, T.; Xu, H.; Chen, J.; Jia, N.; Zhang, Y.; Dou, F.; Shi, L.; Li, Y.; Wen, A.; and Ding, Y. Ultra performance liquid chromatography/quadrupole time-of-flight mass spectrometry-based metabonomics reveal protective effect of *Terminalia chebula* extract on ischemic stroke rats. *Rejuvenation Res*, **2018**, *21*(6), 541–552.

Machado-Goncalves, L.; Tavares-Santos, A.; Santos-Costa, F.; Soares-Diniz, R.; Camara-de Carvalho-Galvao, L.; Martins-de Sousa, E.; and Beninni-Paschoal, M. A. Effects of *Terminalia catappa* Linn. extract on *Candida albicans* biofilms developed on denture acrylic resin discs. *J Clin Exp Dent*, **2018**, *10*(7), e642–e647.

Magalhães, F. E. A.; Batista, F. L. A.; Serpa, O. F.; Moura, L. F. W. G.; Lima, M. D. C. L.; da Silva, A. R. A.; Guedes, M. I. F.; Santos, S. A. A. R.; de Oliveira, B. A.; Nogueira, A. B.; Barbosa, T. M.; Holanda, D. K. R.; Damasceno, M. B. M. V.; de Melo, J. M. A. J.; Barroso, L. K. V.; and Campos, A. R. Orofacial antinociceptive effect of *Mimosa tenuiflora* (Willd.) Poiret. *Biomed Pharmacother*, **2018**, *97*, 1575–1585.

Mahady, G. B.; Pendland, S. L.; Stoia, A.; Hamill, F. A.; Fabricant, D.; Dietz, B. M.; and Chadwick, L. R. *In vitro* susceptibility of *Helicobacter pylori* to botanical extracts used traditionally for the treatment of gastrointestinal disorders. *Phytother Res*, **2005**, *19*(11), 988–991.

Maldini, M.; Sosa, S.; Montoro, P.; Giangaspero, A.; Balick, M. J.; Pizza, C.; and Della, L. R. Screening of the topical anti-inflammatory activity of the bark of *Acacia cornigera* Willdenow, *Byrsonima crassifolia* Kunth, *Sweetia panamensis* Yakovlev and the leaves of *Sphogneticola trilobata* Hitchcock. *J Ethnopharmacol*, **2009**, *122*, 430–433.

Malfertheiner, P.; Megraus, F.; O'morain, C.; Azzoli, F.; El-omar, E.; and Graham, D. Current concepts in the management of *Helicobacter pylori* infection: the Maastricht III consensus report. *Gut*, **2007**, *56*, 772–781.

Mandeville, A.; and Cock, I. E. *Terminalia chebula* Retz. fruit extracts inhibit bacterial triggers of some autoimmune diseases and potentiate the activity of tetracycline. *Indian J Microb*, **2018**, *58*(4), 496–506.

Marcum, Z. A.; and Hanlon, J. T. Recognizing the risks of chronic nonsteroidal anti-inflammatory drug use in older adults. *Ann Longterm Care*, **2010**, *18*(9), 24–27.

Mariutti, L. R. B.; Rodrigues, E.; Chisté, R. C.; Fernandes, E.; and Mercadante, A. Z. The Amazonian fruit *Byrsonima crassifolia* effectively scavenges reactive oxygen and nitrogen species and protects human erythrocytes against oxidative damage. *Food Res Int*, **2014**, *64*, 618–625.

Mazzolin, L. P.; Nasser, A. L. M.; Moraes, T. M.; Santos, R. C.; Nishijima, C. M.; Santos, F. V.; Varanda, E. A.; Bauab, T. M.; Rocha, L. R. M.; Di Stasi, L. C.; Vilegas, W.; and Hiruma-Lima, C. A. *Qualea parviflora* mart.: an integrative study to validate the gastroprotective, antidiarrheal, antihemorragic and mutagenic action. *J Ethnopharmacol*, **2010**, *27*, 508–514.

Mesquita, M. L.; Desrivot, J.; Bories, C.; Fournet, A.; Paula, J. E.; Grellier, P.; and Espindola, L. S. Antileishmanial and trypanocidal activity of Brazilian Cerrado plants. *Mem Inst Oswaldo Cruz*, **2005**, *100*(7), 783–787.

Moghaddam, M. N. *In vitro* Inhibition of *Helicobacter pylori* by some spices and medicinal plants used in Iran. *Global J Pharmacol*, **2011**, *5*, 176–180.

Mohan, G.; Anand, S. P.; and Doss, A. Efficacy of aqueous and methanol extracts of *Caesalpinia sappan* L. and *Mimosa pudica* L. for their potential antimicrobial activity. *South Asian J Biol Sci*, **2011**, *1*, 48–57.

Mohanty, I. R.; Borde, M.; Kumar, C. S.; and Maheshwari, U. Dipeptidyl peptidase IV Inhibitory activity of *Terminalia arjuna* attributes to its cardioprotective effects in experimental diabetes: In silico, *in vitro* and *in vivo* analyses. *Phytomedicine*, **2019**, *57*, 158–165.

Moleiro, F. C.; Andreo, M. A.; Santos Rde, C.; Moraes Tde, M.; Rodrigues, C. M.; Carli, C. B.; Lopes, F. C.; Pellizzon, C. H.; Carlos, I. Z.; Bauab, T. M.; Vilegas, W.; and Hiruma-Lima, C. A. Mouririelliptica: validation of gastroprotective, healing and anti-*Helicobacter pylori* effects. *J Ethnopharmacol*, **2009**, *123*, 359–368.

Monção, N. B. N.; Araújo, B. Q.; Silva, J. D. N.; Lima, D. J. B.; Ferreira, P. M. P.; Airoldi, F. P. S.; Pessoa, C.; and Citó, A. M. G. L. Assessing chemical constituents of *Mimosa caesalpiniifolia* stem bark: possible bioactive components accountable for the cytotoxic effect of *M. caesalpiniifolia* on human tumour cell lines. *Molecules*, **2015**, *20*, 4204–4224.

Mopuri, R.; Ganjayi, M.; Banavathy, K. S.; Parim, B. N.; and Meriga, B. Evaluation of anti-obesity activities of ethanolic extract of *Terminalia paniculata* bark on high fat diet-induced obese rats. *BMC Complement Altern Med*, **2015**, *15*(76), 1–11.

Moraes Tde, M.; Rodrigues, C. M.; Kushima, H.; Bauab, T. M.; Villegas, W.; Pellizzon, C. H.; Brito, A. R.; and Hiruma-Lima, C. A. Hancornia speciosa: indications of gastroprotective, healing and anti-*Helicobacter pylori* actions. *J Ethnopharmacol*, **2008**, *120*, 161–168.

Morais, C. B.; Silva, F. E. K.; Lana, A. D.; Tonello, M. L.; Luciano, S. C.; Fuentefria, A. M.; and Zuanazzi, J. Â. S. Phenolic content of species from Leguminosae family and their antifungal activity. *Planta Med*, **2012**, *78*. DOI: 10.1055/s-0032–1321016

Moreira, L. Q.; Vilela, F. C.; Orlandi, L.; Dias, D. F.; Santos, A. L. A.; da Silva, M. A.; Paiva, R.; Alves-da-Silva, G.; and Giusti-Paiva, A. Anti-inflammatory effect of extract and fractions from the leaves of *Byrsonima intermedia* A. Juss in rats. *J Ethnolopharmacol*, **2011**, *138*, 610–615.

Nagappa A. N.; Thakurdesai P. A.; Venkat Rao, N.; and Singhm J. Anti-diabetic activity of *Terminalia catappa* Linn fruits. *J Ethnopharmacol*, **2003**, *88*, 45–50.

Nair, R. and Chanda S. Antimicrobial activity of *Terminalia catappa*, *Manilkara zapota* and *Piper betel* leaf extract. *Indian J Pharm Sci*, **2008**, *70*, 390–393.

Naitik, P.; Prakash, T.; Kotresha, D.; and Rao, N. R. Effect of *Terminalia catappa* on lipid profile in transplanted fibrosarcoma in rats. *Indian J Pharmacol*, **2012**, 44, 390–392.

Napolitano, D. R.; Mineo, J. R.; De Souza, M. A.; De Paula, J. E.; Espondola, L. S.; and Espindola, F. S. Down-modulation of nitric oxide production in murine macrophages treated with crude plant extracts from the Brazilian Cerrado. *J Ethnopharmacol*, **2005**, *99*(1), 37–41.

Nariman, F.; Eftekhar, F.; Habibi, Z.; Massarra, S. and Malekzadeh, R. Antibacterial activity of twenty Iranian plant extracts against clinical isolates of *Helicobacter pylori. Iran J Basic Med Sci*, **2009**, *12*, 105–111.

NASHMH (National Agency of Supplementary Health, Ministry of Health). Vigitel Brazil 2011: Supplementary Health Surveillance of Risk Factors and Disease Protection Chronicles by Telephone Investigation. Department of Health Surveillance, National Agency of Supplementary Health, Ministry of Health, Brazil, 2011. Accessed on January 29, 2018. URL: http://bvsms.saude.gov.br/bvs/publicacoes/vigitel_brasil_2011.pdf

Ng, S. C.; Lam, Y. T.; Tsoi, K. K.; Chan, F. K.; Sung, J. J.; and Wu, J. C. Systematic review: the efficacy of herbal therapy in inflammatory bowel disease. *Aliment Pharmacol Ther*, **2013**, *38*(8), 854–863.

NHSARRDC (National Health Surveillance Agency Resolution RDC). National Health Surveillance Agency. Resolution RDC No. 26, Dated May 13, 2014. It provides for the registration of herbal medicines and the registration and notification of traditional herbal products. Official Gazette of the Federative Republic of Brazil. Brasília, May 14, 2014.

NHSARRE (National Health Surveillance Agency Resolution RE). National Health Surveillance Agency. Resolution RE No. 899, May 29, 2003. Guide for validation of analytical and bioanalytical methods. Official Journal of the Union, Brasília, DF, June 02, 2003. Accessed on June 24, 2015a. URL: http://www.in.gov.br

Njume, C.; Afolayan, A. J.; Green, E.; and Ndip, R. N. Volatile compounds in the stem bark of *Sclerocarya birrea* (Anacardiaceae) possess antimicrobial activity against drug-resistant strains of *Helicobacter pylori. Int J Antimicrob Agents*, **2011a**, *38*, 319–324.

Njume, C.; Afolayan, A. J.; and Ndip, R. N. Preliminary phytochemical screening and *in vitro* anti-*Helicobacter pylori* activity of acetone and aqueous extracts of the stem bark of *Sclerocarya birrea* (Anacardiaceae). *Arch Med Res*, **2011b**, *42*, 252–257.

Nunes, X. P.; Mesquita, R. F.; Silva, D. A.; Lira, D. P.; Costa, V. C. O.; Silva, M. V. B.; Xavier, A. L.; Diniz, M. F. F. M.; and Agra, M. F. Constituintes químicos, avaliação das atividades citotóxica e antioxidante de *Mimosa paraibana* Barneby (Mimosaceae). *Rev Bras Farmacogn,* **2008**, *18*, 718–723.

Pandey, A. K.; Gupta, P. P.; and Lal, V. K. Hypoglycemic effect of Rhizophora mucronata in streptozotocin induced diabetic rats. *J Complement Integr Med*, **2014**, *11*(3), 179–183.

Pandya, N. B.; Tigari, P.; Dupadahalli, K.; Kamurthy, H.; and Nadendla, R. R. Antitumor and antioxidant status of *Terminalia catappa* against Ehrlich ascites carcinoma in Swiss albino mice. *Indian J Pharmacol*, **2013**, *45*, 464–469.

Paraschos, S.; Magiatis, P.; Mitakou, S.; Petraki, K.; Kalliaropoulos, A.; Maragkoudakis, P.; Mentis, A.; Sgouras, D.; and Skaltsounis, A. L. *In vitro* and *in vivo* activities of Chios mastic gum extracts and constituents against *Helicobacter pylori. Antimicrob Agents Chemother*, **2007**, *51*(2), 551–559.

Patro, G.; Bhattamisra, S. K.; and Mohanty, B. K. Effects of *Mimosa pudica* L. leaves extract on anxiety, depression and memory. *Avicenna J Phytomed*, **2016a**, *6*(6), 696–710.

Patro, G.; Bhattamisra, S. K.; Mohanty, B. K.; and Sahoo, H. B. *In vitro* and *in vivo* antioxidant evaluation and estimation of total phenolic, flavonoidal content of *Mimosa pudica* L. *Pharmacogn Res*, **2016b**, *8*(1), 22–28.

Pawar, S. P.; and Pal, S. C. Antimicrobial activity of extracts of *Terminalia catappa* root. *Indian J Med Sci,* **2002**, *56*, 276–278.

Perez-Gutierrez, R. M.; Muñiz-Ramirez, A.; Gomez, Y. G.; and Ramírez, E. B. Antihyperglycemic, antihyperlipidemic and antiglycation effects of *Byrsonima crassifolia* fruit and seed in normal and streptozotocin-induced diabetic rats. *Plant Foods Hum Nutr*, **2010**, *65*(4), 350–357.

Pérez-Gutiérrez, R. M.; and Ramirez, A. M. Hypoglycemic effects of sesquiterpene lactones from *Byrsonima crassifolia*. *Food Sci Biotechnol*, **2016**, *25*, 1135–1145.

Périco, L. L.; Heredia-Vieira, S. C.; Beserra, F. P.; de Cássia Dos Santos, R.; Weiss, M. B.; Resende, F. A.; Dos Santos Ramos, M. A.; Bonifácio, B. V.; Bauab, T. M.; Varanda, E. A.; de Gobbi, J. I.; da Rocha, L. R.; Vilegas, W.; and Hiruma-Lima, C. A. Does the gastroprotective action of a medicinal plant ensure healing effects? An integrative study of the biological effects of *Serjania marginata* Casar. (Sapindaceae) in rats. *J Ethnopharmacol*, **2015**, 172: 312–324.

Périco, L. L.; Rodrigues, V. P.; Ohara, R.; Bueno, G.; Nunes, V. V. A.; Dos Santos, R. C.; Camargo, A. C. L.; Justulin Júnior, L. A.; de Andrade, S. F.; Steimbach, V. M. B.; da Silva, L. M.; da Rocha, L. R. M.; Vilegas, W.; Dos Santos, C.; and Hiruma-Lima, C. A. Sex-specific effects of *Eugenia punicifolia* extract on gastric ulcer healing in rats. *World J Gastroenterol*, **2018**, *24*(38), 4369–4383.

Périco, L. L.; Rodrigues, V. P.; Ohara, R.; Nunes, V. V. A.; da Rocha, L. R. M.; Vilegas, W.; Dos Santos, C.; and Hiruma-Lima, C. A. Can the gastric healing effect of *Eugenia punicifolia* be the same in male and female rats? *J Ethnopharmacol*, **2019**, 235, 268–278.

Pinheiro Silva, L.; Damacena de Angelis, C.; Bonamin, F.; Kushima, H.; José Mininel, F.; Campaner Dos Santos, L.; Karina Delella, F.; Luis Felisbino, S.; Vilegas, W.; Regina Machado da Rocha, L.; Aparecido Dos Santos Ramos, M.; Maria Bauab, T.; Toma, W.; and Akiko, H.-L. C. *Terminalia catappa* L.: a medicinal plant from the Caribbean pharmacopeia with anti-*Helicobacter pylori* and antiulcer action in experimental rodent models. *J Ethnopharmacol*, **2015**, *159*, 285–295.

Polanco-Hernández, G.; Escalante-Erosa, F.; García-Sosa, K.; Acosta-Viana, K.; Chan-Bacab, M. J.; Sagua-Franco, H.; González, J.; Osorio-Rodríguez, L.; Moo-Puc, R. E.; and Peña-Rodríguez, L. M. *In vitro* and *in vivo* trypanocidal activity of native plants from the Yucatan Peninsula. *Parasitol Res*, **2012**, *110*(1), 31–35.

Puram, S.; Suh, H. C.; Kim, S. U.; Bethapudi, B.; Joseph, J. A.; Agarwal, A.; and Kudiganti, V. Effect of GutGard in the management of *Helicobacter pylori*: a randomized double blind placebo controlled study. *Evid Based Complement Altern Med*, **2013**, *2013*, 1–8.

Quílez, A.; Berenguer, B.; Gilardoni, G.; Souccar, C.; de Mendonça, S.; Oliveira, L. F.; Martín-Calero, M. J.; and Vidari, G. Anti-secretory, anti-inflammatory and anti-*Helicobacter pylori* activities of several fractions isolated from *Piper carpunya* Ruiz & Pav. *J Ethnopharmacol*, **2010**, *128*, 583–589.

Raghupathi, W.; and Raghupathi, V. An empirical study of chronic diseases in the United States: a visual analytics approach to public health. *Int J Environ Res Public Health*, 2018, *15*(431), 1–24.

Rajkumari, J.; Dyavaiah, M.; Sudharshan, S. J.; and Busi, S. Evaluation of *in vivo* antioxidant potential of *Syzygium jambos* (L.) Alston and *Terminalia citrina* Roxb. towards oxidative stress response in *Saccharomyces cerevisiae*. *J Food Sci Technol*, **2018**, *55*(11), 4432–4439.

Rakotomala, G.; Agard, C.; Tonnerre, P.; Tesse, A.; Derbré, S.; Michalet, S.; Hamzaoui, J.; Rio, M.; Cario-Toumaniantz, C.; Richomme, P.; Charreau, B.; Loirand, G.; and Pacaud, P. Extract from *Mimosa pigra* attenuates chronic experimental pulmonary hypertension. *J Ethnopharmacol*, **2013**, *148*(1), 106–116.

Ratnasooriya, W. D.; Dharmasiri, M. G.; Rajapakse, R. A. S.; De Silva, M. S.; Jayawardena, S. P. M.; Fernando, P. U. D.; De Silva, W. N.; Nawela, A. J. M. D. N. B.; Warusawithana,

R. P. Y. T.; Jayakody, J. R. C.; and Digana, P. M. C. B. Tender Leaf Extract of *Terminalia catappa* antinociceptive activity in rats. *Pharm Biol*, **2002**, *40*, 60–66.

Redchits, I. V.; and Petrov, E. E. The age-related characteristics of the clinical picture of duodenal ulcer in women. *Lik Sprava*, **1995,** (5–6): 149–152,.

Rejón-Orantes, J. C.; Suaréz, D. P. P.; Rejón-Rodríguez, A.; Hernández, S. H.; Liévano, O. E. G.; Rodríguez, D. L.; and Mora, M. P. Aqueous root extracts from *Mimosa albida* Humb. & Bonpl. ex Willd display antinociceptive activity in mice. *J Ethnopharmacol*, **2013**, *149*, 522–526.

Robles-Zepeda, R. E.; Velázquez-Contreras, C. A.; Garibay-Escobar, A.; Gálvez-Ruiz, J. C.; and Ruiz-Bustos, E. Antimicrobial activity of Northwestern Mexican plants against *Helicobacter pylori*. *J Med Food*, **2011**, *14*, 1280–1283.

Rodrigues, A. M. S.; Paula, J. E.; Degallier, N.; Molez, J. F.; and Espíndola, L. S. Larvicidal activity of some Cerrado plant extracts against *Aedes aegypti*. *J Am Mosq Control Assoc,* **2006**, *22*(2), 314–317.

Rodrigues, V. P.; Rocha, C. Q. D.; Périco, L. L.; Santos, R. C. D.; Ohara, R.; Nishijima, C. M.; Ferreira Queiroz, E.; Wolfender, J. L.; Rocha, L. R. M. D.; Santos, A. R. S.; Vilegas, W.; and Hiruma-Lima, C. A. Involvement of opioid system, TRPM8, and ASIC receptors in antinociceptive effect of *Arrabidaea brachypoda* (DC) Bureau. *Int J Mol Sci*, **2017**, *18*(11), 1–12.

Saldanha, A. A.; de Siqueira, J. M.; Castro, A. H. F.; Ribeiro, R. I. M. A.; de Oliveira, F. M.; Lopes, D. O.; Pinto, F. C. H.; Silva, D. B.; and Soares, A. C. Anti-inflammatory effects of the butanolic fraction of *Byrsonima verbascifolia* leaves: mechanisms involving inhibition of tumor necrosis factor alpha, prostaglandin E2 production and migration of polymorphonuclear leucocyte *in vivo* experimentation. *Int Immunopharmacol*, **2016a**, *31*, 123–131.

Saldanha, A. A.; do Carmo, L. F.; do Nascimento, S. B.; de Matos, N. A.; Veloso, C. C.; Castro, A. H. F.; De Vos, R. C. H.; Klein, A.; de Siqueira, J. M.; Carollo, C. A.; do Nascimento, T. V.; Toffoli-Kadri, M. C.; and Soares, A. C. Chemical composition and anti-inflammatory activity of the leaves of *Byrsonima verbascifolia*. *J Nat Med*, **2016b**, *70*, 760–768.

Salem, E. M.; Yar, T.; Bamosa, A. O.; Al-Quorain, A.; Yasawy, M. I.; Alsulaiman, R. M.; and Randhawa, M. A. Comparative study of *Nigella sativa* and triple therapy in eradication of *Helicobacter pylori* in patients with non-ulcer dyspepsia. *Saudi J Gastroenterol*, **2010**, *16*, 207–214.

Sales, M. S.; Roy, A.; Antony, L.; Banu, S. K.; Jeyaraman, S.; and Manikkam, R. Octyl gallate and gallic acid isolated from *Terminalia bellarica* regulates normal cell cycle in human breast cancer cell lines. *Biomed Pharmacother*, **2018**, *103*, 1577–1584.

Salih, E. Y. A.; Julkunen-Tiitto, R.; Lampi, A. M.; Kanninen, M.; Luukkanen, O.; Sipi, M.; Lehtonen, M.; Vuorela, H.; and Fyhrquist, P. *Terminalia laxiflora* and *Terminalia brownii* contain a broad spectrum of antimycobacterial compounds including ellagitannins, ellagic acid derivatives, triterpenes, fatty acids and fatty alcohols. *J Ethnopharmacol*, **2018**, *5*(227), 82–96.

Salinas-Sánchez, D. O.; Jiménez-Ferrer, E.; Sánchez-Sánchez, V.; Zamilpa, A.; González-Cortazar, M.; Tortoriello, J.; and Herrera-Ruiz, M. Anti-inflammatory activity of a polymeric proanthocyanidin from *Serjania schiedeana*. *Molecules*, **2017**, *22*(863), 1–19.

Sannomiya, M.; Cardoso, C. R. P.; Figueiredo, M. E.; Rodrigues, C. M.; dos Santos, L. C.; dos Santos, F. V.; Serpeloni, J. M.; Cólus, I. M. S.; Vilegas, W.; and Varanda, E. A. Mutagenic evaluation and chemical investigation of *Byrsonima intermedia* A. Juss. leaf extracts. *J Ethnopharmacol*, **2007**, *112*(2), 319–326.

Sannomiya, M.; Fonseca, V. B.; Da Silva, M. A.; Rocha, L. R. M.; Dos Santos, L. C.; Hiruma-Lima, C. A.; Souza-Brito, A. R. M.; and Vilegas, W. Flavonoids and antiulcerogenic activity from *Byrsonima crassa* leaves extracts. *J Ethnopharmacol*, **2005b**, *97*, 1–6.

Sannomiya, M.; Michelin, D. C.; Rodrigues, C. M.; Dos Santos, L. C.; Salgado, H. R. N.; Hiruma-Lima, C. A.; Souza-Brito, A. R. M.; and Vilegas, W. *Byrsonima crassa* Niedenzu (IK): antimicrobial activity and chemical study. *Rev Cienc Farm Básica Apl*, **2005a**, *26*, 71–75.

Santos, R. C.; Bonamin, F.; Périco, L. L.; Rodrigues, V. P.; Zanatta, A. C.; Rodrigues, C. M.; Sannomiya, M.; Ramos, M. A. S.; Bonifácio, B. B.; Bauab, T. M.; Tamashirog, J.; Rocha, L. R. M.; Vilegas, W.; and Hiruma-Lima, C. A. *Byrsonima intermedia* A. Juss partitions promote gastroprotection against peptic ulcers and improve healing through antioxidant and anti-inflammatory activities. *Biomed Pharmacother*, **2019**, 111, 1112–1123.

Santos, R. C.; Kushima, H.; Rodrigues, C. M.; Sannomiya, M.; Rocha, L. R.; Bauab, T. M.; Tamashiro, J.; Vilegas, W.; and Hiruma-Lima, C. A. *Byrsonima intermedia* A. Juss.: gastric and duodenal antiulcer, antimicrobial and antidiarrheal effects in experimental rodent models. *J Ethnopharmacol*, **2012**, *140*(2): 203–212.

Santos, R. C.; Kushima, H.; Rodrigues, C. M.; Sannomiya, M.; Rocha, L. R. M.; Bauab, T. M.; Tamashiro, J.; Vilegas, W.; and Hiruma-Lima, C. A. *Byrsonima intermedia* A. Juss.: gastric and duodenal antiulcer, antimicrobial and antidiarrheal effects in experimental rodent models. *J Ethnopharmacol*, **2012**, *140*, 203–212.

Schlickmann, F.; Boeing, T.; Mariano, L. N. B.; da Silva, R. C. M. V. A. F.; da Silva, L. M.; de Andrade, S. F.; de Souza, P.; and Cechinel-Filho, V. Gallic acid, a phenolic compound isolated from *Mimosa bimucronata* (DC.) Kuntze leaves, induces diuresis and saluresis in rats. *Naunyn Schmiedebergs Arch Pharmacol*, **2018**, *391*(6), 649–655.

Shaik, A. H.; Shaik, N. R.; Mohammed, A. K.; Omar, S. Y. A.; Mohammad, A.; Mohaya, T. A.; and Kodidhela, L. D. *Terminalia pallida* fruit ethanolic extract ameliorates lipids, lipoproteins, lipid metabolism marker enzymes and paraoxonase in isoproterenol-induced myocardial infarcted rats. *Saudi J Biol Sci*, **2018**, *25*(3), 431–436.

Shang, X.; Tan, Q.; Liu, R.; Kangying, Y.; Li, P.; and Zhao, G. *In vitro* anti-*Helicobacter pylori* effects of medicinal mushroom extracts, with special emphasis on the lion's mane mushroom *Hericium erinaceus* (Higher Basidiomycetes). *Int J Med Mushrooms*, **2013**, *15*, 165–174.

Sheng, Z.; Zhao, J.; Muhammad, I.; and Zhang, Y. Optimization of total phenolic content from *Terminalia chebula* Retz. fruits using response surface methodology and evaluation of their antioxidant activities. *PLoS One*, **2018**, *13*(8), 1–21.

Shi, D. H.; Liu, Y. W.; Liu, W. W.; and Gu, Z. F. Inhibition of urease by extracts derived from 15 Chinese medicinal herbs. *Pharm Biol*, **2011**, *49*, 752–755.

Shin, J. E.; Kim, J. M.; Bae, E. A.; Hyun, Y. J.; and Kim, D. H. *In vitro* inhibitory effect of flavonoids on growth, infection and vacuolation of *Helicobacter pylori*. *Planta Med*, **2005**, *71*, 197–201.

Shinde, S. L.; Junne, S. B.; Wadje, S. S.; and Baig. M. M. The diversity of antibacterial compounds of *Terminalia* species (Combretaceae). *Pak J Biol Sci*, **2009**, *12*, 1483–1486.

Sidahmed, H. M. A.; Abdelwahab, S. I.; Mohan, S.; Abdulla, M. A.; Taha, M. M. E.; Hashim, N. M.; Hadi, A. H. A.; Vadivelu, J.; Fai, M. L.; Rahmani, M.; and Yahayu, M. α-Mangostin from *Cratoxylum arborescens* (Vahl) blume demonstrates anti-ulcerogenic property: a mechanistic study. *Evid Based Complement Altern Med*, **2013**, *2013*, 1–10.

Silva Moreira, S.; Tamashiro, L. K.; Jorge, B. C.; Balin, P. S.; Heredia-Vieira, S. C.; Almeida, G. L.; Cardoso, C. A. L.; Kassuya, C. A. L.; and Arena, A. C. Toxicological safety evaluation in acute and 28-day studies of aqueous extract from *Serjania marginata* Casar. (Sapindaceae) leaves in rats. *J Ethnopharmacol*, **2019**, *231*, 197–204.

Silva, J. L. V.; Carvalho, V. S.; Silva, F. L.; Barbosa-Filho, J. M.; Rigoni, V. L. S.; and Nouailhetas, V. L. A. Gastrointestinal property of *Serjania caracasana* (Jacq.) Willd. (Sapindaceae) on rats. *Pharmacologyonline*, **2012**, *1*(Suppl.), 22–26.

Silva, M. A.; Vilegas, W.; De Moura, C. F. G.; and Ribeiro, D. A.. The anti-inflammatory potential of *Mimosa caesalpiniifolia* following experimental colitis: role of COX-2 and TNF-alpha expression. *Drug Res*, **2018**, *68*(4), 196–204.

Silva, M. J.; Vilegas, W.; da Silva, M. A.; de Moura, C. F.; Ribeiro, F. A.; da Silva, V. H.; and Ribeiro, D. A. Mimosa (*Mimosa caesalpiniifolia*) prevents oxidative DNA damage induced by cadmium exposure in Wistar rats. *Toxicol Mech Methods*, **2014**, *24*(8), 567–574.

Silveira, K.; Aloes, J.; Ferreira, H.; Sawaya, A.; and Florêncio, T. Association between malnutrition in children living in favelas, maternal nutritional status, and environmental factors. *J Pediatr*, **2010**, *86*(3), 215–220.

Sone, Y.; Kumada, T.; Toyoda, H.; Yokoyama, M.; Kato, M.; and Asaka, M. Eradicating *Helicobacter pylori* in peptic ulcer disease reduces medical costs in the community. *Helicobacter*, **2008**, *13*, 346–351.

Souza Mdo, C.; Beserra, A. M.; Martins, D. C.; Real, V. V.; Santos, R. A.; Rao, V. S.; Silva, R. M.; and Martins, D. T. *In vitro* and *in vivo* anti-*Helicobacter pylori* activity of *Calophyllum brasiliense* Camb. *J Ethnopharmacol*, **2009**, *123*, 452–458.

Souza, O. A.; Carneiro, R. L.; Vieira, T. H. M.; Funari, C. S.; and Rinaldo, D. Fingerprinting *Cynara scolymus* L. (Artichoke) by means of a green statistically developed HPLC-PAD method. *Food Anal Methods*, **2018**, *11*, 1977–1985.

Stege, P. W.; Davicino, R. C.; Vega, A. E.; Casali, Y. A.; Correa, S.; and Micalizzi, B. Antimicrobial activity of aqueous extracts of *Larrea divaricata* Cav. (jarilla) against *Helicobacter pylori*. *Phytomedicine*, **2006**, *13*, 724–727.

Tabatabaei-Malazy, O.; Larijani, B.; and Abdollahi, M. Targeting metabolic disorders by natural products. *J Diabetes Metab Disord*, **2015**, *14*, 57. DOI: 10.1186/s40200–015-0184–8

Taganna, J. C.; Quanico, J. P.; Perono, R. M.; Amor, E. C.; and Rivera, W. L. Tannin-rich fraction from *Terminalia catappa* inhibits quorum sensing (QS) in *Chromobacterium violaceum* and the QS-controlled biofilm maturation and LasA staphylolytic activity in *Pseudomonas aeruginosa*. *J Ethnopharmacol*, **2011**, *134*, 865–871.

Tan, G. T.; Pezzuto. J. M.; Kinghorn. A. D.; and Hughes, S. H. Evaluation of natural products as inhibitors of human immunodeficiency virus type 1 (HIV-1) reverse transcriptase. *J Nat Prod*, **1991**, *54*, 143–154.

Tanaka, M.; Kishimoto, Y.; Sasaki, M.; Sato, A.; Kamiya, T.; Kondo, K.; and Iida, K. *Terminalia bellirica* (Gaertn.) Roxb. extract and gallic acid attenuate LPS-induced inflammation and oxidative stress via MAPK/NF-κB and Akt/AMPK/Nrf2 pathways. *Oxid Med Cell Long*, **2018**, 2018, 1–15.

Tang, X. H.; Gao, L.; Gao, J.; Fan, Y. M.; Xu, L. Z.; Zhao, X. N.; and Xu, Q. Mechanisms of hepatoprotection of *Terminalia catappa* L. extract on D-Galactosamine-induced liver damage. *Am J Chin Med*, **2004**, *32*(4), 509–519.

Tang, X.; Gao, J.; Wang, Y.; Fan, Y. M.; Xu, L. Z.; Zhao, X. N.; Xu, Q.; and Qian, Z. M. Effective protection of *Terminalia catappa* L. leaves from damage induced by carbon tetrachloride in liver mitochondria. *J Nutr Biochem*, **2006**, *17*, 177–182.

Toppo, E.; Sylvester Darvin, S.; Esakkimuthu, S.; Buvanesvaragurunathan, K.; Ajeesh Krishna, T. P.; Antony Caesar, S.; Stalin, A.; Balakrishna, K.; Pandikumar, P.; Ignacimuthu, S.; and Al-Dhabi, N. A. Curative effect of arjunolic acid from *Terminalia arjuna* in non-alcoholic fatty liver disease models. *Biomed Pharmacother*, **2018**, *107*, 979–988.

Trevisan, M. T. S.; and Macedo, F. V. V. Selection of plants with anticholinesterase activity for the treatment of Alzheimer's disease. *Quim Nova*, **2003**, *26*, 301–304.

Üstün, O.; Ozçelik, B.; Akyön, Y.; Abbasoglu, U.; and Yesilada, E. Flavonoids with anti-*Helicobacter pylori* activity from *Cistus laurifolius* leaves. *J Ethnopharmacol*, **2006**, *108*, 457–461.

Vasudeva, N.; Yadav, N.; and Sharma, S. K. Natural products: a safest approach for obesity. *Chin J Integr Med*, **2012**, *18*(6), 473–480.

Vinothapooshan, G.; and Sundar, K. Anti-ulcer activity of *Mimosa pudica* leaves against gastric ulcer in rats. *Res J Pharm Biol Chem Sci*, **2010**, *1*, 606–614.

Wang, Y. C.; and Huang, T. L. Screening of anti-*Helicobacter pylori* herbs deriving from Taiwanese folk medicinal plants. *FEMS Immunol Med Microbiol*, **2005**, *43*, 295–300.

Wen, K. C.; Shih, I. C.; Hu, J. C.; Liao, S. T.; Su, T. W.; and Chiang, H. M. Inhibitory effects of *Terminalia catappa* on UVB-induced photodamage in fibroblast cell line. *Evid Based Complement Altern Med*, **2011**. *2011*(904532), 1–9. http://dx.doi.org/10.1155/2011/904532

Wittschier, N.; Faller, G.; and Hensel, A. An extract of *Pelargonium sidoides* (EPs 7630) inhibits in situ adhesion of *Helicobacter pylori* to human stomach. *Phytomedicine*, **2007**, *14*, 285–288.

Yang, S. F.; Chen, M. K.; Hsieh, Y. S.; Yang, J. S.; Zavras, A. I.; Hsieh, Y. H.; Su, S. C.; Kao, T. Y.; Chen, P. N.; Chu, S. C. Anti metastatic effects of *Terminalia catappa* L. on oral cancer via a down-regulation of metastasis-associated proteases. *Food Chem Toxicol*, **2010**, *48*(4), 1052–1058.

Yeh, C. B.; Hsieh, M. J.; Hsieh, Y. S.; Chien, M. H.; Lin, P. Y.; Chiou, H. L.; and Yang, S. F. *Terminalia catappa* exerts antimetastatic effects on hepatocellular carcinoma through transcriptional inhibition of Matrix Metalloproteinase-9 by modulating NF-κB and AP-1 activity. *Evid Based Complement Altern Med*, **2012**, *2012* 595292. DOI: 10.1155/2012/595292.

Zaidi, S. F. H.; Yamada, K.; Kadowaki, M.; Usmanghani, K.; and Sugiyama, T. Bactericidal activity of medicinal plants, employed for the treatment of gastrointestinal ailments, against *Helicobacter pylori*. *J Ethnopharmacol*, **2009**, *121*, 286–291.

Zhang, B. L.; Fan, C. Q.; Dong, L.; Wang, F. D.; and Yue, J. M. Structural modification of a specific antimicrobial lead against *Helicobacter pylori* discovered from traditional Chinese medicine and a structure-activity relationship study. *Eur J Med Chem*, **2010**, *45*, 5258–5264.

Zhou, Y.; Taylor, B.; Smith, T. J.; Liu, Z. P.; Clench, M.; Davies, N. W.; and Rainsford, K. D. A novel compound from celery seed with a bactericidal effect against *Helicobacter pylori*. *J Pharm Pharmacol*, **2009**, *61*, 1067–1077.

Part III

Technological Advances in Phytochemical Study

CHAPTER 6

Phytochemical Alternative for Control of the *Erwinia amylovora*: Extraction Conditions and Phytochemical Source Selection

JOAQUIN HERNANDEZ-ESCAMILLA, KARINA CRUZ,
HELIODORO DE LA GARZA, RAUL RODRIGUEZ,
ANA VERONICA CHARLES, JOSE LUIS MARTINEZ HERNANDEZ,
EMILIO OCHOA, MIGUEL MEDINA, CRISTOBAL NOE AGUILAR[*]

*Bioprocesses Research Group, Food Research Department,
School of Chemistry, Universidad Autonoma de Coahuila,
Unidad Saltillo, 25280, Coahuila, Mexico*

[*]*Corresponding author. E-mail: cristobal.aguilar@uadec.edu.mx*

ABSTRACT

In the present chapter, a comparative study about the polyphenolic contents and antibacterial capacity against *Erwinia amylovora* of plant extracts obtained by three methodologies extraction (reflux, infusion, and ultrasound-assisted extraction) from damiana (*Turnera diffusa*), eucalyptus (*Eucalyptus globulus* Labill), marjoram (*Origanum majorana*), rosemary (*Rosmarinus officinalis*), and rue (*Ruta graveolenes*) using three extracting agents (water, 70% ethanol, and ethyl acetate) was carried out. The results showed that the method of reflux using ethanol as an extractor agent represents a good alternative for obtaining vegetal extracts rich in phenolic compounds. The eucalyptus extract at a concentration of 0.25% is able to control the growth of the bacterium *E, amylovora* (causing the disease of the bacterial fire in fruit trees of apple and pear, up to 30.00%).

6.1 INTRODUCTION

Fruits and vegetables are a great interest by the benefits they bring to intake. Due the content of vitamins; mainly as A and C, mineral elements such as potassium, high soluble and insoluble fiber content, functional compounds, and water. The consumption of these products is essential for a healthy and balanced diet. Vegetables, in addition to fruits and seeds (cereals, legumes, and nuts), inflorescences, tubers, roots, bulbs, stems, leaves, vegetative and floral buds, generally possess the aforementioned elements and compounds.

Food losses due to diseases caused by microorganisms such as fungi, bacteria, and viruses in post-harvest are estimated at 10%–30% of the total agricultural production of rot and in some perishable crops losses of more than 50% in developing countries (Osorio et al., 2010).

The bacteria cause important losses in the world agriculture, these pathogens are important because of devastating diseases, in appropriate environmental conditions are present. Among the gender of agriculture importance are the bacteria *Erwinia, Pseudomona,* and *Xanthomona* (Koduro et al., 2006). The excessive and indiscriminate application of bactericide for the control of agricultural diseases has caused severe problems of resistance, environment damage, and serious complications to human health. The search for strategies, technical methods increase the agricultural productivity and maintain the ecological balance without attacking the ecosystems and without risking human health is nowadays a great challenge for agriculture and development (Gallegos et al., 2003).

In this situation, the new approach to combat against the bacteria tries to integrate new options aimed at protecting and increasing crops but with nonharmful alternatives; in the case of the use of natural substances, it is possible to use phytocompounds that the same plants have to develop through evolution, which can be an alternative that limit the use of agrichemicals (Tanaka and Andomuro, 1993).

Phytochemicals are a diverse group of natural chemical compounds produced by different plants, and are characterized as bioactive components. At present, there are several bio compounds identified and classified; in northwest of Mexico considered as arid zone, there are more than 3500 species of plants identified, the products of these plants are stored in granular fibers (trichomes), and include polyphenols, amines, alkaloids, flavonoids, saponins, terpenes, benzofurans, benzopyrans, vitamins, carotenoids, and organics acids, among others. Some of these components surround the surface of the sheets and prevent water loss through the cuticle and probably protect the plants from excessive radiation damage. It is known that there are many phytomolecules that protect the food from the attacks of the bacteria and fungi; although the antibacterial and antifungal activities in some active compounds are unknown in many of those (Jasso de Rodriguez et al., 2006).

Most of the natural phytochemicals are obtained by extractions; several studies have showed that the extract activity on the microorganisms is variable, those depending on extraction method, extraction solvent used, the section plants used for the extraction (leaves, roots, stems, etc.), plant phenology, the collection season in which is made, as well as the latitude and altitude of where this collection takes place (Hernandez-Castillo et al., 2011).

Currently in Mexico, the expenditure destined to combat agricultural pests and diseases represents up to 20% of the cost of production in the agricultural and food industry. Diseases caused by phytopathogenic microorganisms on fruit trees (apple trees and pear trees) are important for the food; these diseases can be controlled using chemical products such as bactericides, fungicides, nematicides, and insecticides; nevertheless, its efficacy may be short lived and its use has caused chronic and acute poisoning to the population, but also the microorganisms' resistance and ecological damage. The acquired resistance to fungicides is given in response to the repetitive use these, and that chemically or biochemically are related.

Due to the above, the increase interest in finding products that have an advantage over products traditionally used, specifically in efficiency, selectivity and, above all, having a lower impact on the environment has increased. There are antecedents that explain the antimicrobial potential presented in the plant extract components and those are distributed throughout the Mexican semidesert. Some of these species include the creosote bush (*Larrea tridentata*) (Lira, 2003), pecan (*Carya illinoensis*), damiana (*Turnera diffusa*) (Castillo et al., 2010), Mexican oregano (*Lippia berlandieri* Shauer) (Ruiz et al., 2009), these plants are characterized to have high polyphenol concentration and variability, such as gallotannins, ellagitannins, complex tannins, and condensed tannins (Khanbabaee and van Ree, 2001). Plant extracts have proven effective in inhibiting the growth of phytopathogenic microorganisms (Koduro et al., 2006).

The study had an objective obtained and identified the presence of polyphenolic compounds in the extracts of vegetable species of Mexican desert, which can be used to control phytopathogenic microorganisms that attack on the pear trees and apple trees.

6.2 EXPERIMENTAL

6.2.1 RAW MATERIAL

Damiana (*Turnera diffusa*), eucalyptus (*Eucalyptus globulus* Labill), marjoram (*Origanum majorana*), rosemary (*Rosmarinus officinalis*), and rue (*Ruta graveolens*) plants were collected from the Mexican semidesert. The plants were treated according to the method reported by Castillo et al. (2010) and Osorio et al. (2010).

Dry material was ground and stored in plastic dark containers at room temperature and protected from light to prevent oxidation of the compounds.

6.2.2 REACTIVE AND STANDARDS

The extraction mixtures were used distilled water, ethanol, and ethyl acetate. The reagents used in this study were sodium carbonate, the Folin–Ciocalteu reagent (2N), and gallic acid (GA).

6.2.3 REFLUX EXTRACTION METHODOLOGY

In the present study, water, ethanol, and ethyl acetate were selected as solvents because they are found by the Food and Drug Administration for use in sanitizing products within approved food industries.

Reflux extraction was performed using 5 g of dried plants, mixed with solvents (solid/liquid ratio 2 g/10 mL) in Erlenmeyer flasks, and covered with foil paper to prevent oxidation of compounds. A water bath was used at 60 ± 2 °C using different concentrations of ethanol (0.25, 0.50, and 1% v/v) and extraction time was 2 h. Late on extracts were filtered and stored in dark bottles to avoid the oxidation of compounds.

6.2.4 INFUSION EXTRACTION

The extraction of the polyphenols from the plants by extraction of infusion was done using the methodology developed by Ventura-Sobrevilla in 2006 (Ventura-Sobrevilla, 2006). Solvents were heated until boiling point, then added the solid part (powder plant), and infused for a time of 10 min. Later extracts were filtered and were stored in dark bottles to avoid the oxidation of compounds.

6.2.5 ULTRASOUND EXTRACTION

Ultrasound methodology was done using an ultrasonic bath (BRANSON, Model 2510) with a capacity of 10 L. Plastic containers were used with a capacity of 100 mL, which were covered with foil paper to prevent exposing the compounds to light. Ratio of plant material and solvents was 1: 4 (w/v). Solvent mixtures were the same as were used in the extraction by refluxing (0.25, 0.50, and 1% v/v) and sonication time was 10 min (Gao and Liu, 2005). Ultrasound equipment was operated at a frequency of 40 kHz and at room temperature.

The plant extracts were filtered and were stored in amber containers until their analysis. The samples were diluted with water to determine total hydrolysable polyphenols.

6.2.6 TOTAL PHENOLIC COMPOUNDS ASSAY

Total content of hydrolysable polyphenols was analyzed by Folin–Ciocalteu assay modified in microplate. In test tube a 20 μL sample was placed; the same tube was added with 20 μL of Folin–Ciocalteu reagent, stirred and allowed to stand for 5 min. After that, 20 μL of Na_2CO_3 (0.01 M) were added, stirred, and allowed to stand for 5 min. Then it was diluted with 125 μL of distilled water and read on a plate reader (Epoch) at 725 nm to determine hydrolysable tannins. The response variable was the amount of total phenolic compounds in the extracts which were expressed as mg gallic acid equivalents (GAE)/g of plant material using a regression equation and a gallic acid calibration curve (R^2 0.995).

6.2.7 ANTIMICROBIAL ASSAYS WITH ERWINIA AMYLOVORA

It was prepared 1000 mL of King's B and was added 20 g of peptone protease No 3, 10 mL of glycerol, 1.5 g of K_2HPO_4 and 1.5 g of $MgSO_4$. Medium culture was homogenized and heated. Then, it was transferred to 100 mL of medium on Erlemeyer flasks and was sterilized at 120 °C/lb for 15 min. Then 1 mL of the obtained extracts was added.

E. amylovora was inoculated previously on tubes inclined by 24 h at 27 °C. Then, under aseptic conditions, 0.5 mL of inoculum was transferred to the Erlenmeyer flasks with medium and extracts. Flasks were incubated at 27 °C at 150 rpm of stirring by 96 h. Samples were collected in Eppendorf tubes at 0, 12, 24, 48, 72, and 96 h and were analyzed on a spectrophotometer (Spectronic 20 Genesys) at 590 nm.

6.3 RESULTS AND DISCUSSIONS

The evaluations of the extraction methods were determined based on the content of the hydrolysable polyphenols as gallic acid equivalents (mg/L GAE) on the five plants: *T. diffusa* (damiana), *O. majorana* (marjoram), *E. globulus* Labill (eucalyptus), *R. officinalis* (rosemary), and *R. graveolens* (rue).

Tables 6.1–6.5 show the concentrations obtained of the hydrolysable polyphenols in ratio of plant/solvent/extraction method, as well as the solids content of the different extracts.

TABLE 6.1 Polyphenol Concentration in Parts Per Million (ppm) Gallic Acid Equivalents on *T. diffusa*

Plant/Solvent/Method	Total Solids (mg/mL)	Total Hydrolysable Polyphenols (ppm)
T. diffusa/H$_2$O/Reflux	50.3	37.08
T. diffusa/H$_2$O/Infusion	52.8	32.2
T. diffusa/H$_2$O/Ultrasound	47.1	87.67
T. diffusa/EtOH/Reflux	69.5	39.1
T. diffusa/EtOH/Infusion	18.6	50.17
T. diffusa/EtOH/Ultrasound	15.3	53.74
T. diffusa/EA/Reflux	17.1	ND
T. diffusa/EA/Infusion	4.4	ND
T. diffusa/EA/Ultrasound	10.6	ND

ND: Not detected; AE: Ethyl acetate.

TABLE 6.2 Polyphenol Concentration in Parts Per Million (ppm) Gallic Acid Equivalents on *O. majorana*

Plant/Solvent/Method	Total Solids (mg/mL)	Total Hydrolysable Polyphenols (mg/L GAE)
O. majorana/H$_2$O/Reflux	39.7	105.05
O. majorana/H$_2$O/Infusion	108.2	62.1
O. majorana/H$_2$O/Ultrasound	93.7	48.86
O. majorana/EtOH/Reflux	86.2	123.51
O. majorana/EtOH/Infusion	17.6	62.2

TABLE 6.2   *(Continued)*

Plant/Solvent/Method	Total Solids (mg/mL)	Total Hydrolysable Polyphenols (mg/L GAE)
O. majorana/EtOH/Ultrasound	7.2	77.96
O. majorana/EA/Reflux	10.8	ND
O. majorana/EA/Infusion	8.4	ND
O. majorana/EA/Ultrasound	8.5	ND

ND: Not detected; AE: Ethyl acetate

TABLE 6.3   Polyphenols Concentration in Parts Per Million (ppm) Gallic Acid Equivalents on *E. globulus* Labill

Plant/Solvent/Method	Total Solids (mg/mL)	Total Hydrolysable Polyphenols (mg/L GAE)
E. globulus Labill/H$_2$O/Reflux	45.9	55.65
E. globulus Labill/H$_2$O/Infusion	45.9	67.43
E. globulus Labill/H$_2$O/Ultrasound	38.2	72.8
E. globulus Labill/EtOH/Reflux	19.2	117.67
E. globulus Labill/EtOH/Infusion	20.1	78.03
E. globulus Labill/EtOH/Ultrasound	41.6	50.17
E. globulus Labill/EA/Reflux	20.5	ND
E. globulus Labill/EA/Infusion	13.4	ND
E. globulus Labill/EA/Ultrasound	82.2	ND

ND: Not detected; AE: Ethyl acetate

TABLE 6.4   Polyphenols Concentration in Parts Per Million (ppm) Gallic Acid Equivalents on *R. officinalis*

Plant/Solvent/Method	Total Solids (mg/mL)	Total Hydrolysable Polyphenols (mg/L^{-1} GAE)
R. officinalis/H$_2$O/Reflux	65.6	53.51
R. officinalis/H$_2$O/Infusion	69.3	56.13
R. officinalis/H$_2$O/Ultrasound	61.1	30.3
R. officinalis/EtOH/Reflux	53.2	43.87
R. officinalis/EtOH/Infusion	85.4	56.13
R. officinalis/EtOH/Ultrasound	26	56.48
R. officinalis/EA/Reflux	34.5	ND
R. officinalis/EA/Infusion	27.1	ND
R. officinalis/EA/Ultrasound	24.1	ND

ND: Not Detected; AE: Ethyl acetate.

TABLE 6.5 Polyphenols Concentration in Parts Per Million (ppm) Gallic Acid Equivalents on *R. graveolens*

Plant/Solvent/Method	Total Solids (mg/mL)	Total Hydrolysable Polyphenols (mg/L GAE)
R. graveolens/H$_2$O/Reflux	54.3	21.25
R. graveolens/H$_2$O/Infusion	58.1	23.03
R. graveolens/H$_2$O/Ultrasound	54.4	26.01
R. graveolens/EtOH/Reflux	23.5	41.6
R. graveolens/EtOH/Infusion	17.3	37.55
R. graveolens/EtOH/Ultrasound	12.7	41.84
R. graveolens/EA/Reflux	10.6	ND
R. graveolens/EA/Infusion	6.8	ND
R. graveolens/EA/Ultrasound	6.5	ND

ND: Not detected; AE: Ethyl acetate.

Figure 6.1 showed the highest hydrolysable polyphenols concentration using reflux extraction method. The ratio between marjoram/EtOH, marjoram/H$_2$O, and eucalyptus/EtOH was showed, with 123.51, 105.05, and 117.67 ppm, respectively. The lowest concentrations were showed in the ratio between rue/H$_2$O, damiana/H$_2$O, and damiana/EtOH with 21.25, 37.08, and 39.1 ppm, respectively. Ethanol was the best solvent for the reflux extraction and the marjoram and eucalyptus showed the best yield. With ethyl acetate solvent (EA) it was not possible to quantify the hydrolysable polyphenols.

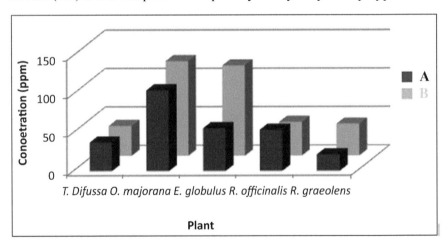

FIGURE 6.1 Extract concentration with reflux method as influenced by plants and solvents: (A) water and (B) ethanol.

Infusion extraction showed better results of hydrolysable polyphenols in the ratios of eucalyptus/EtOH, eucalyptus/H$_2$O, and marjoram/EtOH with 78.03, 67.43, and 62.2 ppm. Ratios with rue/H$_2$O, damiana/EtOH, and rue/EtOH showed low concentrations of hydrolysable polyphenols with 23.03, 32.2, and 37.55 ppm, respectively (Figure 6.2). Eucalyptus and marjoram showed better yield and ethanol was the best solvent from infusion extraction. With EA solvent it was not possible to quantify the hydrolysable polyphenols.

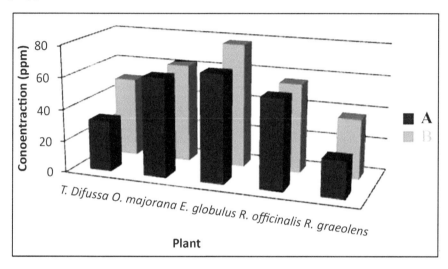

FIGURE 6.2   Extract concentration with infusion method as influenced by plants and solvents: (A) water and (B) ethanol.

Figure 6.3 showed ultrasound extractions of hydrolysable polyphenol concentrations with the ratio between damiana/H$_2$O, marjoram/EtOH, and eucalyptus/H$_2$O that were 87.67, 77.19, and 72.8 ppm, respectively. Furthermore, the hydrolysable polyphenol concentrations with rue/H$_2$O, rosemary/H$_2$O, and rue/EtOH were 26.01, 30.3, and 41.84 ppm, respectively. The damiana and marjoram showed the better yields and the water (H$_2$O) was the better extractant. In the case of ethyl acetate a similar result was obtained as in the previous methods.

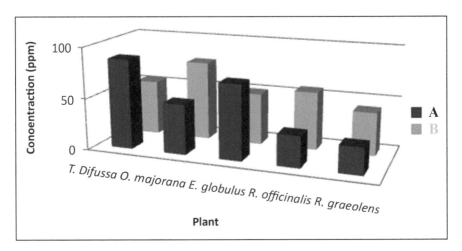

FIGURE 6.3 Extract concentration with ultrasound method as influenced by plants and solvents: (A) water and (B) ethanol.

The better result in hydrolysable polyphenols concentration that was obtained with ratio of plant, solvent, and extraction method was eucalyptus/ EtOH/Reflux with 117.67 ppm and marjoram/EtOH/Reflux with 123.51 ppm. Infusion extraction showed low concentrations with respect to the reflux and ultrasound methods (Figure 6.2).

3.1 EFFECT OF EXTRACTS OF EUCALYPTUS (*E. GLOBULUS* LABILL) AND MARJORAM (*O. MAJORANA*) IN THE GROWTH OF *E. AMYLOVORA*

The evaluation of the growth of *E. amylovora* in liquid medium with the extracts of eucalyptus and marjoram was performed by spectrometry. The extracts of *E. globulus* Labill and *O. majorana* were selected because high concentration of hydrolysable polyphenols which were 117.67 and 123.51 ppm, respectively, with the ethanol solvent and the reflux method.

Figure 6.4(A) showed that *E. globulus* Labill extract at 0.25% concentration retards the growth of *E. amylovora* in 24.52%, being higher than in the concentrations of 0.5% and 1%, which presented a 10.5% and 7.78%, respectively. While Figure 6.4(B) showed that *O. majorana* concentration of 0.5% only retarded the growth of the bacterium by 3.4%, with the concentration of 0.25% the bacteria grew up to 6% more than the control and 1% remained the same as the control.

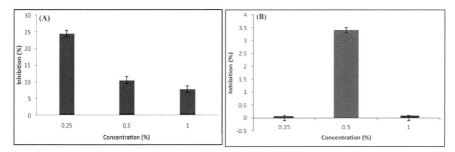

FIGURE 6.4 Percent inhibition of extracts of (A) *Eucaliptus globulus* Labill and (B) *Origanum majorana*.

The results observed with *E. globulus* Labill are similar to those reported by Mosch et al. (1989), who mention that extracts of *Mahonia aguifolium* Nutt, *Berberis vulgaris* L, *Rhus typhina* L., and *Allium sativum* controlled in a 25.6% and 53.2% growth of *E. amylovora*. Mosch et al. (1989) found an inhibition in the growth of *E. amylovora* using aqueous extracts of *Juglans nigra* L, *B. vulgaris*, and *R. typhina* in concentrations of 1.25% and 5.2%, respectively. Zaccheo (1990) reported that extracts from apical meristems of pear. Bartlett observed that 1% had bacteriostatic effects against *E. amylovora*. Effectiveness of the extracts may be according to the plant material from which the extract was obtained, the extraction method employed, the conditions used for the handling of the extract and the microorganism in which it is to be tested.

6.4 CONCLUSIONS

Under the experimental conditions in which the present study was carried out, it is concluded that the reflux method represents a good alternative for obtaining plant extracts rich in phenolic compounds using ethanol as an extractant because it was the solvent that obtained the best results in comparison to the other two methods and solvents studied. The evaluation of the methods of infusion and ultrasound require new studies, because this study presented some factors that need to be analyzed and controlled to obtain better results and thus to obtain higher concentrations of phenolic compounds in plant samples. The plant extract of *E. globulus* Labill at a concentration of 0.25% is capable of retarding the growth of the bacterium *E. amylovora*, which causes bacterial fire disease in apple and pear trees, up to 24.52%.

ACKNOWLEDGMENTS

The authors thank National Council of Science and Technology (CONACYT-Mexico) and Bioingenio LifeTech SA de CV for all financial and technical support.

GLOSSARY FOR TECHNICAL TERMS

Fire blight: Fire blight is a disease of plants in the rose family, especially apple and pear trees, caused by the bacterium *E. amylovora* and characterized by blackened flowers, leaves, and branches.

Infusion extraction: Infusion extraction is a process of extracting chemical compounds or flavors from plant material in a solvent such as water, oil, or alcohol, by allowing the material to remain suspended in the solvent over time.

Percent inhibition: Percent inhibition caused by the plant extract in the *E. amylovora* bacteria.

Reflux extraction: Reflux extraction is a method based on obtaining metabolites according to the solubility of these compounds in the solvent and allows carrying out processes at temperatures above environment, avoiding the loss of solvent and that this leaves to the atmosphere.

Ultrasound-assisted extraction: Ultrasound-assisted extraction is used at high intensity signals that are used to modify a process or a product. In lower frequency and greater power they produce physical and chemical changes in the medium through the generation and collapse of cavitation bubbles, which appear, grow, and collapse in the liquid.

KEYWORDS

- *Eucalyptus globulus*
- **extraction**
- *Origanum majorana*
- **polyphenols**
- *Rosmarinus officinalis*
- *Ruta graveolenes*
- *Turnera diffusa*

REFERENCE

Castillo, F.; Hernandez, D.; Gallegos, G.; Mendez, M.; Rodriguez, R.; Reyes, A. and Aguilar, C. N. *In-vitro* antifungical activity of plant extracts obtained with alternative organic solvents against *Rhizoctonia solani* Kühn. *Industrial Crops Production*, 2010, *32*, 324–328.

Gallegos, M. G.; Cepeda, S. M. and Olayo, P. R. P. *Entomopatogenos*. Editorial Trillas, Mexico, 2003, pages 9–10.

Gao, M. and Liu, C. Comparison techniques for the extraction of flavonoids from cultures cells of *Saussurea medusa* Maxim. *World Journal of Microbiology and Biotechnology*, 2005, *21*, 1461–1463.

Hernandez-Castillo, F. D.; Berlanga, P. A. M.; Gallegos, M. G.; Siller, C. M.; Rodríguez, H. R.; Aguilar, G. C. N. and Castillo, R. R. *In-vitro* antagonist action of *Trichoderma* strains against *Sclerotinia sclerotiorum* and *Sclerotium cepivorum*. *American Journal of Agricultural and Biological Sciences,* 2011, *6* (3), 410–417.

Jasso de Rodriguez, D.; Angulo, S. J. L. and Hernandez C. F. D. An overview of the antimicrobial properties of Mexican medicinal plants. *Advances in Phytomedicine*, 2006, *3*, 325–377.

Khanbabaee, K. and van Ree T. Tannins: Classification and definition. *Natural Products Reports,* 2001, *18*, 641–649.

Koduro, S.; Grierson, D. S. and Alfoloyan, A. J. Antibacterial activity of *Solanum aculeastrum*. *Pharmaceutical Biology*, 2006, *44* (4), 283–286.

Lira, S. R. H. Estado actual del conocimiento sobre las propiedades biosidas de la gobernadora (*Larrea tridentata*). D.C Coville. *Revista Mexicana de Fitopatología*, 2003, *21* (2), 214–221.

Mosch, J.; Klingauf, F. and Zeller, W. On the effect of plant extracts against fireblight (*Erwinia amylovora*). *Acta Horticulturae*, 1989, *273*, 355–361

Osorio, E.; Flores, M.; Hernandez, D.; Ventura, J.; Rodriguez, R. and Aguilar C. N. Biological efficiency of polyphenolic extract from pecan nuts shell (*Carya illinoensis*), pomegranate husk (*Punica granatum*) and creosote bush leaves (*Larrea tridentata* Cov.) against plant pathogenic fungi. *Industrial Crops and Products*, 2010, *31*, 153–157.

Ruiz, B. E.; Velázquez, C.; Garibay, E. A.; García, Z.; Plascencia, J. M.; Cortez, R. M. O.; Hernández, M. J. and Robles, Z. R. E. Antibacterial and antifungical activities of some Mexican medicinal plants. *Journal of Medicinal Food*, 2009, *12*, 1998–1402.

Tanaka, Y. T. and Andomuro, S. Agroactive compound of microbial origin. *Annual Review of Microbiology*, 1993, *47*, 57–87.

Ventura-Sobrevilla, J. M. Degradation of tannins in extracts from governor (*Larrea tridentata* Cov.) and Hojasen (*Fluorencia cernua* DC) by solid state fermentation using *Aspergillus niger* PSH. Bachelor's degree Thesis. Chemical Pharmacist-Biologist. Autonomous University of Coahuila, Mexico. 2006

Zaccheo, A. Growth of *Erwinia amylovora* on extracts of susceptible Rosaceae. *Acta Horticulturae*, 1990, *273*, 339–341.

CHAPTER 7

Isoflavone as a Functional Food and Its Butterfly Model: A Novel Approach

AFROZE ALAM*, SHAILENDRA KUMAR, KAMLESH KUMAR NAIK, UMAR FAROOQ, and K. L. DHAR

Narayan Institute of Pharmacy, Jamuhar, Sasaram (ROHTAS) 821305, Bihar, India

School of Pharmaceutical Sciences, Shoolini University, Bajhol-Solan 173229, Himachal Pradesh, India

*Corresponding author.
E-mail: afrozepharma@gmail.com, afrozalam@niop.in*

ABSTRACT

Soyabean or other plant source isoflavones were used as healthy dietary ingredients and, after menopause, as a component to relieving hormone-related metabolic disorders, such as osteoporosis, cardiac disease, and symptoms. In addition to their anti-inflammatory and antioxidant estrogenic activities, the curative function of isoflavones was extensively studied in heart diseases, diabetes, bone demineralization, or osteoporosis symptoms arose after menopause. In the present chapter, the value of isoflavone as a functional food and the relationship between structure and function as defined in the butterfly model are correlated with it. "As far as we know, our model is the first form/structure-based interaction with colchicine tubulin and estrogens, which shows versatility in pharmacology."

7.1 INTRODUCTION

Currently, researchers have effectively investigated and studied the importance of isoflavone as natural substituents to steroidal drugs commonly employed in hormonal replacement therapy. There is a fact that the diet of Asian women contains plenty of soy food ingredients, hence they are comparatively less influenced by the postmenopausal symptoms such as breast cancer, bone desorption, and heart disease (Adlercreutz et al., 1992). Furthermore, diet enriched with natural isoflavone so-called functional foods are believed to prohibit, postmenopausal symptoms, especially bone desorption or osteoporosis, cancer and cardiovascular disease (Arvanitoyannis et al., 2005). Isoflavone from legumes and nonlegume sources are believed to be traditionally used as functional food products or nutraceuticals. These food ingredients have a measure to mitigate hormone-related pharmacological or physiological imbalance or disorders, such as cancer, bone desorption, and heart disease (Brouns, 2002). The natural phytoestrogen or phytohormones (isoflavones) are greatly recognized and have not showed any adverse reaction, generally observed in traditional therapies with hormone like estrogen.

The researchers have intensively studied and reported that isoflavone can alleviate the degeneration of the skin, especially in postmenopausal women (Lupton, 1996). Due to this matter of fact, isoflavone from different sources could be the attractive compounds for cosmetic formulation (Johnson, 1999). Numerous studies have indicated the inherent relation between diet consumption and appearance of disease conditions led to the identification of a list of bioactive isoflavone, called phytoestrogens (Dillard and German, 2000). Some of these non-nutrient bioactive molecules, such as phytohormones (isoflavone) were shown to produce noteworthy perpetual health benefits (Russo, 2007). Phytohormones, especially isoflavones have shown similar structure and receptor interaction pattern to that of estrogen (Suetsugi et al., 2003). Soybeans are enriched with isoflavones and contain high quantity of genistein and daidzein and their respective β-glycosides (genistin and daidzin). In nonfermented soy products, they appear mostly in form of the polar, water-soluble glycosides, whereas, the biologically active aglycones are essentially found in fermented soy products (Wang and Murphy, 1994). Furthermore, isoflavonoids are important bioactive constituents comprise with polyphenolic structures and are used by humans as functional food (Parr and Bolwell, 2000). Even if, not treated as health food, but necessary for life, many researchers have studied the regular consumption of isoflavonoid may have promising benefits in health and disease (Setchell, 1998).

There is a direct association between isoflavone-rich diet ingestion and mitigation of the incidences of cancer risk, particularly prostate and breast cancer. Some researchers reported that phytoestrogen (isoflavones) can be used to inhibit the multidrug resistance protein (MRP1) transporter by affecting the biochemical and osmotic properties of cell membranes (Setchell and Cassidy, 1999).

The curative role of isoflavones in heart diseases, cancer, symptoms developed after menopause and bone desorption or osteoporosis, in addition to their anti-inflammatory, antioxidant, and estrogenic activities, has largely been studied (Kris-Etherton et al., 2002). Many researchers have investigated the estrogenic activity of genistein, daidzein, and equol at preclinical, clinical, and molecular level to exhibit their significant role for the therapy of chronic diseases, such as osteoporosis, cancer, hormonal imbalance, and heart diseases (Wiseman, 2000).

In general, isoflavones have similar structure to the steroid-related compounds, such as estradiol (Figure 7.1). Thus they can bind at a significant level to the active site of estrogen receptors. The receptor binding rate of isoflavone compared with normal circulating estrogen in human blood is found at satisfactory level (Schmid, 2008) and has capability to compete with active site of the receptors. However, current investigation clearly indicates that the phytoestrogens (isoflavones) have comparatively more affinities toward ERβ than ERα. Isoflavone has been displayed to provide protective mechanism against heart disease and osteoporosis without influencing the ovary, breast, and uterus (Kuiper et al., 1998). Particularly, isoflavone may behave like estrogen receptor (ER) regulator at clinical and preclinical level. Hence, there is a great advantage of the use of isoflavone as phytoestrogen in hormonal disorder over traditional hormonal replacement therapy (Al-Anazi et al., 2011).

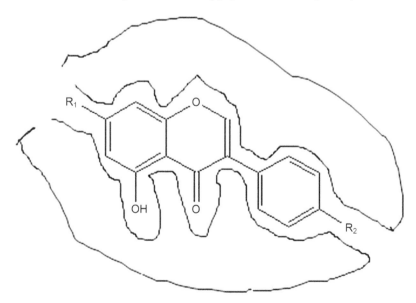

FIGURE 7.1   Isoflavone in ER receptor.

7.2   BUTTERFLY MODEL OF ISOFLAVONE

Butterfly model depicts the arrangement of two aromatic rings with hetero-cyclic ring like two wings of butterfly (Tong et al., 2007). The pharmacophoric distance between the two phenyl rings plays a vital role in the receptor interactions. Many literatures reported that the 17α-estradiol and isoflavone have shown the similar type of interaction pattern with the ER; although, the estrogenic activity of isoflavone has been documented since 1940s in Australian sheep after the identification of "clover disease." That's why isoflavones are considered as a well-known phytoestrogen. The butterfly model significantly attributes the impact of various substitutions pattern on both aromatic rings with receptors; however, the pharmacophoric distance between C-7 and C-4′ augmented a most substantial interaction results (see Figure 7.2). Thus, isoflavones can mimic steroidal activity by filling the stereochemical space that could be possessed by steroidal compounds showing estrogenic activity. This is technically called Butterfly Model (Nepali et al., 2014). Hence, this type of special chemistry helps to identify the effects of many functional food supplements and some topical preparations. A part from the estrogenic potential, isoflavone has shown structural similarity with colchicine combretastatin and phenstatin (all are known marketed anticancer agents) due to their similar spatial orientation between two aromatic rings and is separated by three, two and one carbon atoms, respectively (Table 7.1). Thus, isoflavones also bind to colchicine-tubulin binding site effectively, hence shown prominent anticancer activity against various cancer cell lines. They have shown anticancer activity by means of inhibiting microtubules at G2/M phase (Bhalla, 2003). However, isoflavones are important plant constituents with polyhydroxyl substituted nucleus and are frequently used by humans as food ingredients. Even if not treated health foods and so, indispensable for healthy life, the consumption of isoflavone may illustrate a significant role in health and disease (Setchell and Cassidy, 1999; Rowland et al., 2003). Many literatures documented that there is a direct association of reduction in the occurrence of various type of cancer and regular intake of diet enriched with isoflavone (Williams et al., 1997; Nadaroglu et al., 2007; Wani et al., 2012). It is further revealed that the multidrug resistance transporter (MRP1) could be inhibited by isoflavones affecting the biological physical properties of the membranes (Nadaroglu et al., 2007). The protective measure of isoflavones in cancer (Wu, 1980; Hadfield et al., 2000), heart diseases, postmenopausal imbalance, osteoporosis, including antioxidant (Ali et al., 1983; Van Damme et al., 1997), antimicrobial (Bonfills et al., 2004), anti-inflammatory, and estrogenic activities (García-Lafuente et al., 2009), have been already supported by many literatures. In recent decade, phytoestrogens such as daidzein, genistein, and equol are regularly being studied for their estrogenic activities at different level to identify their prominent role for the treatment of hormone-dependent cancer (Wiseman, 2000). Thus, isoflavones could be used in place of steroidal drugs without any major side effects, as shown by estrogenic compounds (Dweck, 2009). Thus, isoflavones could be used in place of steroidal drugs without any major side effects, as shown by estrogenic compounds (Dweck, 2009). The role of special chemistry itself explains the effects of herbal food supplements specially isoflavone in human health (Dweck, 2006). Hence, butterfly model could be the future target for the detail study of isoflavone showing the estrogen positive, negative, and nonestrogenic activities.

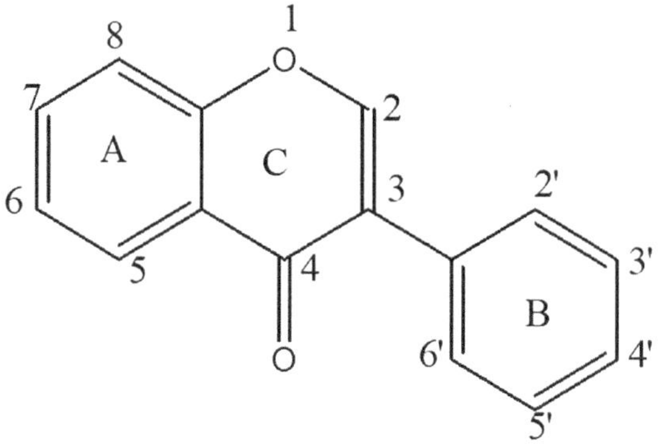

3-phenyl-4*H*-chromen-4-one

FIGURE 7.2   The most common structure of isoflavones.

TABLE 7.1   Structure of Isoflavones from Plant Used as Functional Food

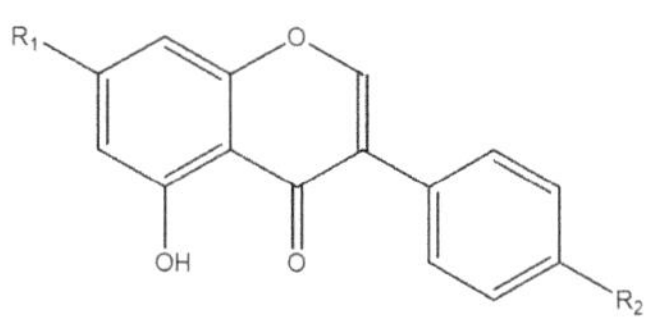

Isoflavones	R_1	R_2
Daidzein	H	OH
Genistein	OH	OH
Biochanin A	OH	OCH_3
Formononetin	H	OCH_3

7.3   OCCURRENCE OF ISOFLAVONE

In general, most of the plants belong to *Fabaceae* family possess indicative quantities of isoflavones (Mazur et al., 1998). The largest quantity of genistein and daidzein has found in *Psoralea corylifolia* after the quantitative analysis of various species (Shinde et al., 2009). Furthermore, various species of legumes such as soybean (*Glycine max* L.), alfalfa sprout (*Medicago sativa* L.), green bean (*Phaseolus vulgaris* L.), mung bean sprout (*Vigna radiata* L.), kudzu root (*Pueraria lobata* L.), cowpea (*Vigna unguiculata* L.), and red clover sprout (*Trifolium pratense* L.) possess isoflavone are investigated for their estrogen positive and estrogen negative activity (Boué et al., 2003). The food generally processed from legumes, for example, tofu, possesses isoflavone in significant quantity (Messina, 2010). Other isoflavone containing food product includes alfalfa (formononetin), chick pea (biochanin A), and peanut (genistein). However, plants of iridaceous family (Iris species) also retain marked quantity of isoflavone. Most of them found as conjugated glycosides or their respective acetyl conjugates or malonates, making them even more polar, hence aqueous solubility has been enhanced (isoflavone-7-O-beta-glucoside 6″-O-malonyltransferase) (Herrmann, 1976; Balasundram et al., 2006). Whenever, leguminous plants are infected with viruses or fungi, the water-soluble transport forms are hydrolyzed at the target site to release respective aglycones.

7.4   ISOFLAVONE AS PHYTOESTROGEN

It is a well-known fact that isoflavones are considered as most proficient plant hormones or phytoestrogens. In 1940s, there was a huge emergence of "clover disease" in Australian sheep led to the identification and investigation of estrogenic activity of isoflavone (Poluzzi et al., 2014). The incidence of reproductive disorders such as abnormal lactation, permanent infertility, change in the sex organs, prolapsed uterus, and mental dystocia were markedly observed to the sheep whose diet mainly contains subterranean clover (*Trifolium subterraneum* L., *Fabaceae*) (Bennetts et al., 1946).

Isoflavones belong to a class of organic compounds, generally found in leguminous plants and classified under flavonoids family, where most of the isoflavone showing estrogenic activity in mammals. Some other pharmacological activities were also reported word wide. Some study clearly showed that diet comprises with soy protein indicated that there is a marked reduction in the emergence of breast cancer and other type of estrogen related cancer, due to the significant and promising role of isoflavone, affecting the metabolism of sex hormones and related biological activity through protein synthesis, intracellular enzymes, growth factor action, angiogenesis, and malignant cell proliferation and differentiation (Omoni and Aluko, 2005).

Furthermore, the low risk of breast and other common cancer emergence from soy isoflavone has been also reported in Asian populations. Earlier, it was reported that isoflavones were only found in the *Fabaceae* or *Leguminosae* family. But, a lot of research has been done on iridaceous family specially Iris species (nonleguminous, monocot) and surprisingly produces large number of isoflavones.

7.5 GENERAL STRUCTURE OF ISOFLAVONE

Isoflavone consists of two aromatic rings (A and B) in conjugation with heterocyclic ring C. B ring attached to position 3 of C-ring (Beecher, 2003). Even they are not steroids; they have the structure similar to estrogens, particularly estradiol. This confers the ability of isoflavone to bind with estrogen receptors, therefore, they are considered as phytoestrogens. In food, isoflavones have been found as secondary metabolites in four different forms as: (1) Aglycone, (2) 7-*O*-glucoside, (3) 6′-*O*-acetyl-7-*O*-glucoside, and (4) 6′-*O*-malonyl-7-*O*-glucoside.

The content of isoflavone may vary from 0.5 to 2.5 mg/g depending upon climate conditions and variety of species. Isoflavones constitute the largest group of natural isoflavonoids with large number of new structures reported in every year. The abundant availability of isoflavonoids in plants of folk or traditional medicine has significantly promoted to enhance the interest in the search for bioactive molecules from both legume and nonlegume plant. Some of the naturally occurring isoflavone found in plants used as functional food.

7.6 ANALYTICAL TECHNIQUES FOR CHARACTERIZATION OF ISOFLAVONE

Studies on isoflavonoids by spectroscopic methods have illustrated that most isoflavones show two important absorption peaks: Band I (315–380 nm) corresponds the B ring absorption, while Band II (240–290 nm) represents to the A ring absorption (de Rijke et al., 2006). Impact of solvent system or shift reagent in isoflavonoid nucleus might have caused a shift in ultraviolet (UV) absorption range from 341 to 371.6 nm of 5,7,8-trihydroxy-4′-methoxy isoflavone in methanol and methanol plus aluminum chloride (shift's reagents) respectively (Alam et al., 2017). Isoflavones show very prominent peak between 275 and 293 nm correspond to Band II absorption maxima, for example, geniestein exhibited at 288 nm and daidzein appear at 285 nm, while only a peak for Band I appears at 325 or 326 nm. Band II exhibits as one peak at 275 nm in molecule comprises with a mono substituted B ring, but has two absorption peaks at 258 and 272 nm when a di-, tri-, or o-substituted B ring is present. Isoflavone iridin exhibits a clear Band I peak in the 445–555 nm regions and Band II peaks in the range of 245–2805 nm because of the presence of cinnamoyl system of the B ring and benzoyl system of the A ring, respectively. Furthermore, isoflavones might have absorption maxima at 265 nm and can be easily identified by reversed-phase high-performance liquid chromatography (RP-HPLC). Hence, the aglycone can be easily eluted by RP-HPLC analysis after the usual process of purification. Isoflavone glycosides such as daidzin and genistin are the major constituents of the analysis. After the hydrolysis of the glycoside by β-glucosidase treatment corresponding aglycones daidzein and genistein are obtained (Setchell, 1998). The genistin (glycoside) from the plant materials can be eluted at 87% as genistein and 55% as daidzein, respectively, after the usual process of isolation. The purity of the product was >80% of the aglycone in alcoholic solution. The white needle-shaped crystals became visible, when appropriate dilution of alcoholic solution was made by the addition of water.

7.7 ISOFLAVONE AS FUNCTIONAL FOOD

Currently, a study has been investigated that isoflavones have promising antioxidant properties, compare to that of the notable antioxidant vitamin E (Soobrattee et al., 2005). The regular consumption of isoflavone-rich diet can enhance the antioxidant ability of biological system; hence, can also reduce the incidence of cancer by inhibiting free radical damage to DNA (Rahman, 2007; Rajendran et al., 2014). Geniestein is the most potent anti-oxidant among the soy isoflavone (from soy food), followed by daidzein. It was assessed that a positive response has been documented for the isofla-vone intake on the prevention of osteoporosis in women. Furthermore, it was found that the regular isoflavone supplements show a 54% increase in bone mineral density and was also associated with a significant lower level of bone resorption (Kreijkamp-Kaspers et al., 2004). Isoflavone has the similar chemical structure to that of female sex hormone estrogen, and can be used as a substituent for postmenopausal women where conventional hormone replacement therapy does not tolerate and also not suitable for the proper treatment (This et al., 2005). Isoflavone exhibits a 40% decrease in menopausal symptoms, such as hot flashes, musculoskeletal pain, and a lower incidence of insomnia and depression (Hachul et al., 2014). Researchers suggested that the isoflavone does not elevate different parameters or markers of breast cancer risk in postmenopausal women. In fact, they may provide a defensive role in most of the women. Even at high doses, there is no evidence that the isoflavones can potentiate cell growth or other markers for cancer risk in breast cell. Even though the protective effect of higher doses of isoflavone has been reported in the literature for the women, who have estrogen hormone at higher level (Anderson et al., 1999). Furthermore, epidemiological studies show that women who consume isoflavone-rich diets may have lower incidence rates of breast cancer. However, isoflavone found in Iris species, legumes, soybeans, and clovers may enhance artery function in stroke patients (Wong and Rabie, 2007). Diet comprises with isoflavone can be used to diminish vasomotor symptoms, such as hot flushes, musculoskeletal pain, lower incidence of insomnia and depression, and enhanced bone density in women. Isoflavone appears to decrease cardiovascular disease through different mechanism. Isoflavone inhibits the deposition and formation of artery clogging plaque. There may be a possibility that isoflavone can be used to enhance hair growth, when the oil of orris was regularly applied. After 12 weeks of regular isoflavone intake, at a dose of 80 mg a day, there was elaborated blood flow in the brachial artery, which is particularly important in patients who have suffered from ischemic stroke which is caused by blood clots or other obstructions (Omura et al., 1996). Nowadays, isoflavone from soybean has been extensively studied for its response on modulation of IL-6 gene expression and is considered as potent candidature for the improved therapy of inflammation and thereby inhibits malignancy progression, aging discomfort, and also restores immune balance (Dijsselbloem et al., 2004). There are some researchers who reported the medicinal use of isoflavone for the relief of airway inflammatory disease as it has capability to bring down mRNA expression of exotoxin (Bellik et al., 2012). It has been found that isoflavone is used to inhibit the lung tissue eosinophil infiltration, collagen deposition, and airways mucus production in lung cell (Bao et al., 2011). Isoflavones are also being estimated to be used in the treatment of cutaneous inflammation by the virtue of preventing the proinflammatory cytokines, expression of COX-2, attenuation of oxidative stress and prohibiting NF-κB activation (Alam et al., 2017) and also rendering the formation of 5-hydroxymethyl-2′-deoxyuridine, a marker for oxidative DNA damage (Davis et al., 2001). Furthermore, it is found to be useful in preventing insulin resistance and hence may be considered as an adjuvant therapy for control of diabetes (Rajasekaran et al., 2008). It is also known to prevent the secretion of inflammatory mediators, such as prostaglandin E_2 and IL-6.

7.8   POTENTIAL HUMAN HEALTH BENFITS

Isoflavones are supposed to retain health benefits in different human conditions, such as menopause, heart disease, osteoporosis, cyclic mastalgia, and endocrine-responsive cancers (Albulescu and Popovici, 2007). It is well-known that isoflavone has estrogen-like activity and has favorable side effect, may be considered as an ideal substituent to hormone replacement therapy. Diet enriched with isoflavone may significantly affect estrogen metabolism by modifying the steroid hormone concentrations and menstrual cycle length, thereby depicting a potential to diminish the risk for breast carcinoma (Kumar et al., 2002).

Isoflavone-rich diet is supposed to have a benefit in cardiovascular conditions because they lower low density lipoprotein (LDL) by inhibiting cholesterol metabolism. The estrogen or estrogen-like isoflavone may reduce the concentration of circulatory inflammatory markers would be the probable mechanism by which postmenopausal women are defended or protected against cardiovascular disease (Sarkar and Li, 2004). Isoflavones improve C reactive protein concentrations as well.

Isoflavones are plant-derived product occur naturally and are well-known as plant hormones or phytoestrogens. Because of the similar chemical structure, isoflavones have pronounced estrogenic activity similar to female sex hormone estrogen (Benachour et al., 2012). Isoflavones are found naturally in soybeans and can be incorporated in several soy-based foods such as, tofu, miso, soy milk, soy sauce, and soy butter. Researchers have investigated that these compounds have some medicinal potential, particularly for women, and continue to study isoflavones for different health benefits. Studies have documented that isoflavone can bind to the same active sites of the receptor as estrogen, hence exhibiting butterfly model. There are multiple targets of isoflavone, such as colchicine-tubulin binding site, chalcone-binding site, estrogenic (ER) β, and ERα, inherently linked with the proposed butterfly model (Nepali et al., 2014). Consequently, isoflavone as functional food and its butterfly model clearly depicted their significance in public health. Soybean is an important dietary source of isoflavones; however, the amount of soy food, necessary to meet the body's requirements can be difficult to add into today's diet.

7.8.1 MECHANISM OF ACTION ON HUMAN HEALTH

Researchers have documented that isoflavone exhibits multiple mode of action on human biological system thereby showing multibiological and pharmacological effects. These include estrogenic positive and negative effect, regulating cell signaling conduction and inducing cell growth and death. Isoflavone can also regulate transcription, modulate transcription factors, behave as antioxidants, as well as influence some enzyme activities.

7.8.1.1 BIOTRANSFORMATION OF ISOFLAVONES

Ingested isoflavones are bio-transformed in the gastrointestinal tract; this particular process is greatly dependent on intestinal microbial or bacterial metabolism. The ingested glycosides daidzin and genistin are not able to absorb in intact form into the peripheral circulation of healthy human; they have to be transformed to the aglycones genistein and daidzein through the action of intestinal β-glucosidases and can be further metabolized into both estrogenic and antiestrogenic metabolites. The process by which isoflavone glycosides are bioavailable is therefore dependent on intestinal microflora (Messina, 2016; Ramdath et al., 2017).

7.9 ECONOMICAL IMPORTANCE OF ISOFLAVONE

The quantitative and qualitative determinations of oils of some Syrian wild Iris species comprise natural isoflavones investigated by Sakamoto et al. (2016). The essential oil was extracted from wild variety of rhizome of Iris species, using hydrodistillation; nearly 0.1%–0.2% of oil yield was achieved. Spectroscopic analyses of essential oil have confirmed the presence of 23 compounds including isoflavone using gas chromatography and mass spectrometry.

These are infamous and very graceful decorative or ornamental plants, cultivated on the eastern Mediterranean region, expanding into Northern India and Northern Africa, and largely grown on the mountain slopes. Iridin an isoflavone is a major component and must contribute to the use that is made of orris root in perfumery.

Orris root was mainly produced and derived from different species of Iris, such as *Iris germanica*, *Iris pallida*, and *Iris florentina*, which is used as chief economical constituents for the production of perfumery.

The powder of orris roots undergoes steam distillation to produce oil of orris, which has an intensified and highly elegant odor with a value of high price. Orris oil can be utilized economically in the manufacturing of the scent and is also combined with artificially manufactured perfumes, the odor of which it delivers more subtle. It enhance the power of reinforcing the odor of other aromatic bodies and also used as a marked adjuvant in perfumery. Oil of orris is known commercially as orris butter (Singab et al 2016).

The fresh juice obtained from the Iris root, mixed with wine is commercially used as a strong purge of high efficiency in dropsy. Sometimes the juice can be utilized as cosmetics and for the suppression of discoloration from the skin. The dried root can be used principally in perfume industry in different dosages form and generally available in sachet powders. These can also be used to flavor dental products and toothpowders. Iridin, an isoflavone has been used in the treatment of liver disorder but has shown milder action on the renal dysfunction. The iridin is preferable over the podophyllin in these conditions. The Iris species, *Iris versicolor*, produces a drug official in United States Pharmacopoeia (USP). However, some of the isoflavone, glabridin, and polyphenolic compounds obtained from *Glycyrrhiza glabra* *prevent* LDL via scavenging free radicals mechanism (Khangholi et al., 2016). Apart from this, iridin is an official drug of USP and is the major source of commerce, used as powdered extract with diuretic and aperient properties, such as bitterness, nauseous, and acrid. The rich source of isoflavone is mainly obtained from soy food, it may contain many type of isoflavones, but the most versatile and beneficial are genistein and daidzein. The major amount of isoflavone is found in soy nuts and tempeh. The other natural source of isoflavone is red clover and *Iris* species.

7.10   CONCLUSION

In this conclusion, isoflavones are compounds showing various biological activities with relevance to the consumption of isoflavone-rich diet and significance of butterfly model. Previously, the role of isoflavone was mostly attributed in terms of their antioxidative properties; however, due to current research, they are also explained as regulatory and signaling molecules. In practice, their influences on various types of chronic diseases are such as cancer, fertility, antifertility, osteoporosis, cardiovascular disease, and post-menopausal hormonal imbalance. The relationship between isoflavone-rich diet and health is rapidly growing of study and increasingly alternative has turned to the role of isoflavone-rich diet in health and disease prevention. More research is required to understand the mechanism that links isoflavone as functional food and health, and weather short-term diet therapy can achieve long-term health benefits.

7.11 SUMMARY

Isoflavones from soybeans or other plant sources were used as healthy dietary ingredients and as a part to mitigate hormone-related metabolic disturbance, such as osteoporosis, heart disease, and symptoms appear after menopause. The plant hormones or phytoestrogen is greatly recognized and has not exhibited any adverse reaction, generally observed in traditional therapies with hormone like estrogen. Some of these non-nutrient bioactive molecules, such as phytohormones (isoflavone) have been shown to exhibit promising perpetual health benefits. Even if, not treated as health food, but necessary for life, many researchers have studied the regular consumption of isoflavonoid may have a promising benefits in health and disease. Researchers have investigated that there is a coherent relation between consumption of isoflavone-containing food products and decrease the risk of appearance of different types of malignancy, especially estrogen-related cancer. The curative role of isoflavones in heart diseases, cancer, bone demineralization, or osteoporosis, symptoms developed after menopause in conjugation to their anti-inflammatory, antioxidant, and estrogenic activities, has largely been studied. In the present study, the importance of isoflavone was focused as functional food and linked/correlate with the structure–function relationship, depicted in butterfly model. The butterfly model inherently deals with ligand–receptor interaction. The two aromatic rings separated by one/two/three carbon atom(s) significantly play a major role to bind with the active site of the receptors. Thus, butterfly model illustrated the arrangement of two aromatic rings with heterocyclic ring like two wings of butterfly. Furthermore, butter fly model significantly attributes the impact of various substitutions pattern on both aromatic rings with receptors; however, the pharmacophoric distance between the two rings (same as the wings of butter fly) augmented the most substantial interaction results. Thus, isoflavones can act as steroidal mimics by filling the stereochemical space that could be occupied by estrogenic compounds. It is this special chemistry that explains the effects of many nutritional herbal supplements and topical preparations. "To our knowledge, our model is the first kind of shape/structure based interactions, deal with colchicine-tubulin and estrogenic binding site showing versatile pharmacological activities."

KEYWORDS

- **butterfly model**
- **cardiovascular diseases**
- **colchicine-tubulin binding site**
- **cytotoxicity**
- **estrogenic receptor**
- **functional food**
- **isoflavone**
- **ligand–receptor interaction**
- **menopausal symptoms**
- **osteoporosis**
- **pharmacophoric distance**
- **phytohormones**
- **topical preparations**

REFERENCES

Adlercreutz, H.; Mousavi, Y.; Clark, J.; Höckerstedt, K.; Hämäläinen, E.; Wähälä, K.; Mäkelä, T.; Hase, T. Dietary phytoestrogens and cancer: *in vitro* and *in vivo* studies. *The Journal of Steroid Biochemistry and Molecular Biology*, 1992, *41* (3), 331–337.

Alam, A.; Naik, K. K.; Upadhaya, N. K.; Kumar, S.; Dhar, K. L. Simple, efficient and economical methods for isolation and estimation of novel isoflavone using RP-HPLC. *Methods X*, 2017, *4*, 128–133.

Alam, A.; Jaiswal, V.; Akhtar, S.; Jayashree, B. S.; Dhar, K. L. Isolation of isoflavones from *Iris kashmiriana* Baker as potential anti proliferative agents targeting NF-kappaB. *Phytochemistry*, 2017, *136*, 70–80.

Al-Anazi, A. F.; Qureshi, V. F.; Javaid, K.; Qureshi, S. Preventive effects of phytoestrogens against postmenopausal osteoporosis as compared to the available therapeutic choices: an overview. *Journal of Natural Science, Biology, and Medicine*, 2011, *2* (2), 154–163.

Albulescu, M.; Popovici, M. Isoflavones-biochemistry, pharmacology and therapeutic use. *Revue Roumaine de Chimie*, 2007, *52* (6), 537–550.

Ali, A. A.; El-Emary, N. A.; El-Moghazi, M. A.; Darwish, F. M.; Frahm, A. W. Three isoflavonoids from *Iris germanica*. *Phytochemistry*, 1983, *22* (9), 2061–2063.

Anderson, J. J.; Anthony, M. S.; Cline, J. M.; Washburn, S. A.; Garner, S. C. Health potential of soy isoflavones for menopausal women. *Public Health Nutrition*, 1999, *2* (4), 489–504.

Arvanitoyannis, I. S.; Van Houwelingen-Koukaliaroglou, M. Functional foods: a survey of health claims, pros and cons, and current legislation. *Critical Reviews in Food Science and Nutrition*, 2005, *45* (5), 385–404.

Balasundram, N.; Sundram, K.; Samman, S. Phenolic compounds in plants and agri-industrial by-products: antioxidant activity, occurrence, and potential uses. *Food Chemistry*, 2006, *99* (1), 191–203.

Bao, Z. S.; Hong, L.; Guan, Y.; Dong, X. W.; Zheng, H. S.; Tan, G. L.; Xie, Q. M. Inhibition of airway inflammation, hyper responsiveness and remodeling by soy isoflavone in a murine model of allergic asthma. *International Immunopharmacology*, 2011, *11* (8), 899–906.

Beecher, G. R. Overview of dietary flavonoids: nomenclature, occurrence and intake. *The Journal of Nutrition*, 2003, *133* (10), 3248S–3254S.

Bellik, Y.; Boukraâ, L.; Alzahrani, H. A.; Bakhotmah, B. A.; Abdellah, F.; Hammoudi, S. M.; Iguer-Ouada, M. Molecular mechanism underlying anti-inflammatory and anti-allergic activities of phytochemicals: an update. *Molecules*, 2012, *18* (1), 322–353.

Benachour, N.; Clair, E.; Mesnage, R.; Séralini, G. E. Endocrine disruptors: new discoveries and possible progress of evaluation. *Advances in Medicine and Biology*, 2012, *29*, 978–981.

Bennetts, H. W.; Uuderwood, E. J.; Shier, F. L. A specific breeding problem of sheep on subterranean clover pastures in Western Australia. *Australian Veterinary Journal*, 1946, *22* (1), 1–12.

Bhalla, K. N. Microtubule-targeted anticancer agents and apoptosis. *Oncogene*, 2003, *22* (56), 9075–9086.

Bonfills, J. P.; Pinguet, F.; Culine, S.; Saurvaire, Y. Cytotoxicity of iridals, triterpenoids from *Iris*. *Planta Medica*, 2004, *67*, 79–81.

Boué, S. M.; Wiese, T. E.; Nehls, S.; Burow, M. E.; Elliott, S.; Carter-Wientjes, C. H.; Shih, B. Y.; McLachlan, J. A.; Cleveland, T. E. Evaluation of the estrogenic effects of legume extracts containing phytoestrogens. *Journal of Agricultural and Food Chemistry*, 2003, *51*(8), 2193–2199.

Brouns, F. Soya isoflavones: a new and promising ingredient for the health foods sector. *Food Research International*, 2002, *35* (2), 187–193.

Davis, J. N.; Kucuk, O.; Djuric, Z.; Sarkar, F. H. Soy isoflavone supplementation in healthy men prevents NF-κB activation by TNF-α in blood lymphocytes. *Free Radical Biology and Medicine*, 2001, *30* (11), 1293–1302.

de Rijke, E.; Out, P.; Niessen, W. M.; Ariese, F.; Gooijer, C.; Udo, A. T. Analytical separation and detection methods for flavonoids. *Journal of Chromatography A*, 2006, *1112* (1), 31–63.

Dijsselbloem, N.; Berghe, W. V.; De Naeyer, A.; Haegeman, G. Soy isoflavone phyto-pharmaceuticals in interleukin-6 affections: multi-purpose nutraceuticals at the crossroad of hormone replacement, anti-cancer and anti-inflammatory therapy. *Biochemical Pharmacology*, 2004, *68* (6), 1171–1185.

Dillard, C. J.; German, J. B. Phytochemicals: nutraceuticals and human health. *Journal of the Science of Food and Agriculture*, 2000, *80* (12), 1744–1756.

Dweck, A. C. Isoflavones, phytohormones and phytosterols. *Journal of Applied Cosmetology*, 2006, *24* (1), 17–33.

Dweck, A. C. The internal and external use of medicinal plants. *Clinics in Dermatology*, 2009, *27* (2), 148–158.

García-Lafuente, A.; Guillamón, E.; Villares, A.; Rostagno, M. A.; Martínez, J. A. Flavonoids as anti-inflammatory agents: implications in cancer and cardiovascular disease. *Inflammation Research*, 2009, *58* (9), 537–552.

Hachul, H.; Monson, C.; Kozasa, E. H.; Oliveira, D. S.; Goto, V.; Afonso, R.; Llanas, A. C.; Tufik, S. Complementary and alternative therapies for treatment of insomnia in women in postmenopause. *Climacteric*, 2014, *17* (6), 645–653.

Hadfield, J. A.; McGown, A. T.; Butler, J. A high-yielding synthesis of the naturally occurring antitumour agent irisquinone. *Molecules*, 2000, *5* (1), 82–88.

Herrmann, K. Flavonols and flavones in food plants: a review. *International Journal of Food Science and Technology*, 1976, *11* (5), 433–448.

Johnson, F. B.; Sinclair, D. A.; Guarente, L. Molecular biology of aging. *Cell*, 1999, *96* (2), 291–302.

Khangholi, S.; Majid, F. A. A.; Berwary, N. J. A.; Ahmad, F.; Aziz, R. B. A. The mechanisms of inhibition of advanced glycation end products formation through polyphenols in hyperglycemic condition. *Planta Medica*, 2016, *82* (01/02), 32–45.

Kreijkamp-Kaspers, S.; Kok, L.; Grobbee, D. E.; De Haan, E. H.; Aleman, A.; Lampe, J. W.; Van Der Schouw, Y. T. Effect of soy protein containing isoflavones on cognitive function, bone mineral density, and plasma lipids in postmenopausal women: a randomized controlled trial. *JAMA*, 2004, *292* (1), 65–74.

Kris-Etherton, P.M.; Hecker, K. D.; Bonanome, A.; Coval, S. M.; Binkoski, A. E.; Hilpert, K. F.; Griel, A. E.; Etherton, T. D. Bioactive compounds in foods: their role in the prevention of cardiovascular disease and cancer. *The American Journal of Medicine*, 2002, *113* (9), 71–88.

Kuiper, G. G.; Lemmen, J. G.; Carlsson, B. O.; Corton, J. C.; Safe, S. H.; Van Der Saag, P. T.; Van Der Burg, B.; Gustafsson, J. A. Interaction of estrogenic chemicals and phytoestrogens with estrogen receptor β. *Endocrinology*, 1998, *139* (10), 4252–4263.

Kumar, N. B.; Cantor, A.; Allen, K.; Riccardi, D.; Cox, C. E. The specific role of isoflavones on estrogen metabolism in premenopausal women. *Cancer*, 2002, *94* (4), 1166–1174.

Lupton, D. Constructing the menopausal body: the discourses on hormone replacement therapy. *Body and Society*, 1996, *2* (1), 91–97.

Mazur, W. M.; Duke, J. A.; Wähälä, K.; Rasku, S.; Adlercreutz, H. Isoflavonoids and lignans in legumes: nutritional and health aspects in humans. *The Journal of Nutritional Biochemistry*, 1998, *9* (4), 193–200.

Messina, M. Impact of soy foods on the development of breast cancer and the prognosis of breast cancer patients. *Complementary Medicine Research*, 2016, *23* (2), 75–80.

Messina, M. Insights gained from 20 years of soy research. *The Journal of Nutrition*, 2010, *140* (12), 2289S–2295S.

Nadaroğlu, H.; Demir, Y; Demir, N. Antioxidant and radical scavenging properties of Iris germanica. *Pharmaceutical Chemistry Journal*, 2007, *41* (8), 409–415.

Nepali, K.; Ojha, R.; Sharma, S.; MS Bedi, P.; L Dhar, K. Tubulin inhibitors: a patent survey. *Recent Patents on Anti-cancer Drug Discovery*, 2014, *9* (2), 176–220.

Omoni, A. O.; Aluko, R. E. Soybean foods and their benefits: potential mechanisms of action. *Nutrition Reviews*, 2005, *63* (8), 272–283.

Omura, Y.; Lee, A. Y.; Beckman, S. L.; Simon, R.; Lorberboym, M.; Duvvi, H.; Heller, S. I.; Urich, C. Cardiovascular risk factors, classified in 10 categories, to be considered in the prevention of cardiovascular diseases: an update of the original 1982 article containing 96 risk factors. *Acupuncture and Electro-Therapeutics Research*, 1996, *21* (1), 21–76.

Parr, A. J.; Bolwell, G. P. Phenols in the plant and in man. The potential for possible nutritional enhancement of the diet by modifying the phenols content or profile. *Journal of the Science of Food and Agriculture*, 2000, *80* (7), 985–1012.

Poluzzi, E.; Piccinni, C.; Raschi, E.; Rampa, A.; Recanatini, M.; De Ponti, F. Phytoestrogens in postmenopause: the state of the art from a chemical, pharmacological and regulatory perspective. *Current Medicinal Chemistry*, 2014, *21* (4), 417–436.

Rahman, K. Studies on free radicals, antioxidants, and co-factors. *Clinical Interventions in Aging*, 2007, *2* (2), 219.

Rajasekaran, A.; Sivagnanam, G.; Xavier, R. Nutraceuticals as therapeutic agents: a review. *Research Journal of Pharmaceutical Technology*, 2008, *1* (4), 328–340.

Rajendran, P.; Nandakumar, N.; Rengarajan, T.; Palaniswami, R.; Gnanadhas, E. N.; Lakshminarasaiah, U.; Gopas, J.; Nishigaki, I. Antioxidants and human diseases. *Clinica Chimica Acta*, 2014, *436*, 332–347.

Ramdath, D. D.; Padhi, E. M.; Sarfaraz, S.; Renwick, S.; Duncan, A. M. Beyond the cholesterol-lowering effect of soy protein: a review of the effects of dietary soy and its constituents on risk factors for cardiovascular disease. *Nutrients*, 2017, *9* (4), 324. DOI:10.3390/nu9040324.

Rowland, I.; Faughnan, M.; Hoey, L.; Wähälä, K.; Williamson, G.; Cassidy, A. Bioavailability of phyto-oestrogens. *British Journal of Nutrition*, 2003, *89* (S1), S45–S58.

Russo, G. L. Ins and outs of dietary phytochemicals in cancer chemoprevention. *Biochemical Pharmacology*, 2007, *74* (4), 533–544.

Sakamoto, S.; Yusakul, G.; Pongkitwitoon, B.; Tanaka, H.; Morimoto, S. Colloidal gold-based indirect competitive immunochromatographic assay for rapid detection of bioactive isoflavone glycosides daidzin and genistin in soy products. *Food Chemistry*, 2016, *194*, 191–195.

Sarkar, F. H.; Li, Y. The role of isoflavones in cancer chemoprevention. *Frontiers in Bioscience*, 2004, *9* (1), 2714–2724.

Schmid, D.; Belser, E.; Meister, S. Use of soy isoflavones for stimulation of skin collagen synthesis. *Switzerland: Mibelle Biochemistry*, 2008, *22* (12), 156–263.

Setchell, K. D. Phytoestrogens: the biochemistry, physiology, and implications for human health of soy isoflavones. *The American Journal of Clinical Nutrition*, 1998, *68* (6), 1333S–1346S.

Setchell, K. D.; Cassidy, A. Dietary isoflavones: biological effects and relevance to human health. *The Journal of Nutrition*, 1999, *129* (3), 758S–767S.

Shinde, A. N.; Malpathak, N.; Fulzele, D. P. Enhanced production of phytoestrogenic isoflavones from hairy root cultures of *Psoralea corylifolia* L. using elicitation and precursor feeding. *Biotechnology and Bioprocess Engineering*, 2009, *14* (3), 288–294.

Singab, A. N. B.; Ayoub, I. M.; El-Shazly, M.; Korinek, M.; Wu, T. Y.; Cheng, Y. B.; Chang, F. R.; Wu, Y. C. Shedding the light on Iridaceae: ethnobotany, phytochemistry and biological activity. *Industrial Crops and Products*, 2016, *92*, 308–335.

Soobrattee, M. A.; Neergheen, V. S.; Luximon-Ramma, A.; Aruoma, O. I.; Bahorun, T. Phenolics as potential antioxidant therapeutic agents: mechanism and actions. *Mutation Research/Fundamental and Molecular Mechanisms of Mutagenesis*, 2005, *579* (1), 200–213.

Suetsugi, M.; Su, L.; Karlsberg, K.; Yuan, Y. C.; Chen, S. Flavone and isoflavone phytoestrogens are agonists of estrogen-related receptors. *Molecular Cancer Research*, 2003, *1* (13), 981–991.

This, P.; De La Rochefordi, A.; Clough, K.; Fourquet, A.; Magdelenat, H. Breast Cancer Group of the Institut Curie, Phytoestrogens after breast cancer. *Endocrine-Related Cancer*, 2001, *8* (2), 129–134.

Tong, H.; Hong, Y.; Dong, Y.; Ren, Y.; Häussler, M.; Lam, J. W.; Wong, K. S.; Tang, B. Z. Color-tunable, aggregation-induced emission of a butterfly-shaped molecule comprising a pyran skeleton and two cholesteryl wings. *The Journal of Physical Chemistry B*, 2007, *111* (8), 2000–2007.

Van Damme, E. J.; Barre, A.; Barbieri, L.; Valbenesi, P.; Rouge, P.; Van Leuven, F.; Stirpe, F.; Peumans, W. J. Type 1 ribosome-inactivating proteins are the most abundant proteins in Iris (*Iris hollandica* var. Professor Blaauw) bulbs: characterization and molecular cloning. *Biochemical Journal*, 1997, *324* (3), 963–970.

Wang, H. J.; Murphy, P. A. Isoflavone content in commercial soybean foods. *Journal of Agricultural and Food Chemistry*, 1994, *42* (8), 1666–1673.

Wani, S. H.; Amin, A.; Rather, M. A.; Parray, J.; Parvaiz, A.; Qadri, R. A. Antibacterial and phytochemical screening of different extracts of five Iris species growing in Kashmir. *Journal of Pharmaceutical Research*, 2012, *5* (6), 3376–3378.

Williams, C. A.; Harborne, J. B. Colasante, M. Flavonoid and xanthone patterns in bearded Iris species and the pathway of chemical evolution in the genus. *Biochemical Systematics and Ecology*, 1997, *25* (4), 309–325.

Wiseman, H. The therapeutic potential of phytoestrogens. *Expert Opinion on Investigational Drugs*, 2000, *9* (8), 1829–1840.

Wong, R.; Rabie, B. Kudzu/Puerarin: medical applications. *Osteoarthritis and Cartilage*, 2007, *15* (8), 894–899.

Wu, Z. X. Pharmacological study of anti-cancer drug irisquinone. *Huanue Xuebao Molecule,* 1980, *38*, 156–159.

CHAPTER 8

Biosynthesis, Bioavailability, and Metabolism of Plant Polyphenols: Biological Activities and Their Potential Benefits in Human Health

KHUSHDEEP KAUR, BAVITA ASTHIR*, and DEEPAK KUMAR VERMA

Department of Biochemistry, College of Basic Sciences and Humanities, Punjab Agriculture University, Ludhiana 141004, Punjab, India

Corresponding author. E-mail: b.asthir@rediffmail.com

ABSTRACT

The chapter explores the plant's polyphenolic compounds, which include their biosynthesis process along with their classification, function, and role as bioactive compounds. Polyphenols are secondary plant metabolites delivering positive effects for humans and animals. They can function as antioxidants, attractants (flavonoids and carotenoids), defensive reaction chemicals (tannins and phytoalexins), signals (salicylic acids and flavonoids), structural polymers (lignin), and ultraviolet (UV) screens (flavonoids). In humans, polyphenols are central in defense responses as they comprise antioxidant, anti-inflammatory, antiproliferative, and antiaging activities. Thus, eating plant foods possessing high polyphenolic content is beneficial, as they will lessen the prevalence of some chronic diseases, such as cancers, cardiovascular diseases, and diabetes. However, high polyphenols doses through pro-oxidative action can lead to unfavorable consequences.

8.1 INTRODUCTION

Polyphenolic compounds (PPCs) are recognized as plant secondary metabolites and are omnipresent in plants (Lin et al., 2016; Tungmunnithum et al.,

2018). They constitute a diverse and large group of compounds. They are mostly the derivatives of phenolic acids, catechins, isoflavones, flavones, and flavonols and are abundantly present in several compounds as in olive oil, vegetables, fruits, beverages, chocolate, and other cocoa products (Raederstorff, 2009; Edirisinghe and Burton-Freeman, 2016; Tungmunnithum et al., 2018). Red wine, tea, and fruit represent the highest sources of polyphenols (Fresco et al., 2010; Pérez-Jiménez et al., 2010; Mojzer et al., 2016). PPCs are usually found as complex mixtures in food systems. Some of them (e.g., quercetin) are present in all plants, plant foods (e.g., cereals, vegetables, wine, tea, fruit, leguminous plants, etc.), and their products, whereas some are specific to particular foods as isoflavones are found in soya, while flavanones are present in citrus fruits (Pérez-Jiménez et al., 2010; Lin et al., 2016; Mojzer et al., 2016; Tungmunnithum et al., 2018). Various sources of polyphenols are discussed in Table 8.1. PPCs are important for reproduction and plant growth. They are found in several parts of the plant, such as fruits, flowers, leaves, seeds, and roots. In general, plant polyphenols play a role in providing a defense mechanism against numerous types of abiotic and biotic stress. They also give protection against other factors, namely, reactive oxygen species (ROS), pathogens, parasites, plant predators, UV light, and reactive nitrogen species (RNS) (Lin et al., 2016; Tungmunnithum et al., 2018). Polyphenols are substantially responsible for pigmentation, astringency, aromas, and oxidative stability (Tungmunnithum et al., 2018). Additionally, polyphenols possess numerous industrial appliances for contributing to the organoleptic properties of plants, cosmetics, food, etc. These can also be used as food preservatives or in the production of paints and paper (Maqsood et al., 2013; Bouarab Chibane et al., 2018; Volf amd Popa, 2018).

8.2 STRUCTURE AND CLASSIFICATION

Approximately 8000 PPCs have been acknowledged in diverse plant varieties with complex and varied chemical structures (Tsao, 2010; Anantharaju et al., 2016). They have an aromatic ring with one or more hydroxyl groups in their chemical structure. These compounds may contain molecules having polyphenolic structure, that is, aromatic rings with numerous hydroxyl groups or molecules with one phenol ring as in phenolic alcohols and phenolic acids. Depending on the number of phenol rings and the structural components that bind these rings to one another, these compounds can be divided into several

TABLE 8.1   Dietary Sources of Polyphenolic Compounds

Polyphenolic Compounds	Dietary Sources
1. *Flavonoids*	
Anthocyanins	Cherries, grapes, strawberries, blueberries, black and red currants, and bilberries
Flavonols	Buckwheat, beans, apples, cranberries, blueberries, olive, onions, tomatoes, and pepper
Flavanols	Onions, lettuce, grapes, blueberries, and apples
Flavanones	Citrus fruits
Flavones	Citrus fruits, spinach, and celery
Isoflavones	Soybeans
2. *Phenolic acids*	
Hydroxycinnamic acid	Cereals, oilseeds, apricots, blueberries, cherries, citrus fruits, peaches, pears, plums, carrots, eggplants, spinach, and tomatoes
Hydroxybenzoic acid	Cereals, oilseeds, blueberries, and cranberries
3. *Tannins*	
Condensed	Plums, pears, peaches, grapes, and apples
Hydrolysable	Pomegranates and raspberries
4. *Stilbenes*	Peanuts, grapes, and red wine
5. *Lignans*	Seeds (e.g., cereals, grains, legumes, linseed, flax, etc.) fruits, and certain vegetables

Sources: Lin et al. (2016); Mojzer et al. (2016).

classes constituting tannins, stilbenes, phenolic acids, lignans, flavonoids, and curcuminoids (Figure 8.1) (Lin et al., 2016; Tungmunnithum et al., 2018).

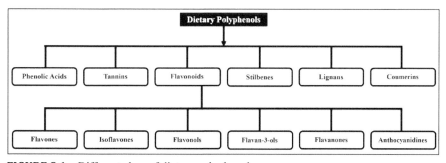

FIGURE 8.1   Different class of dietary polyphenols.

8.2.1 FLAVONOIDS

This is the major group of low molecular weight polyphenols. Individual flavonoids are categorized according to different ring substituents generated during acylation, methylation, hydroxylation, and glycosylation. Flavonoids compose two rings of benzene bonded via a three-carbon bridge forming a C_6–C_3–C_6 structural backbone (Jasinski et al., 2009). In plants, flavonoids occur in free form as aglycones (non-sugar hydrophobic constituents of glycosides) or bonded to sugar residues as glycosides. These are responsible for the varied (blue, red, and yellow) coloration of plants. They are mainly found in soybeans, tea, onions, and berries (Landete, 2013). Flavonoids are considered as important antioxidants due to their high redox potential act as singlet oxygen quenchers, reducing agents, and hydrogen donors. They contain a metal chelating potential as well. These consist of six subclasses: flavones, isoflavones, flavonols, flavanones, flavanols, and anthocyanins.

8.2.2 PHENOLIC ACIDS

They comprise about one-third of the polyphenols and are present inbound (linked through acetal, ether, or ester bonds to various plant components) or free forms in plants. The hydroxybenzoic acids are subgroups of phenolic acids that constitute syringic, gallic, vanillic, protocatechuic, and p-hydroxybenzoic acids that commonly have C_6–C_1 structure (Lin et al., 2016). These are found in very few food crops and their content in edible parts of the plant is usually very small, with the exception of certain red fruits, such as blackberries (Zadernowski et al., 2009). The hydroxycinnamic acids being aromatic compounds contain a three-carbon side chain (C_6–C_3) with p-coumaric, ferulic, sinapic, and caffeic acids as the most common representatives. Ferulic, coumaric, and caffeic acids are mostly found in the bound form. These bound forms are esters of tartaric, quinic, or shikimic acid or glycosylated derivatives. Caffeic and quinic acids together form chlorogenic acid that is found in high amounts in coffee and also in several fruit species (Clifford, 2000).

8.2.3 TANNINS

Tannins are compounds; comparatively, they have high molecular weight and known as the third important group of polyphenols (Lin et al., 2016). There are two subgroups, they are: (1) *Hydrolyzable tannins* and (2) *Condensed tannins*. *Hydrolyzable tannins* are the derivatives of gallic acid, that is, 3,4,5 trihydroxyl benzoic acid. Complex hydrolyzable tannins are produced through the oxidative crosslinking or esterification of gallic acid to a galloyl and the polyol groups (Lin et al., 2016). *Condensed tannins* constitute polymeric flavonoids known as proanthocyanidins. (+)-Catechin and (−)-epicatechin (based on flavan-3-ols) are the most extensively studied condensed tannins (Mojzer et al., 2016). Tannins display several beneficial properties in human health due to their potential biological role, such as antioxidants, protein precipitating agents, and metal ion chelators (Hagerman, 2002).

8.2.4   STILBENES

Stilbenes are obtained from plants in the reaction of different stress conditions or infections by pathogens (Mojzer et al., 2016). Their quantity in the human diet is very low. Peanuts, grapes, and berries are the major sources of stilbenes whereas resveratrol is the primary representative of trans-isomeric and cis-isomeric stilbenes, mostly glycosylated (Delmas et al., 2006).

8.2.5   LIGNANS

Lignans are derived from oxidative dimerization of two units of phenyl propane. Their free form is abundant in nature, while their derivative glycosides are minor. Lignans are of increasing interest as they present potential applications for different pharmacological impacts, such as chemotherapy for cancer and others (Saleem et al., 2005).

8.2.6   CURCUMINOIDS

Curcuminoids belong to the family of polyphenols with a diarylheptanoid carbon skeleton (C_6–C_7–C_6). These compounds are isolated from the rhizome of *Curcuma longa*, a turmeric plant which is being widely used as a dietary spice and as traditional Asian medicine (Osorio-Tobón et al., 2014; Mojzer et al., 2016). Various effects of these compounds on biological systems are attributable to their potential role in preventing and treating various diseases. Curcuminoids are capable of suppressing chronic and acute inflammation. At the molecular level, they are also described to inhibit metastasis and cell proliferation (Palve and Nayak, 2012). Curcumins are characterized by their limited bioavailability. *Curcuma* spp. is the only best natural source of curcuminoids but the plant of *Zingiberales* order has also been described to have curcuminoids and related compounds (Anand et al., 2007; Katsuyama et al., 2008).

8.3   BIOSYNTHESIS OF POLYPHENOLS

Plant polyphenols are synthesized either via phenylpropanoid pathway, shikimic acid pathway, or flavonoid pathway using phenylalanine as the precursor biomolecule (Ma et al., 2016; Sharma et al., 2016) (Figure 8.2). They are phenolic molecules that have one or more hydroxyl substituents that have variation in structure from simple phenols to highly polymerized phenolic compounds, comprising benzene rings. The first phase in polyphenol synthesis is to ensure the glucose in the pentose phosphate pathway (PPP) in which glucose-6-phosphate is transformed by the enzyme G-6-Pdehydrogenase into ribulose-5-phosphate (G-5-P). Then this G-5-P formed either produce by reducing equivalents of nicotinamide adenine dinucleotide phosphate (NADPH) in cellular anabolic reactions or PPP may produce erythrose-4-phosphate along with phosphoenolpyruvate from glycolysis. This erythrose-4-phosphate produces phenylalanine after being channeled to the shikimic acid pathway and is then used to generate phenolic compounds via the phenylpropanoid pathway. The metabolites of the shikimate path are generally regarded to be all phenolic compounds. Biosynthesis of flavonoids (complex polyphenols), which are then exported in the cytoplasm by using intermediates derived from mitochondrial and plastic, is associated with primary metabolism.

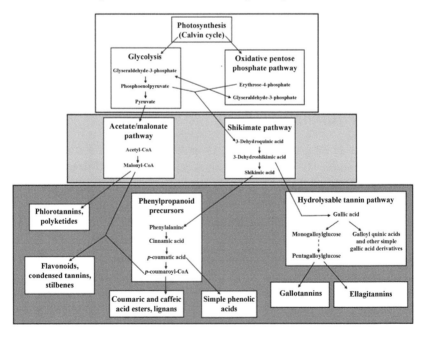

FIGURE 8.2   Pathway of polyphenols biosynthesis in plants (Sharma et al., 2016).

Flavonoid biosynthesis is carried out by various enzyme complexes present on the cytosolic side of endoplasmic reticulum membranes. The deamination of phenylalanine into cinnamic acid is catalyzed by enzyme phenylalanine ammonia-lyase which initiates flavonoid biosynthesis. This cinnamic acid is then oxidized to 4-coumaric acid by cinnamate-4-hydroxylase. In the next step, 4-coumarate: CoA ligase synthesizes 4-coumaroyl-CoA. Chalcone synthase is then used to condense one CoA ester molecule with three malonyl-CoA molecules to form chalcone (Tsao and McCallum, 2009). There are surplus flavonoids about 9000 which are attained from chalcone due to the activity of several enzymes such as oxidoreductases, hydroxylases, isomerases as well as post-modification enzymes like acyltransferases, methyltransferases, and glycosyltransferases (Veitch and Grayer, 2011). The flavonoid pathway synthesizes anthocyanins which belong to phenolic compounds class that is essentially accountable for the red color of wines and grapes. A series of enzymatic modifications in a metabolic pathway yields flavanones → dihydroflavonols → anthocyanins. Various other products are formed along this pathway which may include the proanthocyanidins (condensed tannins), flavan-3-ols and flavonols.

Curcuminoid synthesis is catalyzed through polyketide synthase by condensing two *p*-coumaroyl-CoA molecules with one malonyl CoA molecule. The resulting bisdemethoxycurcumin is transformed to curcumin through demethoxycurcumin by two sequential rounds of hydroxylation, followed by *O*-methylation reactions (Brand et al., 2006). The CoA esters of ferulic acid and *p*-coumaric acid may also be used as substrates by the enzyme curcuminoid synthase. The central pathway could operate in that case. Hydroxylation and the *O*-methylation responses that form the methoxyl functional groups in curcumin can also happen through the same responses as those in the pathway of phenylpropanoid (Chouhan et al., 2017).

8.4   BIOAVAILABILITY AND METABOLISM OF POLYPHENOLS

Polyphenols are characterized by low bioavailability and rapid metabolism which signifies a huge difficulty as very low concentrations of these get to the target organs. Nanoformulation of polyphenols represents a favorable solution to this problem as it has brought some promising results (Tabrez et al., 2013). Another solution is the more practiced one, that is, utilizing the combinations of different polyphenols that provide synergistic effects, ensuing in multitargeted action along with lowering the requirement of therapeutic dose (Mojzer et al., 2016).

Polyphenols' metabolism has not been fully elucidated. In biochemical pathways, a very low amount in which only 5%–10% approximate polyphenols are absorbed and metabolized (Chiva-Blanch and Visioli, 2012). Most polyphenols accumulate in bodily tissues in small quantities as they are not readily absorbed in the small intestine. Aglycones are absorbed by passive diffusion in the small intestine whereas other polyphenols that occur in foods as polymers of higher molecular weight, hydrophilic glycosides, and esters are first broken down to aglycone and sugar by mainly β-glucosidases which are known as an intestinal bacterial enzymes, and then only get absorbed in the large intestine (Surai, 2014). Glycosylated forms with one or more sugar residue conjugated to the aromatic ring or a hydroxyl group are the most common form of dietary polyphenols (one notable exception are the flavanols). However, some isoflavonic aglycones have shown better absorption than their glucosylated forms (Mocanu et al., 2015).

8.5 FACTORS AFFECTING PLANT POLYPHENOLS CONTENT

8.5.1 EFFECT OF ENVIRONMENT

Environmental factors as agronomic (fruit yield per tree, a different type of culture, etc.) or climatic (rainfall, sun exposure) play an important role in determining the polyphenolic content of a plant. For instance, light exposure has an extensive effect on flavonoids. Environmental conditions as water availability, temperature, nutritional status, air, light, soil type, disease incidence, altitude, and other developmental processes significantly influence the synthesis and accumulation of polyphenols (Dai et al., 2011).

8.5.2 EFFECT OF RIPENESS

A series of complex reactions are involved in the maturation of various plant tissues such as fruits resulting in modified phytochemistry of plants. Steady decrease or rise (Pineli et al., 2011) in phenolic contents during maturation represents two distinct phenomena of change. However, their concentration varies at different ripening stages from plant to plant or even in diverse parts of the same plant. The proportions and concentrations of the various polyphenols are differently affected by the degree of ripeness. Generally, anthocyanin concentrations increase during ripening whereas phenolic acid concentrations decrease (Anton et al., 2017). Changed total polyphenolic content was observed during the ripening of *Rosa laevigata Michx* (Xie et al., 2016).

8.5.3 EFFECT OF STORAGE

The content of polyphenols readily oxidized may be influenced by storage. Food quality alters particularly color and organoleptic properties due to the production of more or less polymerized substances as a result of oxidation reactions. Such changes can be harmful (browning of fruit) or beneficial (black tea) to consumer acceptability. Loss of phenolic acids was reported in stored wheat flour (Nissar et al., 2017). However, polyphenolic content remains unaffected in cold storage. Storage studies of the flour blends revealed that the total phenolic content showed a significant decrease with the increase in storage days. This might be due to the oxidation of monohydric or dihydric phenols along with the reduction of active phenols. Also, the antioxidant activity of enzymes like polyphenol oxidase (PPO) may decrease storage due to acidity. This increases the overall potential of flour which is to be used in the preparation of biscuits, cake, etc.

8.5.4 EFFECT OF COOKING

Cooking also imposes a significant effect on the polyphenolic content of various food materials. For instance, tomatoes and onions drop approximately 30% of their initial quercetin content after frying for 15 min, 65% after cooking in a microwave oven, and 75% after boiling. Another example is of potatoes' skin that contains up to 190 mg chlorogenic acid (polyphenol)/kg. So, an extensive loss of polyphenolic content occurs in potato during cooking with no remaining phenolic acids present in French fries (Fares et al., 2010).

8.5.5 EFFECT OF BROWNING

Browning may start off with nonenzymatic and enzymatic oxidation, both leading to the formation of o-quinones. Higher browning degrees are principally associated with monomeric catechins and procyanidins than other phenolics (Oliveira et al., 2011). Polyphenols are found in the vacuoles of a plant cell, whereas plastids contain PPO. Phenolic compounds come in contact with PPO in damaged areas of cells, stimulating the reaction known as enzymatic browning. This enzymatic browning is catalyzed by PPO that oxidizes the phenolic compounds to their corresponding quinones which are then further polymerized with phenolics or other quinones, forming brown pigments (Taranto et al., 2017) (Figure 8.3). Besides, peroxidase (POX) can augment the degradation of polyphenols when coexisting with PPO.

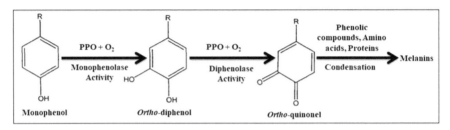

FIGURE 8.3 Mechanism of enzymatic browning (Taranto et al., 2017). [Reprinted from Taranto, F., A. Pasqualone, G. Mangini, P. Tripodi, M. M. Miazzi, S. Pavan, and M. Cinzia. 2017. Polyphenol Oxidases in Crops: Biochemical, physiological and genetic aspects. *International Journal of Molecular Sciences* 18:377. DOI: 10.3390/ijms18020377. https:// creativecommons.org/licenses/by/4.0/

Browning has a negative impact on the commercial value of various agricultural products (apricot, lettuce, fruits, vegetables, and cereals) (Pasqualone et al., 2014). However, in a few cases, browning positively influence the food processing quality related to the formation of flavor compounds, such as in the production of coffee, cocoa, and black tea. The quantity-qualitative composition of phenolic substrates and PPO varies in diverse crop species, leading to varying browning intensities such as chlorogenic acid is the main phenolic compound in potato, sweet potato, eggplant, apple, and sunflower, ferulic acid is abundant in wheat, and catechin is mainly present in grapes and tea (Laddomada et al., 2016).

8.6 BIOLOGICAL ACTIVITIES AND HEALTH BENEFITS OF POLYPHENOLS

The reverse relation between dietary use rich in polyphenols and the risk of chronic human diseases has been continuously revealed in epidemiological studies (Figure 8.4). Disease prevention by phenolic compounds is primarily attributed to their antioxidative characteristics. These compounds besides preventing various diseases (Figure 8.5), also pose a great effect on disease proliferation, suppress progression and play a role in the healing process. Polyphenols are now representing the key target of cancer research due to their potential of becoming superior agents to prevent and cure various malignancies (Wu et al., 2016).

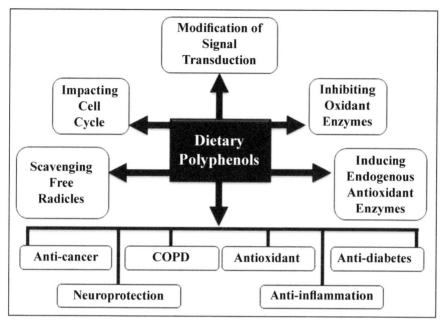

FIGURE 8.4 Various biological activities of dietary polyphenols. [*Note:* COPD refer to chronic obstructive pulmonary disease].

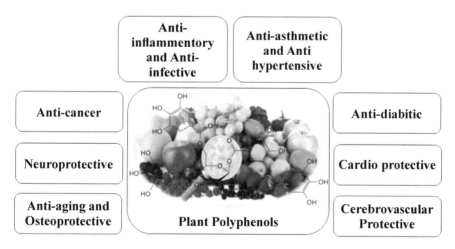

FIGURE 8.5 Potential role of plant polyphenolic compounds in humans health and disease.

Polyphenolic mixtures contribute to a more effective and faster healing due to their synergistic action on different disease pathways (de Kok et al., 2008). These compounds boost up the action of certain therapies like chemotherapy and radiotherapy, used for cancer treatment and also restrain their side effects (Fantini et al., 2015). Alternatively, high doses of polyphenols may result in the problem of toxicity of particular agents, that is, they may act even in the contradictory way leading to cancer formation and progression, instead of preventing it.

8.6.1   POLYPHENOLS AS ANTIOXIDANTS

In homeostasis, ROS and RNS are neutralized by various enzymatic antioxidants (glutathione POX, superoxide dismutase, and catalase) and low-molecular-weight antioxidants as tocopherols and ascorbic acid. During oxidative stress, the body cannot effectively deactivate free radicals as these are produced in excessive quantities. ROS modify amino acids, intensify cell membrane-associated lipid peroxidation, damage entire chromosomes and DNA, and contribute to protein fragmentation, necrosis, and cell apoptosis. Hence, it increases the risk of inflammations and cancer (Durand et al., 2013).

Polyphenols from the first line of defense as antioxidants against the excessive generation of ROS. They protect the components of the cell against oxidative damage caused by free radicals and hence reduce the risk of oxidative stress associated with neurodegenerative diseases. DNA damage induced by free radicals or carcinogenic agents is counteracted by PPCs through various mechanisms: (a) direct radical scavenging, (b) modulation of oxidative stress enzymes (lipooxygenase, superoxide dismutase, xanthine oxidase, glutathione reductase, glutathione POX, nitric oxide synthase, etc.), and (c) chelating divalent cations entailed in Fenton reaction.

Phenolic compounds own both direct and indirect antioxidant activities *in vitro*. Table 8.2 describes the summary of some studies on the antioxidant role of PPCs obtained from plants. *Direct* antioxidants are low molybdate, ubiquinol, lipoic acid, glutathione) that undergo redox reactions and scavenge reactive species (ROS and RNS). These antioxidants are either chemically modified or consumed in the process of their antioxidant action. So, they need to be regenerated or replenished. The *indirect* antioxidants are either redox-active or inactive. These are small molecules that induce antioxidant enzymes or cytoprotective proteins and are not consumed in their antioxidant action (Hu, 2011).

Of all the known polyphenols, most efficient are the flavonoids in eradicating the free radicals generated. This can be due to three factors: (a) the presence of a hydroxyl group at positions 3 and 5, (b) a 4-oxo coupled 2–3 double bond, and (c) an *o*-diphenolic group (Landete, 2013). Additionally, polyphenols curb ROS generation in the cells by restraining the activity of pro-oxidant enzymes, namely, protein kinase C, xanthine oxidase, and membrane-associated NADPH oxidase (Fraga et al., 2010). Furthermore, polyphenols may prevent the chelation of transition metal ions indirectly, for example, copper (Cu) and iron (Fe), consequently retarding the formation of reactive hydroxyl radicals (HO•).

8.6.1.1   *ROLE OF NRF2/KEAP1-ARE SYSTEM*

Nrf2 (nuclear factor-erythroid-2-related factor 2) is a member of the NF-E2 family of basic leucine zipper transcription factors. It controls many phytochemicals which augment the expression of cytoprotective proteins and antioxidant enzymes like NADPH quinone dehydrogenase 1 (NQO1), catalase, glutathione transferase, glutathine peroxidase. *Nrf2* is inactive under physiological conditions due to its binding by Keap1 (Kelch-like ECH-associated protein 1) (skeletal actin-binding protein) that targets *Nrf2* for proteasome degradation (Gopalakrishnan and Kong, 2008). Some phenolic compounds such as sulforaphane and curcumin that contain Michael acceptors (cysteine protease inhibitors) react directly with Keap 1 thiol groups causing conformational changes in Keap 1 protein, hence separating it from *Nrf2* (Surh, 2008). After phosphorylation, *Nrf2* protein translocates into the nuclei and then binds to the antioxidant responsive element (ARE) of antioxidant genes and the result is activated antioxidant enzyme expression. There are numerous upstream kinases such as casein kinase-2, mitogen-activated protein kinases (MAPK), phosphatidylinositol 3-kinase (PI3K)/Akt, and protein kinase C (PKC) that regulate nuclear translocation and transcriptional activation of *Nrf2*. This signaling pathway for *Nrf2/Keap1-ARE* is regarded as a distinctive "redox switch" that can be switched on and off in reaction to oxidative stress.

8.6.1.2   *NF-KB SIGNALING*

NF-κB (nuclear factor-kappa B) controls the immune response, oxidative response, cellular differentiation, inflammation, proliferation, and apoptosis-related gene expression. It is being defined as a redox-regulated transcription factor as it can be inhibited by various antioxidants and activated by oxidative stress. The *NF-κB* dimers (commonly a heterodimer of p50 and p65 proteins) are primarily present in an inactivated form in the cytosol bound to their inhibitors, IκBs. Various agents activate *NF-κB* by degrading IκB through phosphorylation that is carried out by the IκB-kinase complex. Then, *NF-κB* dimer translocates to the nucleus where it connects to particular DNA targets and encourages transcription (Chen and Greene, 2004). Numerous phytochemicals related to anticancer activities have been described to be associated with the inhibition of *NF-κB* (Guo et al., 2009).

8.6.2   POLYPHENOLS AS ANTICANCER AGENTS

Anticancergenic properties of polyphenols comprise several mechanisms as the progression of apoptosis, modifying cell cycle progression and cancer cell signaling, elimination of carcinogenic agents and modulation of enzymatic activities. As anticancer agents, phenolic compounds characterize the specificity of the response, low toxicity, high accessibility, and many other biological effects. Role of polyphenols in carcinogenesis lies in cell signaling cascades regulation and growth factor–receptor interactions that can have an impact on apoptosis of cancerous cells, cell survival, and induce cell cycle arrest (Ramos, 2008). Moreover, these compounds aid to increase the body's immunity by acting as anti-inflammatory agents and inhibiting angiogenesis that is necessary for tumor growth. In the last phases of cancer, polyphenols reduce the invasiveness and adhesiveness of cells and therefore attenuate their metastatic potential (Tabrez et al., 2013). They exercise their biological effects by modulating diverse cellular signaling pathways. Phenolic compounds are particularly capable of affecting PI3K and MAPK, which are involved in cancer cell proliferation. The MAPK signaling pathway plays a crucial role in regulating the growth and survival of diverse cancer cells. So, it can be a striking pathway for anticancer chemotherapy. Apple procyanidins were reported to activate caspase-3, inhibit cell growth and increase PKC activity and MAPK levels in SW620 cells, a colon cancer-derived metastatic cell line (Gosse et al., 2005).

8.6.3   ANTIBACTERIAL EFFECTS

Bacteriostatic and bactericidal properties are composed of PPCs, thereby minimizing the binding of pathogenic bacteria (*Clostridium, Escherichia coli*), inhibiting the digestive tract associated progression of infections and hence improving nutrient utilization (Duenas et al., 2015). Anthocyanins present in berries, cherries, and raspberries exhibit bacteriostatic and bactericidal effects (*Klebsiella, Bacillus, Helicobacter*). The presence of hydroxyl groups in PPCs such as quercetin enables them to increase lipid membranes permeability by integrating into them, hence making pathogens more susceptible to antibacterial compounds (Chiva-Blanch and Visioli, 2012). On the other hand, the pro-oxidant properties of polyphenolic are also accountable for their antimicrobial activity. Oxygen and metal ions promote phenoxyl radicals (possessing cytotoxic effects) formation that damage bacterial DNA (Etxeberria et al., 2013).

8.6.4   ANTIDIABETIC EFFECTS

Glucose metabolism impairment results in physiological imbalance with the onset of hyperglycemia and later on diabetes mellitus. Antidiabetic effects are usually related to attain and maintain glucose homeostasis. Traditionally, medicinal plants with many of its active constituents as polyphenols were used in diabetes treatment (Patel et al., 2012). Polyphenols, namely, catechin, quercetin, kaempferol, rutin, apigenin, and luteolin have antidiabetic roles acting through numerous mechanisms to decrease blood glucose levels.

Polyphenolic antidiabetic mechanisms involve (a) inhibition of facilitated glucose uptake, (b) inhibition of the active transport of glucose, (c) recovering modified antioxidant defenses, (d) restoring pancreatic cells associated insulin-secreting machinery, and (e) inhibiting the activity of carbohydrate hydrolyzing enzymes. For example, green tea polyphenols [Epigallocatechin Gallate and (–)-Epicatechin-3-gallate] inhibit glucose transport, probably by inhibition of sodium-dependent glucose transporter 1. Anthocyanins inhibit the activity of α-glucosidase and α-amylase as well as reducing blood glucose levels after having starch-rich meals (Edirisinghe and Burton-Freeman, 2016).

8.6.5   ANTI-INFLAMMATORY PROPERTIES

Activation of *NF-κB* and AP-1 mediates oxidative stress-induced inflammation. It influences a wide range of cell signaling processes resulting in chromatin remodeling and generation of inflammatory mediators. Phenolic compounds as resveratrol and curcumin and various others (rutin, quercetin, morin, hesperidin, and hesperetin) possessing antioxidant and/or anti-inflammatory characteristics have been reported to combat the undesired effects of oxidative stress (Rahman et al., 2006). These may affect inflammatory processes associated with signaling and enzymatic mechanisms. Tyrosine–protein and serine–threonine kinases are enzymes which can be taken as examples that regulate various cell activation processes like B lymphocyte activation, cytokine production, or T cell proliferation by stimulating monocytes phenolic compounds also have an impact on inflammatory cell secretory procedures (Hussain et al., 2016).

8.6.6   PROTECTION AGAINST CARDIOVASCULAR DISEASES

Cardiovascular diseases (CVDs) are an assembly of diseases including coronary heart disease, a stroke that affects the heart and blood vessels, may be due to age, obesity, hypertension, etc. Numerous studies have reported that consumption of a diet rich with polyphenol is positively related to the amelioration of CVD. Quercetin, the abundant polyphenol in onion, is known to be a potent protector of coronary heart disease by disruption of the atherosclerotic plaques and inhibition of metalloproteinase 1 (MMP1) expression. Polyphenols present in nonalcoholic wine or red wine can inhibit platelet aggregation by exerting antithrombotic effects. Phenolic compounds provide protection against CVDs through mechanisms that confer antioxidant protection, inhibit platelet aggregation, improve endothelial function, lower blood pressure, decrease oxidative stress, reduce inflammatory responses, reduce low-density lipoprotein (LDL) oxidation, and improve coronary vasodilatation (Hossen et al., 2017).

8.6.7   NEUROPROTECTION BY POLYPHENOLS

The oxidative stress and damages of brain macromolecules are caused by neurodegenerative diseases like strokes, Alzheimer's disease (AD), Parkinson's disease (PD), multiple sclerosis, and Huntington's disease. These disorders are the result of dysfunction or death of nerve cells due to increased oxidative stress due to neuroinflammation, glutamatergic excitotoxicity, protein, and mitochondrial dysfunction, genetic alterations, and depletion of antioxidants (Spires and Hannan, 2005). Being antioxidative in nature, PPCs present in honey and other plant food materials can avoid neurodegenerative diseases via enhancement of neuronal function and regeneration, oxidative protection of neurons, hippocampal cells' protection

TABLE 8.2 Summary of Some Studies on the Role of Plant Polyphenols as Antioxidants and their Antioxidant Activities

Year	Study Reports	Polyphenols Substrate from Plants	Findings/Concluding Remarks	References
2013	Phenolic compounds and their bioactivities	Anthocyanins phenolic compound of pigmented rice	Scavenged free radical	Deng et al. (2013)
2010	Antioxidant activities of litchi (*Litchi chinensis*) fruit's polyphenol and their contents	Polyphenol oxidase substrates, namely, (−)-epicatechin and procyanidin from litchi pericarp	Food preservatives for fruit	Sun et al. (2010)
2010	Antioxidant status and their capacity in human volunteers	Green teas polyphenol, namely, gallate, epicatechin, and catechin	Induced a dose-response effect on plasma antioxidant activity	Pecorari et al. (2010)
2010	Relationship between antioxidant capacity and their effect on membrane phospholipid order	Rosemary (*Rosmarinus officinalis*) polyphenols, namely, camosol, as carnosic acid, genkwanin, rosmarinic acid, and rosmadial	Protected the membranes against oxidative damage	Pérez-Fons et al. (2010)
2009	Polyphenols and their antioxidant activity on humans	Olive polyphenols (hydroxytyrosol and its derivatives)	Decreased the oxidized- low-density lipoprotein (LDL) in plasma and affected several biomarkers of oxidative damage	Raederstorff (2009)
2009	Acute effect on plasma total polyphenols, antioxidant capacity and lipid peroxidation	Polyphenols from nut extracts (e.g., walnuts and almonds)	Reduced plasma lipid peroxidation	Torabian et al. (2009)
2007	Beneficial effects on malondialdehyde-modified LDL.	Grape seed extract	Decreased the oxidated LDL in plasma	Sano et al. (2007)
2007	An inhibitory effect on lipid oxidation in fish oil and their radical scavenging and antimicrobial properties	Ethanol extracts of black raspberry seed and Chardonnay	Food preservatives for fish flesh and oil	Luther et al. (2007)
2006	Acute intake effect on healthy with improves antioxidant status	Phenolic-rich extract of grape juice	Reduced oxidative stress in serum	Garcia-Alonso et al. (2006)

against nitric oxide-induced toxicity, protection of neurons from Ab-induced neurotoxicity, and neuronal injury and modulation of neuronal and glial cell signaling pathways (Cirmi et al., 2016; Hossen et al., 2017). Moreover, consumption of high flavonoids diet/beverages daily has been reported to lessen the incidence of dementia (by 50%) and aging. Also, these flavonoids may probably hinder the commencement of AD and decrease the incidence of PD as well (Hussain et al., 2016). Further, PPCs may downregulate NF-κB (transcription factors), that react to p38 signaling and are liable to iNOS induction. This signifies that there might be a link between cytokine production, transcription factors, and signaling pathways in investigating the neuroinflammation response in central nervous system. Furthermore, due to their effect on neuronal signaling, PPCs provide defense in response to advanced glycation end-products induced neurotoxicity (Lee and Lee, 2007).

8.6.8 DEFENSE AGAINST BIOTIC STRESS

Polyphenols offer defense against microbes, viruses, herbivores, or competing plants. For example, coumarins function against insect herbivores and also have a varied range of antimicrobial activity against fungi and bacteria. Physical toughness of lignin prevents herbivorous animals from feeding. This is because of lignin's chemical durability that makes it quite indigestible to herbivores and insect pathogens. Lignifications obstruct the growth of pathogens and are a regular response to wounding or infection. Tannins, being a general toxin, lessen the growth and survival of numerous herbivores. They function as feeding repellents to a vast variety of animals. These defensive properties of tannins are due to their protein binding ability. Caffeic and ferulic acids inhibit the growth of the neighboring plants (*allelopathy*) when released into the soil (Kulbat, 2016).

8.6.9 PRO-OXIDANT EFFECTS OF DIETARY POLYPHENOLS

Polyphenols may exert pro-oxidant effects on cells when their environments are characterized by an increased concentration of oxygen and partial pressure. To facilitate this action, flavonoids possess definite chemical structure, that is, the presence of oxygen (O_2) and copper ions (Cu^{2+}), catechol structures (single OH group at position three on the B-ring or three OH groups) or pyrogallol (Prochazkova et al., 2011). Polyphenols that have pro-oxidant properties can aggravate by a lack of chemical stability in cells, glutathione

(GSH) deficiency, and activation of cellular Cu^{2+} ions that are produced together with oxidized flavonoid (semiquinone radicals) during auto-oxidation. NADH reduces these cytotoxic semiquinone radicals and participates in ROS generation in redox reactions. Cu^{2+} ions lead to an increase in superoxide radical concentration which further gives to the generation of H_2O_2 (hydrogen peroxide) and highly reactive OH^- (hydroxyl radicals) (Halliwell, 2008). Depending upon their concentration, environmental conditions, and target molecules, polyphenols may stimulate apoptosis through pro-oxidative action, instead of their antioxidative action. These compounds are highly susceptible to *in vitro* auto-oxidation and further research is required to study their effects on animal cells.

8.7 ADVANCEMENT AND FUTURE PROSPECTS

A web database on polyphenols known as Phenol-Explorer (http://www.phenol-explorer.eu) has been developed (Phenol-Explorer, 2019). It contains complete polyphenolic compositions of more than 450 foods (Neveu et al., 2010). These available data are valuable primarily for studying associations between health and intake of polyphenol. These data were also used to calculate the intake of polyphenols from dietary questionnaires from cohort study subjects. Phenol-Explorer has also been further improved by data on the effects of food processing on the content of polyphenol in food products (Rothwell et al., 2015).

A better explanation and understanding of the mechanisms concerned with the defensive role of polyphenols in adverse situations may prove to be beneficial. Further chemical, agronomical, and biochemical studies need to be conducted to clarify the role of these compounds reaching from plants to humans. Although many reports indicate the various beneficial effects associated with PPCs, the precise effect of polyphenols as anticancer compounds or in foodstuffs is still a matter of need to be thoroughly investigated especially concerning environmental stresses.

8.8 SUMMARY AND CONCLUSION

Polyphenols are vital compounds of plant-based part of our diet. These compounds defend us from various threats like numerous toxins, various diseases, radiations, and microbes. Absence or low toxicity specificity of the response and omnipresence are the vital advantages of polyphenols.

Therefore, dietary supplements rich in PPCs can provide additional benefits but high-doses may result in toxicity thus establishing a double-edge sword in supplement use. Overall, among all secondary metabolites, polyphenols are the top targets of research, even though their study poses certain challenges.

KEYWORDS

- **bioavailability**
- **biological activities**
- **biosynthesis**
- **dietary sources**
- **flavonoid**
- **human health**
- **polyphenols**
- **secondary metabolites**

REFERENCES

Anand, P., A. B. Kunnunakkara, R. A. Newman, and B. B. Aggarwal. 2007. Bioavailability of curcumin: Problems and promises. *Molecular Pharmaceutics* 4: 807–818. DOI: https://doi.org/10.1021/mp700113r.

Anantharaju, P. G., Gowda, P. C., Vimalambike, M. G., and Madhunapantula, S. V. 2016. An overview on the role of dietary phenolics for the treatment of cancers. *Nutrition Journal* 15(99): 1–16. DOI:10.1186/s12937-016-0217-2

Anton, D., I. Bender, T. Kaart, M. Roasto, M. Heinonen, A. Luik, and T. Pussa. 2017. Changes in polyphenols contents and antioxidant capacities of organically and conventionally cultivated tomato (*Solanum lycopersicum L.*) fruits during ripening. *International Journal of Analytical Chemistry,* 1–11. doi: https://doi.org/10.1155/2017/2367453.

Bouarab Chibane, L., P. Degraeve, H. Ferhout, J. Bouajila, and N. Oulahal. 2018. Plant antimicrobial polyphenols as potential natural food preservatives. *Journal of the Science of Food and Agriculture.* https://doi.org/10.1002/jsfa.9357

Brand, S., D. Holscher, A. Schierhorn, A. Svatos, J. Schroter, and B. Schneider. 2006. A type III polyketide synthase from *Wachendorfia thyrsiflora* and its role in diarylheptanoid and phenylphenalenone biosynthesis. *Planta* 224:413–428. doi: http://doi.org/10.1007/s00425-006-0228-x.

Chen, L. F., and W. C. Greene. 2004. Shaping the nuclear action of NF-kappaB. *Nature Reviews Molecular Cell Biology* 5:392–401. doi: https://doi.org/10.1038/nrm1368.

Chiva-Blanch, G., and F. Visioli. 2012. Polyphenols and health: Moving beyond antioxidants. *Journal of Berry Research* 2:63–71. doi: 10.3233/JBR-2012-02.

Chouhan, S., S. Kanika, J. Zha, S. Guleria, and M. A. G. Koffas. 2017. Recent advances in the recombinant biosynthesis of polyphenols. *Frontiers in Microbiology* 8:1–16. doi: https://doi.org/10.3389/fmicb.2017.02259.

Cirmi, S., N. Ferlazzo, G. E. Lombardo, E. Ventura-Spagnolo, E. Gangemi, and G. Calapai. 2016. Neurodegenerative diseases: Might citrus flavonoids play a protective role? *Molecules* 21(10):E1312. doi: https://doi.org/10.3390/molecules21101312.

Clifford, M. N. 2000. Chlorogenic acids and other cinnamates. Nature, occurrence, dietary burden, absorption and metabolism. *Journal of the Science of Food and Agriculture* 80:1033–1043. DOI: https://doi.org/10.1002/(SICI)1097-0010(20000515)80:7%3C1033.

Dai, Z., W. Ollat, E. Gomes, S. Decroocq, J. P. Tandonnet, L. Bordenave, P. Pieri, G. Hilbert, C. Kappel, C. V. Leeuwen, P. Vivin, and S. Delrot. 2011. Ecophysiological, genetic and molecular causes of variation in grape berry weight and composition: A review. *American Journal of Enology and Viticulture* 62:413–425.

de Kok, T. M., S. G. Van Breda, and M. M. Manson. 2008. Mechanisms of combined action of different chemopreventive dietary compounds. *European Journal of Nutrition* 47:51–59. doi: 10.1007/s00394-008-2006-y.

Delmas, D., A. Lancon, D. Colin, B. Jannin, and N. Latruffe. 2006. Resveratrol as a chemopreventive agent: A promising molecule for fighting cancer. *Current Drug Targets* 7:423–442. doi: https://doi.org/10.2174/138945006776359331.

Deng, G. F., X. R. Xu, Y. Zhang, D. Li, R. Y. Gan, H. B. Li. 2013. Phenolic compounds and bioactivities of pigmented rice. *Critical Reviews in Food Science and Nutrition* 53(3):296–306.

Duenas, M., I. Munoz-Gonzalez, C. Cueva, A. Jimenez-Giron, F. Sanchez-Patan, C. Santos-Buelga, and B. Bartolome. 2015. A survey of modulation of gut microbiota by dietary polyphenols. *BioMed Research International* 1–15. doi: 10.1155/2015/850902.

Durand, D., M. Damon, and M. Gobert. 2013. Oxidative stress in farm animals: General aspects. *Cahiers de Nutrition et de Dietetique* 48:218–224.

Edirisinghe, I., and B. Burton-Freeman. 2016. Anti-diabetic actions of Berry polyphenols—Review on proposed mechanisms of action. *Journal of Berry Research* 6:237–250. doi: 10.3233/JBR-160137.

Etxeberria, U., A. Fernandez-Quintela, F. I. Milagro, L. Aguirre, J. A. Martínez, and M. P. Portillo. 2013. Impact of polyphenols and polyphenol-rich dietary sources on gut microbiota composition. *Journal of Agricultural and Food Chemistry* 61:9517–9533. doi: 10.1021/jf402506c.

Fantini, M., M. Benvenuto, and L. Masuellietal. 2015. *In vitro* and *in vivo* antitumoural effects of combinations of polyphenols or polyphenols and anticancer drugs: Perspectives on cancer treatment. *International Journal of Molecular Sciences* 16:9236–9282. doi: https://doi.org/10.3390/ijms16059236.

Fares, C., C. Platani, A. Baiano, and V. Menga. 2010. Effect of processing and cooking on phenolic acid profile and antioxidant capacity of durum wheat pasta enriched with debranning fractions of wheat. *Food Chemistry* 119:1023–1029. doi: http://dx.doi.org/10.1016/j.foodchem.2009.08.006.

Fraga, C. G., M. Galleano, S. V. Verstraeten, and P. I. Oteiza. 2010. Basic biochemical mechanisms behind the health benefits of polyphenols. *Molecular Aspects of Medicine* 31:435–445. doi: 10.1016/j.mam.2010.09.006.

Fresco, P., F. Borges, M.P.M. Marques, C. Diniz. 2010. The anticancer properties of dietary polyphenols and its relation with apoptosis. *Current Pharmaceutical Design* 16, 114–134.

Garcia-Alonso, J. M. U. E., G. Ros, M. L. Vidal-Guevara, M. J. Periago. 2006. Acute intake of phenolic-rich juice improves antioxidant status in healthy subjects. *Nutrition Research* 26:330–339

Gopalakrishnan, A., and T. A. N. Kong. 2008. Anticarcinogenesis by dietary phytochemicals: cytoprotection by Nrf2 in normal cells and cytotoxicity by modulation of transcription factors NF-kappa B and AP-1 in abnormal cancer cells. *Food and Chemical Toxicology* 46:1257–1270. doi: https://doi.org/10.1016/j.fct.2007.09.082.

Gosse, F., S. Guyot, S. Roussi, A. Lobstein, B. Fischer, N. Seiler, and F. Raul. 2005. Chemopreventive properties of apple procyanidins on human colon cancer-derived metastatic SW620 cells and in a rat model of colon carcinogenesis. *Carcinogenesis* 26:1291–1295. doi: https://doi.org/10.1093/carcin/bgi074.

Guo, W., E. Kong, and M. Meydani. 2009. Dietary polyphenols, inflammation and cancer. *Nutrition and Cancer* 61:807–810. doi: 10.1080/01635580903285098.

Hagerman, A. E. 2002. *Tannin Handbook*, Department of Chemistry and Biochemistry, Miami University, USA.

Halliwell, B. 2008. Are polyphenols antioxidants or pro-oxidants? What do we learn from cell culture and in vivo studies? *Archives of Biochemistry and Biophysics* 476:107–112. doi: 10.1016/j.abb.2008.01.028.

Hossen, M. S., M. Y. Ali, M. H. A. Jahurul, M. M. Abdel-Daim, S. H. Gane, and M. I. Khalil. 2017. Beneficial roles of honey polyphenols against some human degenerative diseases: A review. *Pharmacological Reports* 69:1194–1205.

Hu, M. L. 2011. Dietary polyphenols as antioxidants and anticancer agents: more questions than answers. *Chang Gung Medical Journal* 34:449–460.

Hussain, T., B. Tan, Y. Yin, F. Blachier, M. C. B. Tossou, and N. Rahu. 2016. Oxidative stress and inflammation: What polyphenols can do for us? *Oxidative Medicine and Cell Longevity* 1–9. doi: https://dx.doi.org/10.1155%2F2016%2F7432797.

Jasinski, M., E. Mazurkiewicz, P. Rodziewicz, and M. Figlerowicz. 2009. Flavonoids' structure, properties and particular function for legume plants. *BioTechnologia* 2:81–94.

Katsuyama, Y., M. Matsuzawa, N. Funa, and S. Horinouch. 2008. Production of curcuminoids by *Escherichia coli* carrying an artificial biosynthesis pathway. *Microbiology* 154:2620–2628. doi: 10.1099/mic.0.2008/018721-0.

Kulbat, K. 2016. The role of phenolic compounds in plant resistance. *Biotechnology and Food Sciences* 80(2):97–108.

Laddomada, B., M. Durante, G. Mangini, L. D'Amico, L. S. Marcello, R. Simeone, L. Piarulli, G. Mita, and A. Blanco. 2016. Genetic variation for phenolic acids concentration and composition in a tetraploid wheat (*Triticum turgidum* L.) collection. *Genetic Resources and Crop Evolution* doi: 10.1007/s10722–016-0386-z.

Landete, J. M. 2013. Dietary intake of natural antioxidants: vitamins and polyphenols. *Critical Reviews in Food Science and Nutrition* 53:706–721. doi: 10.1080/10408398.2011.555018.

Lee, S. J., and K. W. Lee. 2007 Protective effect of (−)-epigallocatechin gallate against advanced glycation endproducts-induced injury in neuronal cells. *Biological and Pharmaceutical Bulletin* 30:1369–1373.

Lin, D., M. Xiao, J. Zhao, Z. Li, B. Xing, X. Li, M. Kong, L. Li, Q. Zhang, Y. Liu, H. Chen, W. Qin, H. Wu, and S. Chen. 2016. An overview of plant phenolic compounds and their importance in human nutrition and management of type 2 diabetes. *Molecules* 21(1374): 1–19. DOI:10.3390/molecules21101374.

Luther, M., J. Parry, J. Moore, J. Meng, Y. Zhang, Z. Cheng, L. L. L. U. Yu. 2007. Inhibitory effect of Chardonnay and black raspberry seed extracts on lipid oxidation in fish oil and their radical scavenging and antimicrobial properties. *Food Chemistry* 104:1065–1073.

Ma, D., Y. Li, J. Zhang, C. Wang, H. Qin, H. Ding, Y. Xie, and T. Guo. 2016. Accumulation of phenolic compounds and expression profiles of phenolic acid biosynthesis-related genes in developing grains of white, purple and red wheat. *Frontiers in Plant Science* 7:528. doi: 10.3389/fpls.2016.00528.

Maqsood, S., S. Benjakul, and F. Shahidi. 2013. Emerging role of phenolic compounds as natural food additives in fish and fish products. *Critical Reviews in Food Science and Nutrition* 53(2): 162–179. DOI:10.1080/10408398.2010.518775.

Mocanu, M. M., P. Nagy, and J. Szollosi. 2015. Chemoprevention of breast cancer by dietary polyphenols. *Molecules* 20:22578–22620. doi: 10.3390/molecules201219864.

Mojzer, E. B., M. K. Hrnc, M. Skerget, Z. Knez, and U. Bren. 2016. Polyphenols: extraction methods, antioxidative action, bioavailability and anticarcinogenic effects. *Molecules* 21:1–38. doi:10.3390/molecules21070901.

Neveu, V., J. Perez-Jimenez, F. Vos, V. Crespy, L. du Chaffaut, L. Mennen, C. Knox, R. Eisner, J. Cruz, D. Wishart, and A. Scalbert. 2010. Phenol-Explorer: An online comprehensive database on polyphenol contents in foods. Database, bap024, doi: 10.1093/database/bap024.

Nissar, N., N. A. Qazi, A. H. Rather, H. R. Naik, S. Z. Hussain, L. Masoodi, K. Maqbool, F. Shafi, and R. Monica. 2017. Effect of storage period on total phenolic content, ascorbic acid and titrable acidity of flour blends made from Himalayan variety of wheat, oat and mushroom flour packed in metalized polyester. *International Journal of Chemical Studies* 5:2186–2188.

Oliveira, C.M., A. C. S. Ferreira, V. de Freitas, and A. M. Silva. 2011 Oxidation mechanisms occurring in wines. *Food Research International* 44:1115–1126.

Osorio-Tobón, J. F., P. I. N. Carvalho, M. A. Rostagno, A. J. Petenate, M. A. A. Meireles. 2014. Extraction of curcuminoids from deflavored turmeric (*Curcuma longa* L.) using pressurized liquids: Process integration and economic evaluation. *Journal of Supercritical Fluids* 95, 167–174.

Palve, Y., and P. Nayak. 2012. Curcumin: a wonder anticancer drug. *International Journal of Pharma and Bio Sciences* 3:60–69.

Pasqualone, A., L. N. Delvecchio, G. Mangini, F. Taranto, and A. Blanco. 2014. Variability of total soluble phenolic compounds and antioxidant activity in a collection of tetraploid wheat. *Agricultural and Food Science* 23:307–316.

Patel, D., R. Kumar, D. Laloo, and S. Hemalatha. 2012. Diabetes mellitus: an overview on its pharmacological aspects and reported medicinal plants having antidiabetic activity. *Asian Pacific Journal of Tropical Biomedicine* 2:411–420. doi: https://dx.doi.org/10.1016 %2FS2221-1691(12)60067-7.

Pecorari, M., D. Villaño, M. F. Testa, M. Schmid, and M. Serafini. 2010. Biomarkers of antioxidant status following ingestion of green teas at different polyphenol concentrations and antioxidant capacity in human volunteers. *Molecular Nutrition & Food Research* 54 Suppl 2:S278–83.

Pérez-Fons, L., M. T. Garzón, V. Micol. 2010. Relationship between the antioxidant capacity and effect of rosemary (*Rosmarinus officinalis* L.) polyphenols on membrane phospholipid order. *Journal of Agricultural and Food Chemistry* 58(1):161–71.

Pérez-Jiménez, J., V. Neveu, F. Vos, A. Scalbert. 2010. Identification of the 100 richest dietary sources of polyphenols: An application of the Phenol-Explorer database. *European Journal of Clinical Nutrition* 64:S112–S120.

Phenol-Explorer, Welcome to Phenol-Explorer 3.6. In: *Phenol-Explorer:* Database on Polyphenol Content in Foods. Accessed on 31/09/2019. URL: http://www.phenol-explorer.eu.

Pineli, L. L. O., C. L. Moretti, M. S. Santos, A. B. Campos, A. V. Brasileiro, A. C. Cordova, and M. D. Chiarello. 2011. Antioxidants and other chemical and physical characteristics of two strawberry cultivars at different ripeness stages. *Journal of Food Composition and Analysis* 92:831–838.

Prochazkova, D., I. Bousova, and N. Wilhelmova. 2011. Antioxidant and prooxidant properties of flavonoids. *Fitoterapia* 82:513–523. doi: 10.1016/j.fitote.2011.01.018.

Raederstorff, D. 2009. Antioxidant activity of olive polyphenols in humans: A review. *International Journal for Vitamin and Nutrition Research* 79(3):152–165.

Rahman, I., S. K. Biswas, and P. A. Kirkham. 2006. Regulation of inflammation and redox signaling by dietary polyphenols. *Biochemical Pharmacology* 72:1439–1452. doi: https://doi.org/10.1016/j.bcp.2006.07.004.

Ramos, S. 2008. Cancer chemoprevention and chemotherapy: Dietary polyphenols and signalling pathways. *Molecular Nutrition and Food Research* 52:507–526. doi: 10.1002/mnfr.200700326.

Rothwell, J. A., A. Medina-Remo, J. Perez-Jimenez, V. Neveu, V. Knaze, S. Nadia, and A. Scalbert. 2015. Effects of food processing on polyphenol contents: A systematic analysis using Phenol-Explorer data. *Molecular Nutrition and Food Research* 59:160–170. doi: 10.1002/mnfr.201400494.

Saleem, M., H. J. Kim, M. S. Ali, and Y. S. Lee. 2005. An update on bioactive plant lignans. *Natural Product Reports* 22:696–716. doi: https://doi.org/10.1039/b514045p.

Sano, A., R. Uchida, M. Saito, N. Shioya, Y. Komori, Y. Tho, N. Hashizume. 2007. Beneficial effects of grape seed extract on malondialdehyde-modified LDL. *Journal of Nutritional Science and Vitaminology* (Tokyo) 53(2):174–182.

Sharma, M., R. Sandhir, A. Singh, P. Kumar, A. Mishra, S. Jachak, S. P. Singh, J. Singh, and J. Roy. 2016. Comparative analysis of phenolic compound characterization and their biosynthesis genes between two diverse bread wheat (*Triticum aestivum*) varieties differing for chapatti (unleavened flatbread) quality. *Frontiers in Plant Science* 7:1870. DOI: 10.3389/fpls.2016.01870.

Spires, T. L., and A. J. Hannan. 2005. Nature, nurture and neurology: Gene-environment interactions in neurodegenerative disease. *The FEBS Journal* 272:2347–2361. DOI: https://doi.org/10.1111/j.1742-4658.2005.04677.x.

Sun, J., Y. Y. S. A. Jiang, J. Shi, X. Wei, S. J. Xue, J. Shi, C. Yi. 2010. Antioxidant activities and contents of polyphenol oxidase substrates from pericarp tissues of litchi fruit. *Food Chemistry* 119:753–757.

Surai, P. F. 2014. Polyphenol compounds in the chicken/animal diet: From the past to the future. *Journal of Animal Physiology and Animal Nutrition* 98:19–31. DOI: 10.1111/jpn.12070.

Surh, Y. J. 2008. NF-kappa B and Nrf2 as potential chemopreventive targets of some anti-inflammatory and antioxidative phytonutrients with anti-inflammatory and antioxidative activities. *Asia Pacific Journal of Clinical Nutrition* 17(SI):269–272.

Tabrez, S., M. Priyadarshini, M. Urooj, S. Shakil, G. M. Ashraf, M. S. Khan, M. A. Kamal, Q. Alam, N. R. Jabir, and A. M. Abuzenadah. 2013. Cancer chemoprevention by polyphenols and their potential application as nanomedicine. *Journal of Environmental Science and Health Part C, Environmental Carcinogenesis and Ecotoxicology Reviews* 31:67–98. doi: 10.1080/10590501.2013.763577.

Taranto, F., A. Pasqualone, G. Mangini, P. Tripodi, M. M. Miazzi, S. Pavan, and M. Cinzia. 2017. Polyphenol oxidases in crops: Biochemical, physiological and genetic aspects. *International Journal of Molecular Sciences* 18:377. DOI: 10.3390/ijms18020377.

Torabian, S., E. Haddad, S. Rajaram, J. Banta, J. Sabaté. 2009. Acute effect of nut consumption on plasma total polyphenols, antioxidant capacity and lipid peroxidation. *Journal of Human Nutrition and Dietetics* 22(1):64–71.

Tsao, R. 2010. Chemistry and biochemistry of dietary polyphenols. *Nutrients* 2(12):1231–1246. DOI:10.3390/nu2121231.

Tsao, R., and J. McCallum. 2009. Chemistry of flavonoids. In *Fruit and Vegetable Phytochemicals: Chemistry, Nutritional Value and Stability*, Eds. L. A. de la Rosa, E. Alvarez-Parrilla, and G. Gonzalez-Aguilar, pp. 131–153. Blackwell Publishing, Ames, IA, USA. doi: https://doi.org/10.1002/9780813809397.ch5.

Tungmunnithum, D., A. Thongboonyou, A. Pholboon, and A. Yangsabai. 2018. Flavonoids and other phenolic compounds from medicinal plants for pharmaceutical and medical aspects: An overview. *Medicines (Basel, Switzerland)* 5(3):93. DOI:10.3390/medicines5030093.

Veitch, N. C., and R. J. Grayer. 2011. Flavonoids and their glycosides, including anthocyanins. *Natural Product Reports* 28:1626–1695. doi: 10.1039/c1np00044f.

Volf, I., V. I. Popa. 2018. Integrated processing of biomass resources for fine chemical obtaining: Polyphenols. In: *Biomass as Renewable Raw Material to Obtain Bioproducts of High-Tech Value*, Eds. Volf, I., and Popa, V. I. Elsevier, pp. 113–160, ISBN 9780444637741, https://doi.org/10.1016/B978-0-444-63774-1.00004-1.

Wu, J. C., C. S. Lai, P. S. Lee, C. T. Ho, W. S. Liou, Y. J. Wang, and M. H. Pan. 2016. Anti-cancer efficacy of dietary polyphenols is mediated through epigenetic modifications. *Current Opinion in Food Science* 8:1–7. doi: http://dx.doi.org/10.1016%2Fj.cofs.2016.01.009.

Xie, G., J. Wang, X. Xu, R. Wang, X. Zhou, and Z. Liu. 2016. Effect of different ripening stages on bioactive compounds and antioxidant capacity of wild *Rosa laevigata Michx. Food Science and Technology* 36:396–400. doi: http://dx.doi.org/10.1590/1678-457X.00715.

Zadernowski, R., S. Czaplicki, and M. Naczk. 2009 Phenolic acid profiles of mangosteen fruits (*Garcinia mangostana*). *Food Chemistry* 112:685–689. doi: http://dx.doi.org/10.1016/j.foodchem.2008.06.030.

CHAPTER 9

Scientific Exploration and Exploitation of Tannins

SANKHADIP BOSE*, SUBHASH C. MANDAL, and SUBHAJIT DUTTA

NSHM Knowledge Campus, Kolkata—Group of Institutions, 124 B. L. Saha Road, Kolkata, India

Corresponding author. E-mail: sankha.bose@gmail.com

ABSTRACT

Tannins, the polyphenolic polymers, both in their hydrolyzable and condensed forms possess high molecular weight and being there with immense number of phenolic hydroxyl groups imparts these tannins their potentiality in forming complexes with proteins. Throughout the world, both forms of tannins are broadly distributed in shrubs, legumes, forage trees, grains, and cereals. Many potent healing properties like antidiarrheal, hemostatic, anti-inflammatory, and antihemorrhoidal are observed in tannins as their scientific explorations and simultaneously their impact in specific bitter taste accompanied by strong astringency in fruits and drinks, and this may also be counted as exploitations of tannins. Tannins play a role in protection from predation, and perhaps also as pesticides. The astringency taste of tannins creates dry and puckery feeling in the mouth when tea, red wine, or unripened fruit is consumed. The modification and destruction of tannins may occur any time during harvesting and other preparation of foods and drugs. The addition of tannins in the food can develop the nutritional quality of the food and improve body weight. Different scientific explorations and exploitations of tannins generally depend upon stereochemistry and carbon–carbon bonding of tannins, their degree of polymerization, conversion of procyanidins to prop delphinidins, and finally on the concentrations of tannins in diets.

9.1   INTRODUCTION

Tannins come under the heterogeneous group of high molecular weight polyphenolic compounds. These are water soluble with many hydroxyl groups. Their molecular weight is around 500–3000 Daltons and widely available in plants and food additives (de Jesus et al., 2012). As phenolic compounds, they contains inter and intramolecular hydrogen bonds which after reaction precipitate some macromolecules like carbohydrates and proteins. Astringent taste of many foods is due to presence of these tannins (de Jesus et al., 2012; Lamy et al., 2016). With increasing number of hydroxyl groups (1–5) the astringency increases in the tannins but more than seven hydroxyl groups decrease the same property due to steric hindrance which lowers the power of the hydrogen bonds (Zou et al., 2015).

Condensed tannins and hydrolyzable tannins are two major groups to classify tannins. Another two subclasses of hydrolyzable tannins are gallotannins and ellagitannins. The former one on hydrolysis produces sugar and gallic acid. But the later one with same reaction gives ellagic acid too with sugar and gallic acid (Lamy et al., 2016). Hydrolyzable tannins when getting hydrolyzed by weak acids produce a hepatotoxic and highly irritant compound called pyrogallol (Jiménez et al., 2014). Proanthocyanidins, another group of condensed tannins, are the most copious polyphenols obtained from the plant. They are generally oligomers of flavan-3,4-diol and flavan-3-ol. Both of them containing C–C (4–8 or 6–8) and sometime C–O–C bonds are also visible in their structure (de Jesus et al., 2012; Lamy et al., 2016). These compounds are also known as oligomeric proanthocyanidins. Unlike hydrolyzable tannins, condensed tannins are not hydrolyzed but they get decomposed when treated with acidic or alcoholic conditions and on decomposition give phlobaphenes, a red-colored pigment. Except their abundance in our diet, tannins are also very important due to their polymeric nature (Serrano et al., 2016). These basic structures of different tannins control their properties like binding to proteins, antioxidant activities, and pigments.

Presently, proanthocyanidins have been proved to have great medicinal value on human health as antioxidant, cardioprotective, antithrombotic, immunomodulatory, anti-inflammatory, and anticancer (Nile and Park, 2014; Smeriglio et al., 2014; Sieniawska, 2015). Besides these, proanthocyanidins, obtained from many plants, are also used as nutritional supplements for humans and animals (Berry et al., 2016). These features also show the main qualitative and quantitative analytical dissimilarity between tannins and other polyphenols. Constancy in the chemical structure and composition of tannins is essential for distinguishing the biological and pharmacological properties of them toward the target compounds.

This entitled chapter focuses on the exploration of different types of tannins in terms of their medicinal values with special reference to exploration of condensed tannins and on the exploitation of tannins to show their impact in producing specific bitter taste accompanied by strong astringency in fruits and drinks. Moreover, a detailed account of the chemistry on tannins is presented along with a table showing variable content of different types of tannins present to occur in different plant parts. In short, the aim of this chapter is to show the properties of tannins as their scientific exploration and exploitation that show potentiality to be beneficial toward mankind and human society.

9.2   CHEMISTRY OF TANNINS

In plants, the complicated phenolic metabolism yields a range of compounds starting from flower pigments like anthocyanidins to the complex components of plant cell walls like lignin. But the special group of these phenolic compounds known as tannins can be separated easily from other polyphenolic compounds according to their chemical and biological activities. The common sources of the tannins are tea, cacao beans, nuts, cereal grains, legumes, fruit juices, chocolates, and red wines (Table 9.1) (Okuda and Ito, 2011). The structure of important tannins commonly found in several/various parts of plant is shown in Figure 9.1. As proanthocyanidins contain monomeric units linked by C-4 to C-8 bonds, they are mainly called as B-type proanthocyanidins but with a supplementary bond betwixt C-2 to C-7 of the basic flavan-3-ol units, the compound is called as A-type proanthocyanidins.

These specific condensed tannins are structured of several flavan-3-ol subunits, named as proanthocyanidin catechins or monomers. In between them, the greatest important and easily available monomeric units are the diastereomers of (epi)gallocatechin, (epi)afzelechin, and (epi)catechin. One heterocyclic ring and two aromatic homocyclic rings are present in these compounds. These are generally connected by a three-atom carbon bridge. Their carbon ring attributes a hydroxyl group at the C-3 position with absence of a double bond between C-2 and C-3. The most popular and therapeutically important proanthocyanidins of vegetables are constructed of epicatechin and catechin units but at the same time very less important are prodelphinidin or propelargonidin with (epi)gallocatechin or (epi)afzelechin basic

TABLE 9.1 Plant Parts Containing Different Types of Tannins

Fruits and Nuts	Proanthocyanidins (mg/100g)	Ellagitannins (mg/100g)	Gallotannins (mg/100g)	Reference
Cranberries (*Vaccinium oxycoccus*)	194–496	—	—	Liwei et al., 2004; Smeriglio c, 2017
Chokeberries (*Aronia melanocarpa* (Michx.) Elliott)	553–2106	—	—	Borowska and Brzóska, 2016; Smeriglio et al., 2017
Plums (*Prunus domestica*)	32–334	—	—	Smeriglio et al., 2017
Black diamond (*Prunus* spp.)	210–267	—	—	Smeriglio et al., 2017
Blueberries (*Vaccinium myrtillus*)	87–274	—	—	Burdulis et al., 2007; Smeriglio et al., 2017
Black currants (*Ribes nigrum*)	105–255	3–6	—	Butnariu, 2014; Smeriglio et al., 2017
Red currant (*Ribes rubrum*)	30–61	—	—	Butnariu, 2014; Smeriglio et al, 2017
Blackberries (*Rubus fructicosus*)	5–46	150–270	—	Burdulis et al., 2007; Smeriglio et al., 2017
Crowberries (*Empetrum nigrum*)	153–173	—	—	Burdulis et al., 2007; Smeriglio et al., 2017
Lingonberries (*Vaccinium vitis-idaea*)	175–545	—	—	Burdulis et al., 2007; Smeriglio et al., 2017
Red Grapes (*Vitis labrusca*)	8–75	—	—	Ortega-Regules et al., 2008; Smeriglio et al., 2017
Grape seeds (*Vitis vinifera*)	2180–6050	—	—	Ortega-Regules et al., 2008; Smeriglio et al., 2017
Peaches (*Prunus persica*)	29–110	-	—	Smeriglio et al., 2017
Apricot (*Prunus armeniaca*)	8–73	—	—	Smeriglio et al., 2017
Raspberries (*Rubus occidentalis*)	3–74	160–326	—	Burdulis et al., 2007; Smeriglio et al., 2017
Pears (*Pyrus communis* L)	5–81	—	—	Smeriglio et al., 2017
Apple (*Malus domestica* Borkh)	46–278	—	—	Martin et al., 2017; Smeriglio et al., 2017
Pomegranate (*Punica granatum*)	–	58–170	—	Hussein et al., 1997; Smeriglio et al., 2017

TABLE 9.1 *(Continued)*

Fruits and Nuts	Proanthocyanidins (mg/100g)	Ellagitannins (mg/100g)	Gallotannins (mg/100g)	Reference
Guava (*Psidium guajava*)	–	20–25	–	Smeriglio et al., 2017
Mango (*Mangifera indica*)	–	–	32–165	Smeriglio et al., 2017
Almonds (*Prunus dulcis*)	67–257	–	25–35	Chung et al., 1998; Smeriglio et al., 2017
Hazelnuts (*Corylus* spp.)	125–645	–	–	Chung et al., 1998; Smeriglio et al., 2017
Pecans (*Carya illinoinensis*)	238–695	11–33	–	Smeriglio et al., 2017
Pistachio nuts (*Pistacia vera*)	113–271	–	–	Chung et al., 1998; Smeriglio et al., 2017
Walnuts (*Juglans regia* L.)	35–87	36–59	–	Chung et al., 1998; Smeriglio et al., 2017

units. The biological sources of these compounds are red kidney beans, pinto beans, redcurrants, broad beans, barley, cinnamon, and black tea (Landete, 2011; de Jesus et al., 2012; Mateos-Martín et al., 2012; Lamy et al., 2016). Procyanidins are available naturally in different forms like dimeric, trimeric, tetrameric, and oligomeric structures. Procyanidin B1–B8 and procyanidin A1–A2 are the examples of dimeric structures and procyanidin C1 and C2, selligueain A and B structures are trimeric. The tetrameric and oligomeric forms of tannins are observed with polymerization degree (5 to 11). Here, the galloyl group of acyl substituent is combined with hydroxyl group at C-3 position. In glycosylated proanthocyanidin oligomers, the carbohydrate moieties are normally attached at the C-5 or C-3 position (Smeriglio et al., 2017).

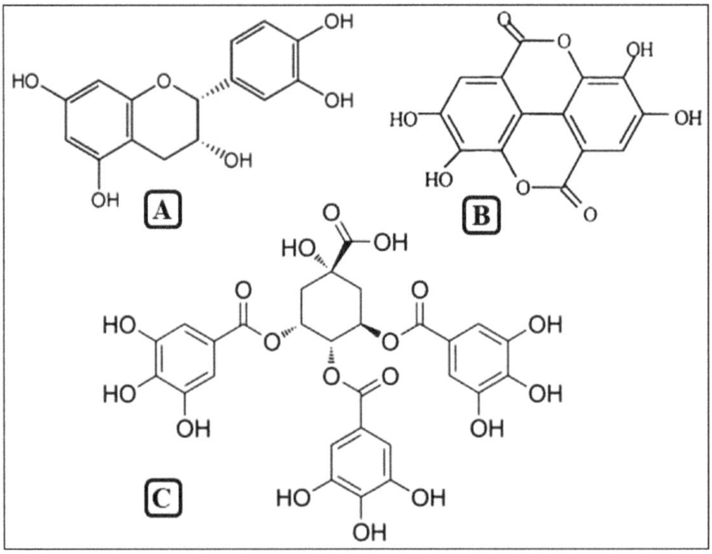

FIGURE 9.1   Structure of varieties of tannins found in all parts of plant. (A) Proanthocyanidin, (B) ellagitannin, and (C) gallotannin.

9.3   TYPES OF TANNINS USED FOR SCIENTIFIC EXPLORATION

As said earlier, according to the chemical structure and therapeutic activity, tannins are generally categorized into two major groups and they are condensed tannin and hydrolyzable tannin. In between them, condensed tannins have high-binding capability for dietary protein that is very important for decreasing the degradability of protein diet. Some plants like forage birds-foot trefoil (*Lotus corniculatus*) containing the condensed tannins improve the bodyweight of the cattle and sheep (Wang et al., 1996; Waghorn, 2008) but the total metabolizable protein in the small intestine is generally not increased. The reason for that is the undegraded feed protein will be decreased by lower level of microbial crude protein synthesis (Wang et al., 1996; MacAdam and Villalba, 2015). The presence of condensed tannins also lowers the enteric methane (CH_4) production (Carulla et al., 2005; Grainger et al., 2009) but the combining power of the same may also minimize fiber digestibility (Reed, 1995). Like this the application of tannins as a medicine for human beings and as a food for animals is very much variable on some factors like source, estimated amount, chemical structure, and the dose of the desired tannins.

Compared to condensed tannins, hydrolyzable tannins have smaller molecular weight. Where the molecular weights of hydrolyzable tannins are in the range of 500 to 3000, the same of the condensed tannins are 1900 to 28,000. Similarly, the affinity to proteins is more in condensed tannins than hydrolyzable tannins and so it absorbed from the digestive tract more easily thereby enhancing the potential toxicity to the animal (McLeod, 1974). Although the scientists' interest is more in condensed tannins due to above factors but many in vitro studies also mentions that in case of protein degradation there are no differences from the sources of the tannins (Getachew et al., 2008). When the hydrolyzable tannins are used as supplement, at 3% of dry matter, no toxicity was observed and the CH_4 releases was also minimized by 24% compared with control (Liu et al., 2011). Generally, hydrolyzable tannins penetrate the rumen protozoa by interrupting their association with methanogens (Patra and Saxena, 2011). About 0.6% dietary dry matter of both groups of tannins shows no effect on growth of animals but when combination of both hydrolyzable and condensed tannins has been applied in the dose of 0.3% each, the average daily gain is increased (Rivera-Méndez et al., 2016). Due to the cellular toxicity produced by the tannins, a low dose can be used to get the desired application. It can also be used as a supplement and in this case the combinations of both the tannins are more beneficial for humans and animals. It will be more helpful to the lactating dairy cattle and report showed a straight enhancement in dry matter intake with no harmful result on milk production. Uses of both the tannins improve nitrogen use and minimize hydrogen accessible for methanogens (Reed, 1995; Jayanegara et al., 2015). Besides these, the combination of both the tannins may decrease rumen ammonia concentration and also CH_4 emissions (Isaac et al., 2015; Aboagye et al., 2018).

9.4 SCIENTIFIC EXPLORATION OF TANNINS

The medicinal explorations of tannins are mainly their anti-inflammatory, hemostatic, antihemorrhoidal, antidiarrheal, and antidiabetic properties (Table 9.2) (Kumarappan and Mandal, 2015). The treatment of digestive disorders like irritating bowel disorders, esophagitis, enteritis, and gastritis may also be different parts of these scientific explorations. In wound healing, tannins not only stop bleeding and heal burns but also heal the wound and treat the infections internally. A preventive layer over the exposed tissue has been prepared by tannins to control the further infections. Other scientific explorations of tannins are the properties that give protection on kidneys, regression of tumors, antibacterial, antiviral, and antiparasitic effects. When tannins have been administered with red wines and red grape juice various enteric viruses, poliovirus and the herpes simplex virus get disabled (Figure 9.2) (Kraus et al., 2003; Schweitzer et al., 2008; Barbehenn and Constabel, 2011).

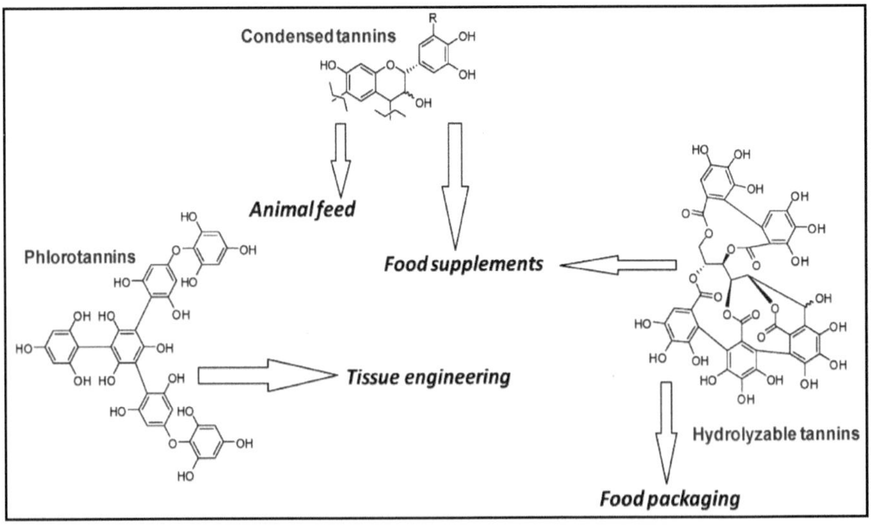

FIGURE 9.2   Scientific exploration of tannins (Kraus et al., 2003; Schweitzer et al., 2008; Barbehenn and Constabel, 2011).

9.5 SCIENTIFIC EXPLORATION OF CONDENSED TANNINS

Condensed tannins can be biosynthesized in many plant species. In its structure, flavan-3-ols is either connected between C4 and C6′ or between C4 and C8′. Occasional C2 to O to C7′ linkages also can be observed (Yoshida et al., 2005). Around 25–35 species of ephemeral flowering plants under genus *Populus* in the family Salicaceae are native to most of the Northern Hemisphere. This genus contains condensed tannins 25% dry mass in its leaves (Kraus et al., 2003; Sibley, 2019). The condensed tannins control the biotic and abiotic interactions of these plants (Kraus et al., 2003; Schweitzer et al., 2008; Barbehenn and Constabel, 2011). The estimated amount of these tannins depends on genetics, environment, and definitely interlinkage between genetics and environment (Schweitzer et al., 2008; Barbehenn and Constabel, 2011; Lindroth and St Clair, 2013). They can influence the chemical and molecular structures and structure-related activity like polymer size, hydroxylation, and stereochemistry (Scioneauxet al., 2011; Decker et al., 2017) and also biochemical properties (Ayres et al., 2007; Makkar et al., 2007; Mueller-Harvey et al., 2019). Comparing with other plants, *Populus* shows a less relationship between concentrations of condensed tannins, ecological effects, and biological properties (Table 9.3). The differences in stereochemistry, polymer size, and hydroxylation of condensed tannins are also observed in *Populus*. This is evaluated by a reversed-phase high-performance liquid chromatography (HPLC) followed by electrochemical, photodiode array or mass spectrometry detection (Guyot et al., 2001; Karonen et al., 2006; Karonen et al., 2007; Kardel et al., 2013; Li and Meng, 2016). Thiolytic depolymerization of condensed tannins by using benzyl mercaptan under acidic environment liberates terminal units and produces thioether derivatives of extender units (Guyot et al., 1998; Guyot et al., 2001; Gu et al., 2003; Karonen et al., 2007; Hümmer and Schreier, 2008; Mouls et al., 2011). In *Populus* foliage, structural investigation of condensed tannins is plainer because the polymers are reportedly straight and embraced of proportionately some dissimilar types of repeating units like gallocatechin, catechin, and their stereoisomers (Scioneaux et al., 2011). These reports revealed differences in stereochemistry, hydroxylation, foliar polymer size, and total concentration of condensed tannins among *Populus tremuloides* genotypes which will be ecologically pertinent (Kennedy et al., 2019).

9.6   SCIENTIFIC EXPLORATION OF OTHER SPECIFIC TANNINS

9.6.1   *PREPARATION OF THIOETHER DERIVATIVES FROM CONDENSED TANNIN MIXTURE*

The biological properties of tannins depend upon their molecular structure. Mainly polymer size, hydroxylation, and stereochemistry of tannins show a clear idea about the pharmacological properties. Although, the ecological effect of the tannins influenced by genetical and environmental properties but the molecular structure has an important role in its activity. Condensed tannin mixtures are generally used to produce thioether derivatives of monomeric flavanols (Figure 9.3).

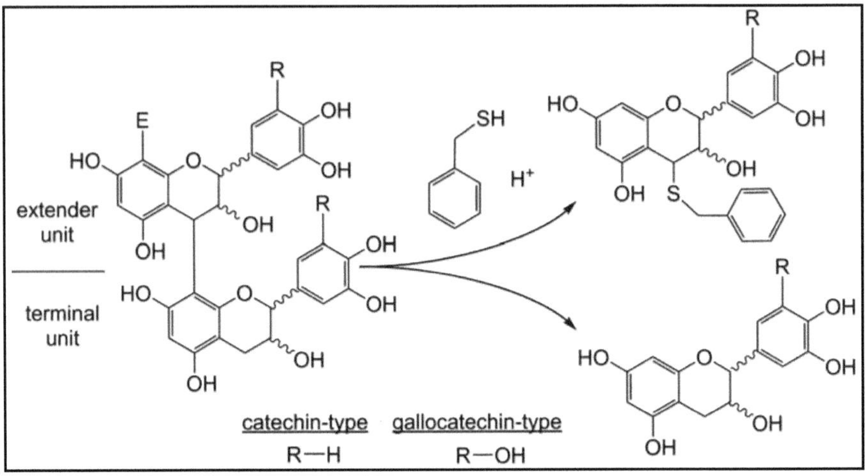

FIGURE 9.3   The extender units of condensed tannin polymers are transformed to thioethers when terminal units are emancipated without conjugation to benzyl mercaptan (Kennedy et al., 2019) [Reprinted with permission from Rubert-Nason, K. F.; Lindroth, R. L.. Analysis of condensed tannins in Populus spp. using reversed phase UPLC-DA-(−)esi-MS following thiolytic depolymerisation. Phytochemical Analysis, 2018, 1–11. © 2018 John Wiley & Sons.]

According to the various reports, a bulk extraction of the same can be done from *P. tremuloides* and from that thioether derivatives can be produced. The mixtures of gallocatechins, catechins, and their thioethers can be then separated by ultra-performance liquid chromatography (UPLC) and perceived by photodiode array (PDA) and electrospray ionization mass spectrometry. If different plants have been selected, the thiolysis-UPLC–PDA-(−)esi-MS showed a considerable differences in tannin concentrations and their molecular structures (Table 9.4) (Kennedy et al., 2019).

9.6.2   ENZYME-INHIBITORY ACTIVITY OF ELLAGITANNINS

N-myristoylation is a eukaryotic *N*-terminal co- or post-translational protein (Thinon et al., 2014). In this protein modification, one enzyme called *N*-myristoyltransferase (NMT) conveys a fatty acid toward *N*-terminal glycine residues of assorted cellular lead proteins (Landete, 2011; Apel et al., 2018). On the basis of the cellular context, NMT acts as a molecular target in anti-infectious and anticancer treatment. Generally some drugs impede this

TABLE 9.2 Medicinal Exploration of Tannin to Solve the Risk of Major Problem of Human Health.

Human Health Problem	Tannins	Molecular Structure	Botanical Sources	Finding and Concluding Remark	Reference
Antidiabetic					
Diabetes	Catechins (Flavan-3,4- diols)		Centaurea maculosa, Malus domestica, Prunus armeniaca, Phaseolus vulgaris, Camellia sinensis, Rubus fructicosus, Prunus avium, Vitis vinifera, Prunus persica, Rubus idaeus	Centaurea maculosa, the spotted knapweed often studied for this behavior, releases catechin isomers into the ground through its roots, potentially having effects as an antibiotic or herbicide. The same function has also been observed in other plants containing catechins.	Bais et al., 2003
	Gallic acid		Rheum rhabarbarum, Vitis vinifera, Oenothera biennis, Corylus avellana, Camellia sinensis	The amount of gallic acid emancipated by tannase categorized from 5 to 309 mg/g with the maximum amount resoluted in the tannin fraction of the bearberry-leaf extract. It is used as antidiabetic durg due its hypoglycaemic property.	Karamać et al., 2006
	Chlorogenic acid		Coffea arabica and Coffea robusta	Using in vitro studies, reported that CGA increased glucose uptake in L6 muscular cells, an effect only observed in the presence of stimulating concentrations of insulin. CGA has been described as a potential antidiabetic agent	Tousch et al., 2008

TABLE 9.2 *(Continued)*

Human Health Problem	Tannins	Molecular Structure	Botanical Sources	Finding and Concluding Remark	Reference
Antidiarrheal					
Diarrhoea	Catechins (Flavan-3,4- diols)		*Centaurea maculosa, Malus domestica, Prunus armeniaca L., Phaseolus vulgaris, Camellia sinensis, Rubus fruticosus L., Prunus avium, Vitis vinifera, Prunus persica,* and *Rubus idaeus*	*Centaurea maculosa*, the spotted knapweed often studied for this behavior, releases catechin isomers into the ground through its roots, potentially having effects as an antibiotic or herbicide. The same function has also been observed in other plants containing catechins	(Bais et al., 2003)
Antihemorrhoidal					
Hemorrhoida	Chinese gallotannin		*Magnifera indica, Ceratonia siliqua, Lithocarpus densiflorus, Vitis rotundifolia, Arbutus unedo,* and *Oenothera paradoxa*	This compound is used as antihemorrhoidal drug. It is available in many plants	Bais et al., 2003
Anti-inflammatory					
Inflammation	Ellagitannins		*Juglans regia*	In vivo: inhibition of macrophage recruitment and infiltration and inflammatory markers (TNF-α, IL-6, IL-10) in epididymal adipose tissues of mice	Choi et al., 2016

TABLE 9.2 *(Continued)*

Human Health Problem	Tannins	Molecular Structure	Botanical Sources	Finding and Concluding Remark	Reference
	Hexahydroxydiphenic acid (Ellagitannin)		*Pimenta racemosa*	In vivo: inhibition of macrophage recruitment and infiltration and inflammatory markers (TNF-α, IL-6, IL-10) in epididymal adipose tissues of mice	Choi et al., 2016
	Tellimagrandin (Ellagitannin)		*Cornus canadensis, Eucalyptus globulus, Melaleuca styphelioides,* and *Rosa rugosa*	In vivo: inhibition of macrophage recruitment and infiltration and inflammatory markers (TNF-α, IL-6, IL-10) in epididymal adipose tissues of mice	Choi et al., 2016
	Gallic acid		*Rheum rhabarbarum, Vitis vinifera, Oenothera biennis, Corylus avellana,* and *Camellia sinensis*	The amount of gallic acid emancipated by tannase categorized from 5 to 309 mg/g with the maximum amount resoluted in the tannin fraction of the barberry-leaf extract This compound is used as anti-inflammatory drug. It is available in many plants	Karamać et al., 2006
	Catechins (Flavan-3,4-diols)		*Centaurea maculosa, Malus domestica, Prunus armeniaca* L., *Phaseolus vulgaris, Camellia sinensis, Rubus fruticosus* L., *Prunus avium, Vitis vinifera, Prunus persica,* and *Rubus idaeus*	Epigallocatechin-3-gallate was reported as anti-inflammatory drug in modifying the IL-I E-induced activation of mitogen-activated protein kinase in human chondrocytes	Suzuki and Takahashi, 1975

TABLE 9.2 *(Continued)*

Human Health Problem	Tannins	Molecular Structure	Botanical Sources	Finding and Concluding Remark	Reference
	Gallotannins		*Magnifera indica, Ceratonia siliqua, Lithocarpus densiflorus, Vitis rotundifolia, Arbutus unedo,* and *Oenothera paradoxa*	Oral administration inhibited tumor necrosis factor alpha (TNF-α) serum levels in both models of inflammation (AA and PMA)	Garrido et al., 2004
Hemostatic					
Bleeding	Gallic acid		*Rheum rhabarbarum, Vitis vinifera, Oenothera biennis, Corylus avellana,* and *Camellia sinensis*	The amount of gallic acid emancipated by tannase categorized from 5 to 309 mg/g with the maximum amount resoluted in the tannin fraction of the bearberry-leaf extract	Karamać et al., 2006
				This compound is used as hemostatic. It is available in many plants.	
Other Human Health Problem					
Antibacterial activity	Catechins (Flavan-3,4-diols)		*Centaurea maculosa, Malus domestica, Prunus armeniaca* L., *Phaseolus vulgaris, Camellia sinensis, Rubus fruticosus* L., *Prunus avium, Vitis vinifera, Prunus persica,* and *Rubus idaeus*	The tannin portion was very potent against *Escherichia coli, Pseudomonas aeruginosa,* and *Staphylococcus aureus* on agar plate method	Riso et al., 2002
Anticancer activity				Catechin, controlled to pheochromocytoma cells in cell culture.	Akagi et al., 1997
Anti-cataract activity				Tea, executed in culture to amplified rat lens, decreased the occurrence of selenite cataract in vivo	Chaudhuri et al., 1997

TABLE 9.2 *(Continued)*

Human Health Problem	Tannins	Molecular Structure	Botanical Sources	Finding and Concluding Remark	Reference
Antifungal activity				Synergic antifungal activity of the combination of EGCG and anti-mycotics against *Candida albicans*	Hirasawa and Takada, 2004
Anti-hypercholesterolemic activity				Inhibited the inclusion of cholesterol within micelles in the intestine, encouraging its exudation into the feces	Matsui et al., 2006
Antimutagenic activity				(–)-Epicatechin is indicated to be a better antimutagenic agent	Geetha et al., 2004
Antioxidative effect				Epigallocatechin gallate, tea polyphenols, and tea extract were appended to human plasma and lipid peroxidation induces by the water-soluble radical generator 2,2-azobis (2-amidinopropane) dihydrochloride	Finger et al., 1991
Antiproliferative activity				Flavan-3-ols, epigallocatechin gallate and gallocatechin gallate reported their maximum potency.	Finger et al., 1991
Antiviral activity				Epigallocatechin-3-gallate, administered to Hep2 cells in culture, generated a therapeutic index of 22 and an IC50 of 25M	Davis et al., 1997

TABLE 9.3 Medicinal Exploration of Condensed Tannins to Solve the Risk of Human Health

Human Health Problem	Tannins	Molecular Structure	Botanical Sources	Finding and Concluding Remark	Reference
Low level of oxytocin and various menstrual problems	Catechol		*Saraca indica*	It is used as uterine tonic. It stimulates the uterus by the prolonged and frequent uterine contractions. It is reported to have a stimulant effect on the endometrium and ovarian tissue and useful in menorrhagia.	Kokate et al., 2009; Baskerville et al., 2010
Low level of oxytocin and various menstrual problems	Ketosterol		*Saraca indica*	It is used as uterine tonic. It stimulates the uterus by the prolonged and frequent uterine contractions. It is reported to have a stimulant effect on the endometrium and ovarian tissue and useful in menorrhagia	Kokate et al., 2009; Baskerville et al., 2010
Used as astringent to minimize pores and drying up oily skin	Acacatechin		*Acacia catechu*	It is used as an astringent externally for boils, skin eruptions, and ulcers	Abbe and Amin, 2008; Kokate et al., 2009
Used as astringent to minimize pores and drying up oily skin	Quercetin		*Acacia catechu*	It is used as an astringent externally for boils, skin eruptions, and ulcers	Abbe and Amin, 2008; Kokate et al., 2009

TABLE 9.3 (Continued)

Human Health Problem	Tannins	Molecular Structure	Botanical Sources	Finding and Concluding Remark	Reference
Diarrhoea	Catechin		Uncaria gambier	It is used as astringent in the treatment of diarrhoea	Abbe and Amin, 2008; Kokate et al., 2009
Free radicals formation in the human body	Epicatechin		Centaurea maculosa, Malus domestica, Prunus armeniaca L., Phaseolus vulgaris, Camellia sinensis, Rubus fruticosus L., Prunus avium, Vitis vinifera, Prunus persica, Rubus idaeus, etc.	It is used as antioxidant to scavenge the free radicals formed in the human body	Pushp et al., 2013
Diarrhoea	Catechu tannic acid		Uncaria gambier	It is used as astringent in the treatment of diarrhoea	Abbe and Amin, 2008; Kokate et al., 2009
Diabetes	Kino tannic acid		Pterocarpus marsupium	The aqueous infusion and alcoholic extracts are used in the treatment of diabetes	Kokate et al., 2009; Mishra et al., 2013
Diabetes	K-pyrocatechol		Pterocarpus marsupium	The aqueous infusion and alcoholic extracts are used in the treatment of diabetes	Kokate et al., 2009; Mishra et al., 2013
Fungal and bacterial infections, tumor	Phlobaphenes		Cinchona officinalis, Zea mays	It has antibacterial, antifungal, and antitumor properties	Rehman et al., 2014

enzyme and those drugs are also useful in the treatment of infectious diseases or cancer (Selvakumar et al., 2007; Wright et al., 2010). Condensed tannin mixtures contain ellagitannins, punicalagin, and isoterchebulin. In addition to these, eschweilenol C and ellagic acid are also included (Chung et al., 1998; Kraus et al., 2003; Yoshida et al., 2005; Ayres et al., 2007). According to the report, they can be easily isolated from the bark of *Terminalia bentzoe* (L.) (Apel et al., 2018; Chandrasekhar et al., 2018). In between the above constituents, punicalagin and isoterchebulin have also potent inhibitory activity to the HsNMT1. They can also act against *Plasmodium falciparum* NMT (PfNMT) both in vitro and *in cellulo* (Muganga et al., 2014; Apel et al., 2018). This mechanism opens different paths for new NMT encumber blossoming. Although, the inhibitory effects of both the compounds on PfNMT in vitro and *in cellulo* are in the micromolar range, but this report is very much important to treat the malarial fevers traditionally (Apel et al., 2018).

9.6.3 TANNIN–IRON HYBRID MICROCAPSULES AS ANTITUBERCULOSIS AGENT

Another scientific exploration of tannins is the ferric tannin microcapsules. It can be prepared throughout a liquid, non-sacrificial core. In the ultrasonic treatment, this creation becomes complete very easily and successfully. In this strategy, the addition of ferric ions occurred into the embryonic emulsion (Figure 9.4). It encourages shell formation showing stable complexation effects. The formations of microcapsule assemblies of monomeric tannins like epigallocatechin-3-O-gallate are impotent to structure without a templating metal. The effectiveness of these microcapsules as a hydrophobic molecule is active against *Mycobacterium tuberculosis* (Elisavet et al., 2018). Like this, the scientific exploration of tannin can also be elaborated in microcapsule formation to treat tuberculosis.

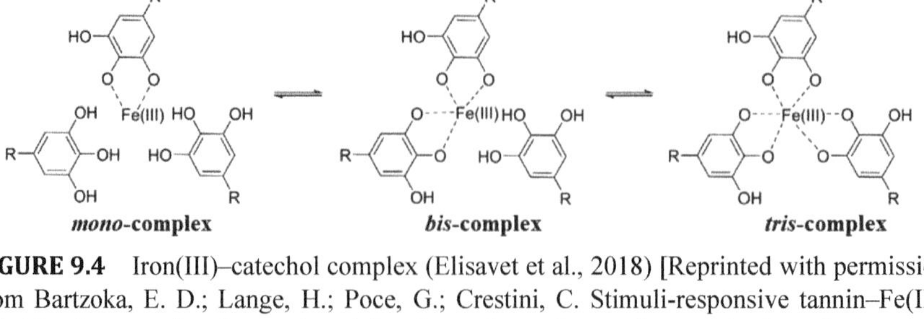

FIGURE 9.4 Iron(III)–catechol complex (Elisavet et al., 2018) [Reprinted with permission from Bartzoka, E. D.; Lange, H.; Poce, G.; Crestini, C. Stimuli-responsive tannin–Fe(III) hybrid microcapsules demonstrated by the active release of an anti-tuberculosis agent. ChemSusChem, 2018, 11(22): 3975–399. © 2018 John Wiley & Sons.].

9.6.4 TANNINS ATTENUATES ANXIETY

"A state of extreme trepidation, uncertainty and a fear resulting from antici-pation of a future threat" is termed as Anxiety (O'Donovan et al., 2013). In psychopharmacology, it is very important portion because 90% population of the earth is suffering from anxiety nowadays (Ingale and Gandhi, 2016). The disturbance in the balance of neurotransmitters is due to the etiopathogenesis of several psychosomatic disorders (Kathleen, 2009). To treat anxiety among several drugs, the first-line drug of choice is benzodiazepines (Cloos and Ferreira, 2009). But, slow heart rate, sedation, nausea and vomiting, respira-tory depression, skin rash, and double vision are different side effects that can be observed when using anxiolytic drugs. In long-term use of these drugs, the dependency and tolerance are visible in the patient body (Chatterjee et al., 2013). The hydrolyzable tannins isolated from hydroalcoholic extract of fruits of *Terminalia chebula* (Combretaceae) can be used as anxiolytic drug according to its properties and mechanism of action. A neurotoxic chemical called picrotoxin (PTX) acts via interaction with the convulsant site of the Gamma Aminobutyric Acid-gated chlorine channel (Manayi et al., 2016). When tested on different sets of animal models, it has been observed that PTX is used everywhere to produce consistent pro-anxiety effects (Stankevi-cius et al., 2008; Shekhar, 1993). For anxiety disorders the most important drugs are serotonin inhibitors, norepinephrine reuptake inhibitors, serotonin, and benzodiazepines (Ravindran and Stein, 2010). The hydrolyzable tannins isolated from the above said plant showed promising result as anxiolytic drug in PTX-induced anxiety via GABAergic system and modulation of other neurotransmitters compared with diazepam (Chandrasekhar et al., 2018). The exploration of tannin in anxiety is also very much helpful to treat this disease that is very common nowadays in almost all countries.

9.6.5 EFFECT OF TANNIN ON DIETARY NITROGEN EFFICIENCY, METHANE EMISSION, AND MILK FATTY ACID COMPOSITION

Tannin extracts alone or in combination with other foods always influence the daily enteric CH_4 production (Grainger et al., 2009; Aboagye et al., 2018; Isaac et al., 2015). For domestic animals, the normal diet is deficient of palmitic acid and fatty acids but at the same time it is rich source of rumenic acid, vaccenic acid, oleic acid, stearic acid, and α-linolenic acid in milk fat. When tannin mixtures (tannins mixed with other food materials) mixed with the normal diet of the pet animals, it ameliorates fatty acid composition of

TABLE 9.4 Thioether Derivatives Prepared From Condensed Tannin Mixture

Thioether Derivatives Preparation	Botanical Sources	Separation Method	Specific Properties	Application	Finding and Concluding Remark	Reference
(−)-Epigallocathechin gallate-(2,4,6-trimethyl) benzylthioether	Air-dried roots of grape seeds, *Rhodiola cremulata* and *Rhodiola kirilowii*	Ethanol portions of epigallocatechin gallate is separated by HP-20 macroporous adsorbent resin (4000 g, dried weight) column (HPLC) then it is derivatized by thiolysis in acidic media. The purified derivative product was obtained using reverse-phase PHPLC.	Identified as an autophagic flux activator using the autophagy-screening system	Melanoma As an antitumor and novel anticancer	Preferentially induces cell death in B16 melanoma cells. Selectively induces ROS accumulation in cancer cells. Induced autophagy promotes the apoptotic cell death but does not affect ROS generation	Jing et al., 2017
6,8-Bis(octylthiomethyl)-epigallocatechin 3-O-gallate and 6,8-bis(octylthiomethyl)-413-(2-hydroxyethylthio) epigallocatechin 3-O-gallate	Leaves of green tea, *Camellia sinensis*	Separation by column chromatography on Sephadex LH-20 eluting with ethanol.	Anti-lipid peroxidative	Antioxidant	Inhibited lipid peroxidation in liposome lipid bilayer caused by both AAPH [2,20-azobis(2-amidinopropane) dihydrocholoride] and AMVN [2,20-azobis (2,4-dimethylvaleronitrile)]	Tanaka et al., 1998

the milk. Uptake of tannins in single form or in mixture form, the amount of α-linolenic acid has been increased by more than 17%. This special diet with good amount of tannin extract is decreasing the urinary nitrogen excretion (Focant et al., 2018).

9.6.6 PHYTOGENIC FEED ADDITIVES IN TANNINS, SAPONINS, AND ESSENTIAL OILS

When animals cannot get proper nutrition from the regular feeds, feed additives has to be given as nutritional supplement for their good health. These feed additives are used for the development of the health of animals, as well as their productivity. These additives also expand the standard of foods from animal genesis. Many chemical constituents as defaunation (Van Nevel and Demeyer 1996), microbial feed additives and prebiotics (Mutsvangwa et al., 1992), supplementation of unsaturated fatty acids (Johnson and Johnson 1995), and ionophores have been attempted to build livestock more feed efficient. In many cases, few tannins of both types, that is, condensed and hydrolyzable, have the property to provide nutritional supplements. These are called phytogenic feed additives. Mainly, saponins, tannins, and few essential oils are used as phytogenic feed additives that can be used in many places with the feeds of the animals (Lakhani et al., 2019). Thus the scientific explorations of tannin in animal food also show a significant role in the modern society. It takes important part to develop the animal feed and supplements for development of their health and of course human society.

9.6.7 TANNIN-RICH DIETS IN RABBIT PRODUCTION

Infection occurred by the genus *Eimeria* of monoxenous coccidian is very common at the time of rabbit breeding. This creates maximum health problems in those rabbits. The livestock building cladding same restriction like gastrointestinal nematodes' infections in small ruminants, condensed tannin rich plants have been broadly used due to their antihelmintic activity (Arroyo-Lopez et al., 2014; Hoste et al., 2015). Many reports suggest that plants containing tannins have shown potentiality against Emeria infection in lambs (Burke et al., 2012; Saratsis et al., 2016) and kids (Fraquelli et al., 2015). In the southern Europe, two different plants namely *Onobrychis viciifolia* (common name: sainfoin) and *Cerotonia siliqua* (common name: carob pods) are the rich source of tannins and for this reason these plants are generally added in the feeds of rabbit (Abu-Hafsa et al., 2017; Legendre et al., 2017; Legendre et al., 2018). Again, as mentioned earlier, in maintenance of animal health and to cure their diseases, especially in rabbits, the scientific exploration of tannin plays an important and major role.

9.6.8   EFFECT OF TANNIN ON RED WINE COLOR

Wine color is the first attractive feature according to consumer's require-ments. As the color of the wine improves the acceptance of the wine, simultaneously, the age, quality, and present preservation condition can be gained from this color. Anthocyanins are the most important constituents responsible for the proper color of the wine (Figure 9.5). At the start of the preparation of a wine, it shows the exact color but with time the deterioration of the anthocyanins takes place and the color of the wine changes. Both flavonols and anthocyanins get condensed straight forward. Sometimes these two compounds became condensed by mediation of acetaldehyde or other compounds (He et al., 2012).

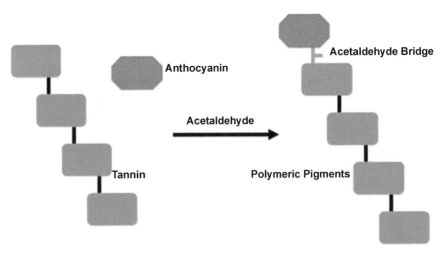

FIGURE 9.5   Polymeric pigment formation by reaction with acetaldehyde (He et al., 2012).

These reactions give a bathochromical shift to the compound and due to that the changes of absorption maxima of the anthocyanins have been observed. This bathochromical shift is responsible for the bluish-red hue in the wine (Salas et al., 2004; Escribano-Bailón et al., 2001). After these reactions, the produced anthocyanin-derived pigments constructed from the cycloaddition of wine nucleophiles at C-4 and at the hydroxyl group attached to C-5 of the anthocyanin flavylium nucleus. This is also accompanied by aromatization through autoxidation. This pigment leads to an additional pyran ring in the pigment skeletal (Fulcrand et al., 1998). All the compounds present in the wine are responsible to react with anthocyanins to produce these types of pigments. In between them the most important are acetone (Benab-deljalil et al., 2000), vinylcatechol (Quijada-Morín et al., 2010; Håkansson et al., 2003), monomeric and dimericprocyanidins (Francia-Aricha et al., 1997; Rivas-Gonzalo et al., 1995), pyruvicacid (Fulcrand et al., 1998; Fulcrand et al., 1996), vinylphenol (Fulcrand et al., 1996), acetaldehyde (Bakker and Timberlake, 1997; Benabdeljalil et al., 2000), vinylguaiacol (Quijada-Morín et al., 2010; Hayasaka and Asenstorfer, 2002), hydroxycinnamic acids (Schwarz et al., 2003), diacetyl (Blanco-Vega et al., 2011), and aceto-acetic acid that are present in the wine. On the other hand, the cycloaddition reaction occurs due to a hypsochromical shift of anthocyanins. This is the reason for another color change of the wine toward orange hues (Fulcrand et al., 1996; Benabdeljalil et al., 2000; Quijada-Morín et al., 2010; Francia-Aricha et al., 1997; Rivas-Gonzalo et al., 1995). It is now well observed that in different fields the exploration of tannins activity improves the human health and social life.

9.6.9   QUEBRACHO AND TARA TANNINS IN FUNGAL BIOREACTORS

Tannins obtained from the different sources are generally used in the tanning of leather in industries. Tara tannin and Quebracho tannin are two different types of tannins that are very important for the tanning industry (Falcão and Araújo, 2018). Many reports suggest that the effect of condensed and hydrolyzable tannins on the fungal biomass can be developed in the bioreactors with Tara tannin and Quebracho tannin (Peng et al., 2018; Spennatia et al., 2019). Fungi were surpassed by bacteria through biomolecular analysis as a chief component to a stable culture of suspended biomass in the long run. Fungi show greater resistance to inhibit Quebracho tannin than bacteria (Peng et al., 2018). So, this tannin concentration is allowed for the preservation of a stable fungal biofilm in nonsterile conditions (Figure 9.6). This explorative report of tannin is really important for the industry to develop the products (Spennatia et al., 2019).

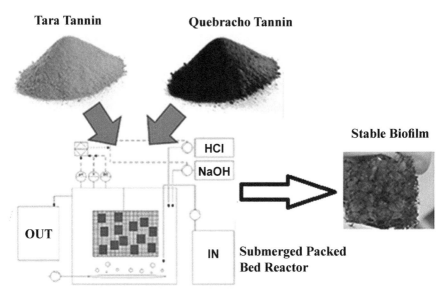

FIGURE 9.6   Preparation of stable biofilm by *Tara tannin* and *Quebracho tannin* (Reprinted with permission from Spennatia et al., 2019). © Elsevier.)

9.7   EXPLOITATION OF TANNINS

9.7.1   *UNPLEASANT TASTE AND ASTRINGENT FEEL OF TANNINS*

The fruits of *Fructus chaenomeles* (Rosaceae), commonly known as Mugua fruit (Shanga et al., 2019), are very potent traditional Chinese medicine used for the treatment of various inflammation, dyspepsia, cholera gastrointestinal spasms, and infectious diseases. Although tannins have many pharmacological properties like anti-asthmatic, antioxidant, anti-inflammatory, antimicrobial, and anticancer properties (Lu et al., 2004; Shanga et al., 2019; Xu et al., 2019). Huge amount of tannins show physical properties as unpleasant taste and as an astringent feel. Different methods like physical, chemical, and biological can be carried out to remove the excess tannins from the plant parts. Mugua fruit is very much important in the health science as a medicine, but it consists of a large amount of tannins. Due to this fact the unpleasant taste and an astringent feel of that fruit may cause the patient's avoidance toward this drug. Several methods like crosslinking polyvingypyrrolidone and activated carbon are carried out to remove the excess tannins from the different foods like Mugua fruits (Shanga et al., 2019).

9.7.2 APPLICATION OF TANNINS AS ADSORBENT

The widely distributed tannins obtained from Bayberry are available in very low cost in the market. It naturally shows a very good chelating affinity toward metal ions because it consists of huge number of adjacent phenolic hydroxyls (Xu et al., 2017). Although it is widely available, it cannot be used as an adsorbent due to its easy solubility in the water and many organic solvents. To bypass this problem, many research works have been carried out to immobilize tannins on various materials. According to many reports and reviews, mesoporous silica (Huang et al., 2010), activated carbon (Wang et al., 2013), and collagen fiber (Bacelo et al., 2016) can be used as tannins carriers. In between them, the most common material is collagen fiber. This collagen fiber has been selected in many cases to immobilize tannins (Sun et al., 2011; Huang et al., 2009). The reason of this is the presence of several functional groups like –OH, –COOH, and $-NH_2$. These functional groups react with uranium and produce chelates. Actually, the adsorption capacity of collagen fiber, which is immobilized with tannins, is not very high, because fewer amounts of tannins can be immobilized with the collagen. Besides this, the diameter of collagen fiber is limiting the surface area that can contact as active sites between collagen fiber, tannins, and uranium (Menga et al., 2019).

9.8 CONCLUSION

Many plants are containing tannins in their different parts either in the form of condensed or hydrolyzable tannins. The scientific exploration and exploitation of tannins are two major directions that are really important for the pharmaceutical industry and also to the researchers working with secondary metabolites especially tannins. Tannins showed multidisciplinary scientific explorations in development of human health and their society. The effects of tannins are important in curing several diseases. Tannins play important roles not only in humans, but also in case of animal food supplements, food ingredients, and also in the development of their health. To treat the diseases of domestic animals tannin is a well-known drug. These important polyphenolic compounds play their job in protection of plants from predation. It is also as pesticides and might assist in controlling plant growth and metabolism. Tannin's use in world's leather production is also vast range more than 90%. With all these potential properties, the pungency test of tannins is not suitable for many drugs and not accepted by the patients. The astringency from the tannins is the main reason of the dry and puckery sensation in the mouth at the time of consumption of tea, red wine, or unripened fruit. Similarly, the demolition or moderation of tannins with time plays a foremost task when determining harvesting times. This chapter shows both scientific exploration and exploitation of tannins in case of their various properties in the beneficial to mankind.

9.9 SUMMARY

Tannins are polyphenolic compounds and classified as condensed tannins and hydrolyzable tannins. Hydrolyzable tannins when getting hydrolyzed by weak acids produce a hepatotoxic and highly irritant compound called pyrogallol. Condensed tannins are not hydrolyzed but they get decomposed when treated with acidic or alcoholic conditions and on decomposition give phlobaphenes, a red-colored pigment. The affinity to proteins is more in condensed tannins than hydrolyzable tannins and so it absorbed from the digestive tract more easily thereby enhancing the potential toxicity to the animal. The hydrolyzable tannins are also used as food supplement. Due to the cellular toxicity produced by the tannins, a low dose can be used to get the desired application. The scientific explorations of tannins are the properties that give protection on kidneys, regression of tumors, antibacterial, antiviral, and antiparasitic effects. The condensed tannins control the biotic and abiotic interactions of the plant. Condensed tannin mixtures are also generally used to produce thioether derivatives of monomeric flavanols. These tannin mixtures contain ellagitannins, punicalagin, and isoterchebulin. They have a potent inhibitory activity to the HsNMT1. In formulation, the formations of microcapsule assemblies of monomeric tannins like epigallo-catechin-3-O-gallate can also be structured without a templating metal. The hydrolyzable tannins isolated from hydroalcoholic extract of different plants can be used as anxiolytic drug according to their properties and mechanism of action. The special diet for the domestic animals with good amount of tannin extract decreases the urinary nitrogen excretion. Saponins, tannins, and few essential oils are used as phytogenic feed additives that can be used in many places with the feeds of the animals. Except these, the color of wine is also dependent on the presence of tannins in it. Like these a vast scientific exploration of tannin has been observed in various fields as foods and drugs. On the other hand, tannins have an unpleasant taste and astringent feel. Due to this fact the unpleasant taste and an astringent feel may cause the patient's avoidance toward this drug. In addition, tannins cannot be used as an adsorbent due to its easy solubility in the water and many organic solvents. These different scientific explorations and exploitations of tannin generally depend upon stereochemistry and C–C bonding of tannins, their degree of polymerization, conversion of procyanidins to prop delphinidins, and finally on the concentrations of tannins in diets.

KEYWORDS

- **condensed tannin**
- **ellagitannins**
- **exploitation**
- **exploration**
- **gallotannins**
- **hydrolysable tannin**
- **oligomeric proanthocyanidins**
- **phlobaphenes**
- **polyphenolic polymer**
- **proanthocyanidins**
- **prop delphinidins**

REFERENCES

Abbe, M. M. J.; Amin I. Polyphenols in cocoa and cocoa products: is there a link between antioxidant properties and health? *Molecules* 2008, *13*, 2190–2219.

Aboagye, I. A.; Oba, M.; Castillo, A. R.; Koenig, K. M.; Iwaasa, A. D.; Beauchemin, K. A. Effects of hydrolyzable tannin with or without condensed tannin on methane emissions, nitrogen use and performance of beef cattle fed a high-forage diet, *Journal of Animal Science*, 2018, *96*(12): 5276–5286.

Abu-Hafsa, S. H.; Ibrahim, S. A.; Hassan, A. A. Carob pods (*Ceratonia siliqua* L.) improve growth performance, antioxidant status and caecal characteristics in growing rabbits. *Journal of Animal Physiology and Animal Nutrition*, 2017, *101*(6): 1307–1315.

Akagi, M.; Fukuishi, N.; Kan, T.; Sagesaka, Y. M.; Akagi, R. Anti-allergic effect of tea-saponin (TLS) from tea leaves (*Camellia sinensis* L.). *Biological and Pharmaceutical Bulletin*, 1997, *20*(5): 565–567.

Apel, C.; Bignon, J.; Garcia-Alvarez, M. C.; Ciccone, S.; Clerc, P.; Grondin, I.; Girard-Valenciennes, E.; Smadja, J.; Lopes, P.; Frédérich, M.; Roussi, F.; Meinnel, T.; Giglione, C.; and Litaudon, M. N-myristoyltransferases inhibitory activity of ellagitannins from *Terminalia bentzoë* (L.) L. f. subsp. bentzoë. *Fitoterapia*, 2018, 131: 91–95. DOI: 10.1016/j.fitote.2018.10.014

Arroyo-Lopez, C.; Manolaraki, F.; Saratsis, A.; Saratsi, K.; Stefanakis, A.; Skampardonis, V.; Voutzourakis, N.; Hoste, H.; Sotiraki, S. Anthelmintic effect of carob pods and sainfoin hay when fed to lambs after experimental trickle infections with *Haemonchus contortus* and *Trichostrongylus colubriformis*. *Parasite*, 2014, 21: 71.

Ayres, M. P.; Clausen, T. P.; MacLean, S. F.; Redman, A. M.; Reichardt, P. B. Diversity of structure and antiherbivore activity in condensed tannins. *Ecology*, 1997, 78(6): 1696–1712.

Bacelo, H.; Santos, S.; and Botelho, C. Tannin-based biosorbents for environmental applications–a review. *Chemical Engineering Journal*, 2016, 303: 575–587.

Bais, H. P.; Vepachedu, R.; Gilroy, S.; Callaway, R. M.; Vivanco, J. M. Allelopathy and exotic plant invasion: from molecules and genes to species interactions. *Science*, 2003, 301(5638): 1377–1380.

Bakker, J.; Timberlake, C. F. Isolation, identification, and characterization of new color-stable anthocyanins occurring in some red wines. *Journal of Agricultural and Food Chemistry*, 1997, 45(1): 35–43.

Barbehenn, R. V.; Constabel, C. P. Tannins in plant–herbivore interactions. *Phytochemistry*, 2011, 72(13): 1551–1565.

Baskerville, T. A.; Douglas, A. J. Dopamine and oxytocin interactions underlying behaviors: potential contributions to behavioral disorders, 2010, 16(3): e92–e123.

Benabdeljalil, C.; Cheynier, V.; Fulcrand, H.; Hakiki, A.; Mosaddak, M.; Moutounet, M. Evidence of new pigments resulting from reaction between anthocyanins and yeast metabolites. *Sciences des Aliments*, 2000, 20: 203–219.

Berry, A. C.; Nakshabendi, R.; Abidali, H.; Atchaneeyasakul, K.; Dholaria, K.; Johnson, C. Adverse effects of grape seed extract supplement: a clinical case and long-term follow-up. *Journal of Dietary Supplements*, 2016, 13(2): 232–235.

Blanco-Vega, D.; López-Bellido, F. J.; Alia-Robledo, J. M.; Hermosin-Gutierrez, I. HPLC-DAD-ESI-MS/MS Characterization of pyranoanthocyanins pigments formed in model wine. *Journal of Agricultural and Food Chemistry*, 2011, 59: 9523–9531.

Borowska, S.; Brzóska, M. M.. Chokeberries (*Aronia melanocarpa*) and their products as a possible means for the prevention and treatment of noncommunicable diseases and unfavorable health effects due to exposure to xenobiotics, *Comprehensive Review in Food Science and Food Safety*, 2016, 15: 982–1017.

Burdulis, D.; Ivanauskas, L.; Jakstas, V.; Janulis, V. Analysis of anthocyanin content in bilberry (*Vaccinium myrtillus* L.) fruit crude drugs by high-performance liquid chromatography method. *Medicina (Kaunas)*, 2007, 43(7): 568–574.

Burke, J. M.; Miller, J. E.; Mosjidis, J. A.; Terrill, T. H. Use of a mixed Sericea lespedeza and grass pasture system for control of gastrointestinal nematodes in lambs and kids. *Veterinary Parasitology*, 2012, 186(3–4): 328–336.

Butnariu, M. Detection of the polyphenolic components in *Ribes nigrum* L. *Annals of Agricultural and Environmental Medicine*, 2014, 21(1): 11–14.

Carulla, J. E.; Kreuzer, M.; Machmüller, A.; Hess, H. D. Supplementation of *Acacia mearnsii* tannins decreases methanogenesis and urinary nitrogen in forage-fed sheep. *Australian Journal of Agricultural Research*, 2005, 56: 961–970.

Chandrasekhar, Y.; Garlapati, P. K.; Katram, N.; Edavalath, M. R.; Kandangath, R. A. Tannins from *Terminalia chebula* fruits attenuates GABA antagonist-induced anxiety-like behaviour via modulation of neurotransmitters. *Journal of Pharmacy and Pharmacology*, 2018, *70*(12): 1662–1674.

Chatterjee, M.; Verma, R.; Lakshmi, V.; Sengupta, S.; Verma, A. K.; Mahdi, A. A.; Palit, G. Anxiolytic effects of *Plumeriarubra* var. acutifolia (Poiret) L. flower extracts in the elevated plus-maze model of anxiety in mice. *Asian Journal of Psychiatry*, 2013, *6*(2): 113–118.

Chaudhuri, T.; Das, S. K.; Vedasiromoni, J. R.; Ganguly, D. K. Phytochemical investigation of the roots of *Camellia sinensis* L. (O. Kuntze). *Journal of the Indian Chemical Society*, 1997, *74*: 166.

Choi, Y.; Abdelmegeed, M. A.; Akbar, M.; Song, B. J. Dietary walnut reduces hepatic triglyceride content in high-fat-fed mice via modulation of hepatic fatty acid metabolism and adipose tissue inflammation. *Journal of Nutritional Biochemistry*, 2016, *30*: 116–125.

Chung, K. T.; Wong, T. Y.; Wei, C. I.; Huang, Y. W.; Lin, Y. Tannins and human health: a review. *Critical Reviews in Food Science and Nutrition*, 1998, *38*(6): 421–464.

Cloos, J. M.; Ferreira, V. Current use of benzodiazepines in anxiety disorders. *Current Opinion in Psychiatry*, 2009, *22*(1): 90–95.

Davis, A. L.; Lewis, J. R.; Cai, Y.; Powell, C.; Davis, A. P.; Wilkins, J. P. G.; Pudney, P.; Clifford, M. N. A polyphenolic pigment from black tea. *Phytochemistry*, 1997, *46*(8): 1397–1402.

de Jesus, N. Z.; de Souza Falcão, H.; Gomes, I. F.; de Almeida Leite, T. J.; de Morais Lima, G. R.; Barbosa-Filho, J. M. Tannins, peptic ulcers and related mechanisms. *International Journal of Molecular Sciences*, 2012, *13*(3): 3203–3228.

Decker, V. H. G.; Bandau, F.; Gundale, M. J.; Cole, C. T.; Albrechtsen, B. R. Aspen phenylpropanoid genes' expression levels correlate with genets' tannin richness and vary both in responses to soil nitrogen and associations with phenolic profiles. *Tree Physiology*, 2017, *37*(2): 270–279.

Elisavet, D. B.; Heiko, L.; Giovanna, P.; Claudia, C. Stimuli-responsive tannin–FeIII hybrid microcapsules demonstrated by the active release of an anti-tuberculosis agent. *ChemSusChem*, 2018, *11*(22): 3975–3991.

Escribano-Bailón, T.; Álvarez-García, M.; Rivas-Gonzalo, J. C.; Heredia, F. J.; Santos-Buelga, C. Colour and stability of pigments derived from the acetaldehyde-mediated condensation between malvidin 3-O-glucoside and (+)-catechin. *Journal of Agricultural and Food Chemistry*, 2001, *49*(3): 1213–1217.

Falcão, L.; and Araújo, M. E. M. Vegetable tannins used in the manufacture of historic leathers. *Molecules*, 2018, 23(1081): 2–20. DOI:10.3390/molecules23051081

Finger, A.; Engelhadt, U. H.; Wray, V. Flavonol triglycosides containing galactose in tea. *Phytochemistry*, 1991, *30*(6): 2057–2060.

Focant, M.; Froidmont, E.; Archambeau, Q.; Dang Van, Q. C.; and Larondelle, Y. The effect of oak tannin (*Quercus robur*) and hops (*Humulus lupulus*) on dietary nitrogen efficiency, methane emission, and milk fatty acid composition of dairy cows fed a low-protein diet including linseed. *Journal of Dairy Science*, 2018, *102*(2):1144–1159.

Francia-Aricha, E. M.; Guerra, M. T.; Rivas-Gonzalo, J. C.; Santos-Buelga, C. New anthocyanin pigments formed after condensation with flavanols. *Journal of Agricultural and Food Chemistry*, 1997, *45*(6): 2262–2266.

Fraquelli, C.; Zanzani, S. A.; Gazzonis, A. L.; Rizzi, R.; Manfredi, M. T. Effects of condensed tannin on natural coccidian infection in goat kids. *Small Ruminant Research*, 2015, *126* (1): 19–24.

Fulcrand, H.; Benabdeljalil, C.; Rigaud, J.; Cheynier, V.; Moutounet, M. A new class of wine pigments generated by reaction between pyruvic acid and grape anthocyanins. *Phytochemistry*, 1998, *47*(7): 1401–1407.

Fulcrand, H.; dosSantos, P. J. C.; SarniManchado, P.; Cheynier, V.; Favre Bonvin. J. Structure of new anthocyanin-derived wine pigments. *Journal of the Chemical Society*, 1996, *7*: 735–739.

Garrido, G.; González, D.; Lemusa, Y.; García, D.; Lodeiro, L.; Quintero, G.; Delporte, C.; Núñez-Sellés, A. J.; Delgado, R. *In vivo* and *in vitro* anti-inflammatory activity of *Mangifera indica* L. Extract, *Pharmacological Research*, 2004, *50*(2): 143–149.

Geetha, T.; Garg, A.; Chopra, K.; Kaur, I. P. Delineation of antimutagenic activity of catechin, epicatechin and green tea extract. *Mutation Research*, 2004, *556*(1–2), 65–74.

Getachew, G.; Pittroff, W.; Putnam, D. H.; Dandekar, A.; Goyal, S.; DePeters, E. J. The influence of addition of gallic acid, tannic acid or quebracho tannins to alfalfa hay on *in vitro* rumen fermentation and microbial protein synthesis. *Animal Feed Science and Technology*, 2008, *140*(3–4): 444–461.

Grainger, C.; Clarke, T.; Auldist, M. J.; Beauchemin, K. A.; McGinn, S. M.; Waghorn, G. C.; Eckard, R. J. Potential use of *Acacia mearnsii* condensed tannins to reduce methane emissions and nitrogen excretion from grazing dairy cows. *Canadian Journal of Animal Science*, 2009, *89*(2): 241–251.

Gu, L.; Kelm, M. A.; Hammerstone, J. F. Screening of foods containing proanthocyanidins and their structural characterization using LC-MS/ MS and thiolytic degradation. *Journal of Agricultural and Food Chemistry*, 2003, *51*(25): 7513–7521.

Gu, L.; Kelm, M. A.; Hammerstone, J. F.; Beecher, G.; Holden, J.; Haytowitz, D.; Gebhardt, S.; Prior, R. L. Concentrations of proanthocyanidins in common foods and estimations of normal consumption. *Journal of Nutrition*, 2004, *134*(3): 613–617.

Guyot, S.; Marnet, N.; Drilleau, J. Thiolysis-HPLC characterization of apple procyanidins covering a large range of polymerization states. *Journal of Agricultural and Food Chemistry*, 2001, *49*(1): 14–20.

Guyot, S.; Marnet, N.; Laraba, D.; Sanoner, P.; Drilleau, J. Reversed-phase HPLC following thiolysis for quantitative estimation and characterization of the four main classes of phenolic compounds in different tissue zones of a French cider apple variety (*Malus domestica* Var. Kermerrien). *Journal of Agricultural and Food Chemistry*, 1998, *46*(5): 1698–1705.

Håkansson, A. E.; Pardon, K.; Hayasaka, Y.; de Sa, M.; Herderich, M. Structures and colour properties of new red wine pigments. *Tetrahedron Letters*, 2003, *44*(26): 4887–4891.

Hayasaka, Y.; Asenstorfer, R. E. Screening for potential pigments derived from anthocyanins in red wine using nano electrospray tandem mass spectrometry. *Journal of Agricultural and Food Chemistry*, 2002, *50*(4): 756–761.

He, F.; Liang, N. N.; Mu, L.; Pan, Q. H.; Wang, J.; Reeves, M. J.; Duan, C. Q. Anthocyanins and their variation in red wines II. Anthocyanin derived pigments and their colour evolution. *Molecules*, 2012, *17*(2): 1483–1519.

Hirasawa, M.; Takada, K. Multiple effects of green tea catechin on the antifungal activity of antimycotics against *Candida albicans*. *Journal of Antimicrobial Chemotherapy*, 2004, *53*(2): 225–229.

Hoste, H.; Torres-Acosta, J. F. J.; Sandoval-Castro, C. A.; Mueller-Harvey, I.; Sotiraki, S.; Louvandini, H.; Thamsborg, S. M.; Terrill, T. H. Tannin containing legumes as a model for nutraceuticals against digestive parasites in livestock. *Veterinary Parasitology*, 2015, *212*(1–2): 5–17.

Huang, X.; Wang, Y. P.; Liao, X. P. Adsorptive recovery of Au^{3+} from aqueous solutions using bayberry tannin-immobilized mesoporous silica. *Journal of Hazardous Materials*, 2010, *183*(1–3): 793–798.

Hümmer, W.; Schreier, P. Analysis of proanthocyanidins. *Molecular Nutrition & Food Research*, 2008, *52*(12): 1381–1398.

Hussein, S. A. M.; Barakat, H. H.; Merfort, I.; Nawwar, M. A. M. Tannins from the leaves of *Punica granatum*, *Phytochemistry*, 1997, *45*(4): 819–823.

Ingale, S. P.; Gandhi, F. P. Effect of aqueous extract of *Moringa oleifera* leaves on pharmacological models of epilepsy and anxiety in mice. *International Journal of Epilepsy*, 2016; *3*(1): 12–19.

Isaac, A. A.; Masahito, O.; Alejandro R. C.; Karen, M. K.; Alan, D. I.; Jayanegara, A. Divergence between purified hydrolysable and condensed tannin effects on methane emission, rumen fermentation and microbial population *in vitro*. *Animal Feed Science and Technology*, 2015, *209*: 60–68.

Jiménez, N.; Esteban-Torres, M.; Mancheño, J. M.; de las Rivas, B.; Muñoz, R. Tannin degradation by a novel tannase enzyme present in some *Lactobacillus plantarum* strains. *Applied and Environmental Microbiology*, 2014, *80*(10): 2991–2997.

Jing, X.; Ju-ping, Y.; Ya-nan, Y.; Fang, H.; Xiao-wei, Z.; Heng, L.; Xiao-xi, L.; Ke, L.; Pei-cheng, Z.; Zhuo-wei, H. A novel ECG analog 4-(S)(2,4,6-trimethylthiobenzyl) epigallocatechin gallate selectively induces apoptosis of B16-F10 melanoma via activation of autophagy and ROS. *Scientific Reports*, 2017, *7*: 42194.

Johnson, K. A.; Johnson, D. E. Methane emissions from cattle. *Journal of Animal Science*, 1995, *73*(8): 2483–2492.

Karamać, M.; Kosinska, A.; Pegg, R. B. Content of Gallic acid in selected plant extracts. *Journal of Food and Nutrition Sciences*, 2006, *15*(1): 55–58.

Kardel, M.; Taube, F.; Schulz, H.; Schütze, W.; Gierus, M. Different approaches to evaluate tannin content and structure of selected plant extracts—review and new aspects. *Journal of Applied Botany and Food Quality*, 2013, 86: 154–166.

Karonen, M.; Leikas, A.; Loponen, J.; Sinkkonen, J.; Ossipov, V.; Pihlaja, K. Reversed-phase HPLC-ESI/MS analysis of birch leaf proanthocyanidins after their acidic degradation in the presence of nucleophiles. *Phytochemical Analysis*, 2007, *18*(5): 378–386.

Karonen, M.; Ossipov, V.; Sinkkonen, J.; Loponen, J.; Haukioja, E.; Pihlaja, K. Quantitative analysis of polymeric proanthocyanidins in birch leaves with normal-phase HPLC. *Phytochemical Analysis*, 2006, 17(3): 149–156.

Kathleen, A.; Gregory, S. K. Nutrients and botanicals for treatment of stress: adrenal fatigue, neurotransmitter imbalance, anxiety, and restless sleep. *Alternative Medicine Review*, 2009, *14*(2): 114–140.

Kennedy, F. R.; Richard, L. L. Analysis of condensed tannins in *Populus* spp. using reversed phase UPLC-PDA-(−)esi-MS following thiolytic depolymerisation. *Phytochemical Analysis*, 2019, *30*: 257–267. https://doi.org/10.1002/pca.2810

Kokate, C. K.; Purohit, A. P.; Gokhale, S. B. *Pharmacognosy*. Nirali Prakashan: Pune, 2009, pages 9.1–9.19.

Kraus, T. E. C.; Dahlgren, R. A.; Zasoski, R. J. Tannins in nutrient dynamics of forest ecosystems—a review. *Plant and Soil*, 2003, *256*(1): 41–66.

Kumarappan, C.; Mandal, S. C. Antidiabetic effect of polyphenol enriched extract of *Ichnocarpus frutescens* on key carbohydrate metabolic enzymes. *International Journal of Diabetes in Developing Countries*, 2015, *35*(4): 425–431.

Lakhani, N.; Kamra, D. N.; Lakhani, P.; Alhussien, M. N. Immune status and haemato-biochemical profile of buffalo calves supplemented with phytogenic feed additives rich in tannins, saponins and essential oils. Tropical animal health and production, 2019, *51*(3), 565–573.

Lamy, E.; Pinheiro, C.; Rodrigues, L.; Capelae Silva F.; Lopes O. S.; Tavares, S.; Gaspar, R. Determinants of tannin-rich food and beverage consumption: oral perception vs. psychosocial aspects. In: Combs, C. A. Ed., *Tannins: Biochemistry. Food Sources and Nutritional Properties.* Nova Science Publishers: New York, USA, 2016, pages 29–58.

Landete, J. M. Ellagitannins, ellagic acid and their derived metabolites: a review about source, metabolism, functions and health. *Food Research International*, 2011, *44*(5): 1150–1160.

Legendre, H.; Hoste, H.; Gidenne, T. Nutritive value and anthelmintic effect of sainfoin pellets fed to experimentally infected growing rabbits. *Animal*, 2017, *11*(9): 1464–1471.

Legendre, H.; Saratsi, K.; Voutzourakis, N.; Saratsis, A.; Stefanakis, A.; Gombault, P.; Hoste, H.; Gidenne, T.; Sotiraki, S. Coccidiostatic effects of tannin-rich diets in rabbit production. *Parasitology Research*, 2018, *117*(12): 3705–3713.

Li, D.; Meng, X.; Li, B. Profiling of anthocyanins from blueberries produced in China using HPLC-DAD-MS and exploratory analysis by principal component analysis. *Journal of Food Composition and Analysis*, 2016, *47*: 1–7.

Lin, L.; Sun, S.; Chen, P.; Monagas, M. J.; Harnly, J. M. UHPLC-PDA-ESI/HRMSn profiling method to identify and quantify oligomeric proanthocyanidins in plant products. *Journal of Agricultural and Food Chemistry*, 2014, *62*(39): 9387–9400.

Lindroth, R. L.; St Clair, S. B. Adaptations of quaking aspen (*Populus tremuloides* Michx.) for defence against herbivores. *Forest Ecology and Management*, 2013, *299*: 14–21.

Liu, H.; Vaddella, V.; and Zhou, D. Effects of chestnut tannins and coconut oil on growth performance, methane emission, ruminal fermentation, and microbial populations in sheep. *Journal of Dairy Science*, 2011, *94*(12): 6069–6077.

Lu, A. P., Jia, H. W., Xiao, C.; and Lu, Q. P. Theory of traditional Chinese medicine and therapeutic method of diseases. *World Journal of Gastroenterology,* 2004, *10*(13): 1854–1856. DOI:10.3748/wjg.v10.i13.1854

MacAdam, J. W.; Villalba, J. J. Beneficial effects of temperate forage legumes that contain condensed tannins. Agriculture, 2015, *5*: 475–491.

Makkar, H. P. S.; Siddhuraju, P.; Becker, K. Plant secondary metabolites. In: *Methods in Molecular Biology*. Vol. 393, Humana Press: New York, USA, 2007, pages 67–81.

Manayi, A.; Nabavi, S. M.; Daglia, M.; Jafari, S. Natural terpenoids as a promising source for modulation of GABAergic system and treatment of neurological diseases. *Pharmacological Reports*, 2016, *68*(4): 671–679.

Martin, M.; Padilla-Zakour, O. I.; Gerling, C. Tannin additions to improve the quality of hard cider made from dessert apples. *Fruit Quarterly*, 2017, *25*(1): 25–28.

Mateos-Martín, M. L.; Fuguet, E.; Quero, C.; Pérez-Jiménez, J.; Torres, J. L. New identification of proanthocyanidins in cinnamon (*Cinnamomum zeylanicum* L.) using MALDI-TOF/TOF mass spectrometry. *Analytical and Bioanalytical Chemistry*, 2012, *402*(3): 1327–1336.

Matsui, Y.; Kumagai, H.; Masuda, H. Antihypercholesterolemic activity of catechin-free saponin-rich extract from green tea leaves. *Food Science and Technology Research*, 2006, *12*(1): 50–54.

McLeod, M. N. Plant tannins—their role in forage quality. *Nutrition Abstracts and Reviews*, 1974, *44*: 803–815.

Menga, J.; Xiaoyan, L.; Jian, Z.; Ruigang, Z.; Yan, C.; Xiaoyan, L.; Ran, S.; Xuegang, L. Preparation of tannin-immobilized gelatin/PVA nanofiber band for extraction of uranium (VI) from simulated seawater. *Ecotoxicology and Environmental Safety*, 2019, *170*: 9–17.

Mishra, A., Srivastava, R.; Srivastava, S. P.; Gautam, S.; Tamrakar, A. K.; Maurya, R.; Srivastava, A. K. Antidiabetic activity of heart wood of *Pterocarpus marsupium* Roxb. and analysis of phytoconstituents. *Indian Journal of Experimental Biology*, 2013, *51*(5): 363–74.

Mouls, L.; Mazauric, J. P.; Sommerer, N.; Fulcrand, H.; Mazerolles, G. Comprehensive study of condensed tannins by ESI mass spectrometry: average degree of polymerisation and polymer distribution determination from mass spectra. *Analytical and Bioanalytical Chemistry*, 2011, *400*(2): 613–623.

Mueller-Harvey, I.; Bee, G.; Dohme-Meier, F.; Hoste, H; Karonen, M.; Kölliker R.; Lüscher A.; Niderkorn V.; Pellikaan, W. F.; Salminen J. P.; Skøt, L.; Smith, L. M. J.; Thamsborg, S. M.; Totterdell, P.; Wilkinson, I.; Williams, A. R.; Azuhnwi, B. N.; Nicolas, B.; Brinkhaus, A. G.; Giuseppe, C.; Olivier, D.; Chris, D.; Marica, E.; Christos, F.; Marion, G.; Nguyen, T. H.; Katharina, K.; Carsten, M.; Marina, M. O.; Jessica, Q.; Aina, R.; Honorata, M. R.; Garry, C. W. Benefits of condensed tannins in forage legumes fed to ruminants: importance of structure. *Crop Science*, 2019, *59*: 1–25.

Muganga, R.; Angenot, L.; Tits, M.; and Frederich, M. *In vitro* and *in vivo* antiplasmodial activity of three Rwandan medicinal plants and identification of their active compounds. *Planta Medica*, **2014**, *80*: 482–489.

Mutsvangwa, T.; Edwards, I. E.; Topps, J. H.; Paterson, G. F. M. The effect of dietary inclusion of yeast culture (Yea-Sacc) on patterns of rumen fermentation, food intake and growth of intensively fed bulls. *Animal Science*, 1992, *55*: 35–40.

Nile, S. H.; Park, S. W. Edible berries: bioactive components and their effect on human health. *Nutrition*, 2014, *30*(2): 134–144.

O'Donovan, A.; Slavich, G. M.; Epel, E. S.; Neylan, T. C. Exaggerated neurobiological sensitivity to threat as a mechanism linking anxiety with increased risk for diseases of aging. *Neuroscience and Biobehavioral Reviews*, 2013, *37*(1): 96–108.

Okuda, T.; Ito, H. Tannins of constant structure in medicinal and food plants—hydrolyzable tannins and polyphenols related to tannins. *Molecules*, 2011, *16*(3): 2191–2217.

Ortega-Regules, A.; Romero-cascales, I.; Ros garcía, J. M.; Bautista-ortín, A. B.; López-roca, J. M.; Fernández-fernández, J. I.; Gómez-plaza, E. Anthocyanins and tannins in four grape varieties (*Vitis vinifera* l.) evolution of their content and extractability. *Journal International des Sciences de la Vigne et du Vin*, 2008, *42*(3): 147–156.

Patra, A. K.; Saxena, J. Exploitation of dietary tannins to improve rumen metabolism and ruminant nutrition. *Journal of the Science of Food and Agriculture*, 2011, *91*(1): 24–37.

Peng, K., Jin, L., Niu, Y. D., Huang, Q., McAllister, T. A., Yang, H. E.; Denise, H.; Xu, Z.; Acharya, S.; Wang, S.; and Wang, Y. Condensed tannins affect bacterial and fungal microbiomes and mycotoxin production during ensiling and upon aerobic exposure. *Applied and Environmental Microbiology*, 2018, 84(5): e02274–17. DOI:10.1128/AEM.02274–17

Pushp, P.; Sharma, N.; Joseph, G. S, Singh, R. P. Antioxidant activity and detection of (−) epicatechin in the methanolic extract of stem of *Tinospora cordifolia, Journal of Food Science and Technology*, 2013, *50*(3): 567–572.

Quijada-Morín, N.; Dangles, O.; Rivas-Gonzalo, J. C.; Escribano-Bailón, M. T. Physico-chemical and chromatic characterization of malvidin 3-glucoside-vinylcatechol and malvidin 3-glucoside-vinylguaiacol wine pigments. *Journal of Agricultural and Food Chemistry*, 2010, *58*(17): 9744–9752.

Rahman, A.; Ullah, N.; Ullah, H.; Ahmed, I. Antibacterial and antifungal study of *Cichorium intybus*. *Asian Pacific Journal of Tropical Disease*, 2014, *4*(2): S943–S945.

Ravindran, L. N.; Stein, M. B. The pharmacologic treatment of anxiety disorders: a review of progress. *Journal of Clinical Psychiatry*, 2010, *71*(7): 839–854.

Reed, J. D. Nutritional toxicology of tannins and related polyphenols in forage legumes. *Journal of Animal Science*, 1995, *73*(5): 1516–1528.

Riso, P.; Erba, D.; Criscuoli, F.; Testolin, G. Effect of green tea extract on DNA repair and oxidative damage due to H_2O_2 in Jurkat T cells. *Nutrition Research*, 2002, *22*(10): 1143–1150.

Rivas-Gonzalo, J. C.; Bravo-Haro, S.; Santos-Buelga, C. Detection of compounds formed through the reaction of malvidin 3-monoglucoside and catechin in the presence of acetaldehyde. *Journal of Agricultural and Food Chemistry*, 1995, *43*(6): 1444–1449.

Rivera-Méndez, C.; Plascencia, A.; Torrentera, N.; Zinn, R. A. Effect of level and source of supplemental tannin on growth performance of steers during the late finishing phase. *Journal of Applied Animal Research*, 2016, *45*: 199–203.

Salas, E.; Le Guerneve, C.; Fulcrand, H.; Poncet-Legrand, C.; Cheynier, W. Structure determination and colour properties of a new directly linked flavanol-anthocyanin dimer. *Tetrahedron Letter*, 2004, *45*(47): 8725–8729.

Saratsis, A.; Voutzourakis, N.; Theodosiou, T.; Stefanakis, A.; Sotiraki, S. The effect of sainfoin (*Onobrychis viciifolia*) and carob pods (*Ceratonia siliqua*) feeding regimes on the control of lamb coccidiosis. *Parasitology Research*, 2016, *115*(6): 2233–2242.

Schwarz, M.; Wabnitz, T. C.; Winterhalter, P. Pathway leading to the formation of anthocyanin-vinylphenol adducts and related pigments in red wines. *Journal of Agricultural and Food Chemistry*, 2003, *51*(12): 3682–3687.

Schweitzer, J. A.; Madritch, M. D.; Bailey, J. K.; Carri, J. L.; Dylan, G. F.; Brian, J. R.; Richard, L. L.; Ann, E. H.; Stuart, C. W.; Stephen, C. H.; Thomas, G. W. From genes to ecosystems: the genetic basis of condensed tannins and their role in nutrient regulation in a Populus model system. *Ecosystems*, 2008, *11*(6): 1005–1020.

Scioneaux, A. N.; Schmidt, M. A.; Moore, M. A.; Lindroth, R. L.; Wooley, S. C.; Hagerman, A. E. Qualitative variation in proanthocyanidin composition of *Populus* species and hybrids: genetics is the key. *Journal of Chemical Ecology*, 2011, *37*(1): 57–70.

Selvakumar, P. et al. Potential role of *N*-myristoyltransferase in cancer. *Progress in Lipid Research*, 2007, 46: 1–36.

Serrano, J.; Casanova-Martí, À.; Gil-Cardoso, K.; Blay, M. T.; Terra, X.; Pinent, M.; Anna, A. Acutely administered grape-seed proanthocyanidin extract acts as a satiating agent. *Food and Function*, 2016, 7: 483–490.

Shanga, Y. F.; Heng, C.; Yi-Long, M.; Chen, Z.; Fei, M.; Chun-Xian, W.; Xiao-Long, N.; Won-Jong, L.; Zhao-Jun, W. Effect of lactic acid bacteria fermentation on tannins removal in Xuan Mugua fruits. *Food Chemistry*, 2019, *274*: 118–122.

Shekhar, A. GABA receptors in the region of the dorsomedial hypothalamus of rats regulate anxiety in the elevated plus-maze test. I. Behavioral measures. *Brain Research*, 1993, *627*(1): 9–16.

Sibley, D. A. *The Sibley Guide to Trees*. First ed. Alfred A. Knopf: New York, USA, 2009.

Sieniawska, E. Activities of tannins—from *in vitro* studies to clinical trials. *Natural Product Communications*, 2015, *10*(11): 1877–1884.

Smeriglio, A.; Barreca, D.; Bellocco, E.; Trombetta, D. Proanthocyanidins and hydrolysable tannins: occurrence, dietary intake and pharmacological effects. *British Journal of Pharmacology*, 2017, *174*(11): 1244–1262.

Smeriglio, A.; Monteleone, D.; Trombetta, D. Health effects of *Vacciniummyrtillus* L.: evaluation of efficacy and technological strategies for preservation of active ingredients. *Mini-Reviews in Medicinal Chemistry*, 2014, *14*(7): 567–584.

Spennatia, F.; Mora, M.; Tigini, V.; LaChina, S.; DiGregorio, S.; Gabriel, D.; Munza, G. Removal of Quebracho and Tara tannins in fungal bioreactors: performance and biofilm stability analysis. *Journal of Environmental Management*, 2019, *231*: 137–145.

Stankevicius, D.; Rodrigues-Costa, E. C.; Camilo, F. J.; Palermo-Neto, J. Neuroendocrine, behavioral and macrophage activity changes induced by picrotoxin effects in mice. *Neuropharmacology*, 2008; *54*(2): 300–308.

Sun, X.; Huang, X.; Liao, X.; Shi, B. Adsorptive removal of Cu(II) from aqueous solutions using collagen-tannin resin. *Journal of Hazardous* Materials, 2011, *186*(2–3): 1058–1063.

Suzuki, T.; Takahashi, E. Metabolism of xanthine and hypoxnthine in the tea plant (*Thea sinensis*). *Biochemical Journal*, 1975, *146*(1): 79–85.

Tanaka, T.; Kusano, R.; Kouno, I. Synthesis and antioxidant activity of novel amphipathic derivatives of tea polyphenol. *Bioorganic & Medicinal Chemistry Letters*, 1998, *8*(14): 1801–1806.

Thinon, E.; Serwa, R. A.; Broncel, M.; Brannigan, J. A.; Brassat, U.; Wright, M. H.; Heal, W. P.; Wilkinson, A. J.; Mann, D. J.; and Tate, E. W. Global profiling of co- and post-translationally *N*-myristoylated proteomes in human cells. *Nature Communications*, 2014, 5(4919): 1–13. DOI: 10.1038/ncomms5919

Tousch, D.; Lajoix, A. D. Chicoric acid, a new compound able to enhance insulin release and glucose uptake. *Biochemical and Biophysical Research Communications*, 2008, *377*(1): 131–135.

Van Nevel, C. J.; Demeyer, D. I., Control of rumen methanogenesis, *Environmental Monitoring and Assessment*, 1996, *42*: 73–97.

Waghorn, G. Beneficial and detrimental effects of dietary condensed tannins for sustainable sheep and goat production—progress and challenges. *Animal Feed Science and Technology*, 2008, *147*: 116–139.

Wang, Y.; Waghorn, G. C.; McNabb, W. C.; Barry, T. N.; Hedley, M. J.; Shelton, I. D. Effect of condensed tannins in *Lotus corniculatus* upon the digestion of methionine and cysteine in the small intestine of sheep. *Journal of Agricultural Science*, 1996, *127*(3): 413–421.

Wang, Y.; Wang, F.; Wan, T.; Cheng, S.; Xu, G.; Cao, R.; Gao, M. Enhanced adsorption of Pb(II) ions from aqueous solution by persimmon tannin-activated carbon composites. *Journal of Wuhan University of Technology*, 2013, *28*(4): 650–657.

Wright, M. H., Heal, W. P., Mann, D. J.; and Tate, E. W. Protein myristoylation in health and disease. *Journal of Chemical Biology*, 2010, 3: 19–35.

Xu, H. Y., Zhang, Y. Q., Liu, Z. M., Chen, T., Lv, C. Y., Tang, S. H. et al. ETCM: an encyclopaedia of traditional Chinese medicine. *Nucleic Acids Research*, 2019, 47(D1): D976–D982. DOI:10.1093/nar/gky987

Xu, X.; Jiang, X.Y.; Jiao, F.P.; Chen, X.Q.; Yu, J.G. Tunable assembly of porous three-dimensional graphene oxide—corn zein composites with strong mechanical properties for adsorption of rare earth elements. *Journal of the Taiwan Institute of Chemical Engineers*, 2018, *85*: 106–114.

Yoshida, T.; Hatano, T.; Ito, H. High molecular weight plant polyphenols (tannins): prospective functions. In: *Recent Advances in Phytochemistry,* John T. Romeo (Ed.). Springer: New York, USA, 2005, pages 163–190.

Zou,Y.; Guo, J.; Yin, S.W.; Wang, J. M.; Yang, X. Q. Pickering emulsion gels prepared by hydrogen-bonded zein/tannic acid complex colloidal particles. *Journal of Agricultural and Food Chemistry*, 2015, *63*(33): 7405–7414.

Index